THE AMERICAN PSYCHIATRIC ASSOCIATION PUBLISHING
TEXTBOOK OF
SUICIDE RISK ASSESSMENT AND MANAGEMENT

THIRD EDITION

The American Psychiatric Association Publishing

TEXTBOOK OF
SUICIDE RISK ASSESSMENT AND MANAGEMENT

THIRD EDITION

EDITED BY

Liza H. Gold, M.D.
Richard L. Frierson, M.D.

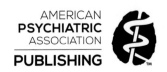

AMERICAN
PSYCHIATRIC
ASSOCIATION
PUBLISHING

If you wish to buy 50 or more copies of the same title, please go to www.appi.org/specialdiscounts for more information.

Copyright © 2020 American Psychiatric Association Publishing

ALL RIGHTS RESERVED

Third Edition

Manufactured in the United States of America on acid-free paper
24 23 22 21 20   5 4 3 2 1

American Psychiatric Association Publishing
800 Maine Avenue SW
Suite 900
Washington, DC 20024-2812
www.appi.org

Library of Congress Cataloging-in-Publication Data
Names: Gold, Liza H., 1958- editor. | Frierson, Richard L., editor. | American Psychiatric Association Publishing, publisher.
Title: The American Psychiatric Association Publishing textbook of suicide risk assessment and management / edited by Liza H. Gold, Richard L. Frierson.
Other titles: American Psychiatric Publishing textbook of suicide assessment and management. | Textbook of suicide risk assessment and management
Description: Third edition. | Washington : American Psychiatric Association Publishing, [2020] | Preceded by The American Psychiatric Publishing textbook of suicide assessment and management / edited by Robert I. Simon, Robert E. Hales. 2nd ed. c2012. | Includes bibliographical references and index.
Identifiers: LCCN 2019039725 (print) | LCCN 2019039726 (ebook) | ISBN 9781615372232 (hardcover) | ISBN 9781615372843 (ebook)
Subjects: MESH: Suicide—prevention & control | Suicide—psychology | Risk Assessment—methods | Mental Disorders—complications
Classification: LCC RC569 (print) | LCC RC569 (ebook) | NLM WM 165 | DDC 616.85/8445—dc23
LC record available at https://lccn.loc.gov/2019039725
LC ebook record available at https://lccn.loc.gov/2019039726

British Library Cataloguing in Publication Data
A CIP record is available from the British Library.

Contents

Liza H. Gold, M.D.
Richard L. Frierson, M.D.

PART I

Suicide Risk Assessment and Treatment

Liza H. Gold, M.D.

Robert L. Trestman, Ph.D., M.D.
Anita S. Kablinger, M.D., CPI, FAAP, FAPA, FACRP

Amy Wenzel, Ph.D., ABPP
Abby Adler, Ph.D.

Andreea L. Seritan, M.D.
Katherine A. Straznickas, Ph.D.
Glen O. Gabbard, M.D.

Richard Balon, M.D.

PART II

Major Mental Disorders

PART III

Treatment Settings

PART IV

Special Populations

PART V

Special Topics

PART VI

Prevention

PART VII

Aftermath of Suicide

Contributors

Abby Adler, Ph.D.
Associate, Main Line Center for Evidence-Based Psychotherapy, Bryn Mawr, Pennsylvania; Assistant Professor, The Catholic University, Washington, DC

Peter Ash, M.D.
Professor and Director, Psychiatry and Law Service, Emory University School of Medicine, Atlanta, Georgia

Claudia Avina, Ph.D.
Assistant Professor, Harbor-UCLA Medical Center and David Geffen School of Medicine at UCLA, Los Angeles, California

Alaina Baker, B.S.
Research Assistant, Department of Psychiatry and Behavioral Sciences, Stanford University School of Medicine, Stanford, California

Richard Balon, M.D.
Departments of Psychiatry and Behavioral Neurosciences and Anesthesiology, Wayne State University School of Medicine, Detroit, Michigan

Michele Berk, Ph.D.
Assistant Professor, Stanford University School of Medicine, Stanford, California

Kimberly Brandt, D.O.
Assistant Professor, Department of Psychiatry, University of Missouri, Columbia, Missouri

Beth S. Brodsky, Ph.D.
New York State Psychiatric Institute and Vagelos College of Physicians and Surgeons, Columbia University, New York, New York

Juan José Carballo, M.D.
Department of Child and Adolescent Psychiatry, Hospital General Universitario Gregorio Marañón, CIBERSAM, Instituto de Investigación Sanitaria Gregorio Marañón (IiSGM), School of Medicine, Universidad Complutense, Madrid, Spain

Stephanie Clarke, Ph.D.
Clinical Instructor, Stanford University School of Medicine, Stanford, California

Victoria Cosgrove, Ph.D.
Clinical Associate Professor, and Director, Prevention and Intervention Laboratory, Department of Psychiatry and Behavioral Sciences, Stanford University School of Medicine, Stanford, California

Katrina DeBonis, M.D.
Assistant Clinical Professor, and Director of Residency Education, Geffen School of Medicine at UCLA, Los Angeles, California

Nathan Fairman, M.D., M.P.H.
Director, Supportive Oncology and Survivorship, Comprehensive Cancer Center; Assistant Clinical Professor, Department of Psychiatry and Behavioral Sciences, University of California, Davis School of Medicine, Sacramento, California

Antonio Fernando, M.D., ABPN
Consultant Psychiatrist, Senior Lecturer in Psychological Medicine, University of Auckland, Auckland, New Zealand

Susan Hatters Friedman, M.D.
The Phillip Resnick Professor of Forensic Psychiatry, Professor of Reproductive Biology, Adjunct Professor of Law, and Professor of Pediatrics, Case Western Reserve University, Cleveland, Ohio; Associate Professor of Psychological Medicine, University of Auckland, New Zealand

Richard L. Frierson, M.D.
Alexander G. Donald Professor and Vice Chair for Education, Department of Neuropsychiatry and Behavioral Science, University of South Carolina School of Medicine, Columbia, South Carolina

Rachel Funk-Lawler, Ph.D.
Assistant Professor, Department of Psychiatry and Behavioral Sciences and Stephenson Cancer Center, University of Oklahoma Health Sciences Center, Oklahoma City, Oklahoma

Glen O. Gabbard, M.D.
Clinical Professor of Psychiatry, Baylor College of Medicine, Houston, Texas

Michael Gitlin, M.D.
Distinguished Professor of Clinical Psychiatry, Geffen School of Medicine at UCLA, Los Angeles, California

Liza H. Gold, M.D.
Clinical Professor of Psychiatry, Georgetown University School of Medicine, Washington, DC

Derrick A. Hamaoka, M.D.
Associate Professor of Psychiatry, and Scientist, Center for the Study of Traumatic Stress, Department of Psychiatry, Uniformed Services University, School of Medicine, Bethesda, Maryland

Annette Hanson, M.D.
Assistant Clinical Professor, and Director, Forensic Psychiatry Fellowship, University of Maryland School of Medicine, Baltimore, Maryland

Lindsay M. Hayes, M.S.
Project Director, National Center on Institutions and Alternatives, Mansfield, Massachusetts

Ryan Holliday, Ph.D.
Advanced Postdoctoral Fellow, Rocky Mountain MIRECC; Instructor of Psychiatry, University of Colorado Anschutz Medical Campus, Aurora, Colorado

Poh Choo How, M.D., Ph.D.
Health Sciences Assistant Clinical Professor, Department of Psychiatry and Behavioral Sciences, University of California, Davis, Sacramento, California

Pamela Howard, M.D., M.B.A.
President, Howard Medical Corporation; and President, World Health Information Network, San Clemente, California

Ashley Blackmon Jones, M.D.
Associate Professor of Clinical Psychiatry, and Director, General Psychiatry Residency, Department of Neuropsychiatry and Behavioral Science, University of South Carolina School of Medicine, Columbia, South Carolina

Kaustubh G. Joshi, M.D.
Associate Professor of Clinical Psychiatry, Department of Neuropsychiatry and Behavioral Science, University of South Carolina School of Medicine, Columbia, South Carolina

Anita S. Kablinger, M.D., CPI, FAAP, FAPA, FACRP
Professor, and Program Director, Clinical Trials Research, Department of Psychiatry and Behavioral Medicine, Virginia Tech/Carilion School of Medicine and Carilion Clinic, Roanoke, Virginia

Kieran Kennedy, M.B.Ch.B., B.Sc.
Senior Psychiatry Registrar, Department of Consultation-Liaison and Emergency Psychiatry, The Alfred Hospital, Melbourne, Australia

Christine Kho, M.D.
Resident Physician, Combined Internal Medicine/Psychiatry Residency Training Program, University of California, Davis, Sacramento, California

Nicole Kramer, M.S.
Research Assistant, Department of Psychiatry and Behavioral Sciences, Stanford University School of Medicine, Stanford, California

John Lauriello, M.D.
Robert J. Douglas, MD, and Betty Douglas Distinguished Professor in Psychiatry, Department of Psychiatry, University of Missouri, Columbia, Missouri

Benjamin Liu, M.D.
Resident in Psychiatry, Department of Psychiatry, University of California, Davis, Sacramento, California

Dexter Louie, M.D.
Resident Psychiatrist, Department of Psychiatry and Behavioral Sciences, Stanford University School of Medicine, Stanford, California

Jeffrey L. Metzner, M.D.
Clinical Professor of Psychiatry, School of Medicine, University of Colorado, Denver, Colorado

Lindsey L. Monteith, Ph.D.
Clinical Research Psychologist, Rocky Mountain MIRECC; Assistant Professor of Psychiatry, University of Colorado Anschutz Medical Campus, Aurora, Colorado

Sarra Nazem, Ph.D.
Clinical Research Psychologist, Rocky Mountain MIRECC; Assistant Professor of Psychiatry and Physical Medicine and Rehabilitation, University of Colorado School of Medicine, Aurora, Colorado

Maria A. Oquendo, M.D.
Perelman School of Medicine, University of Pennsylvania, Philadelphia, Pennsylvania

Britta Klara Ostermeyer, M.D., M.B.A., FAPA
Professor and Chairman, The Paul and Ruth Jonas Chair in Mental Health; Chief of Psychiatry, OU Medicine; and Mental Health Authority, Oklahoma City Detention Center, Oklahoma City, Oklahoma

Paula Padierna, M.D.
Department of Psychiatry, Hospital La Princesa, Madrid, Spain

Rebecca A. Payne, M.D.
Associate Professor, Department of Neuropsychiatry and Behavioral Science, University of South Carolina, Columbia, South Carolina

Jedidiah Perdue, M.D., M.P.H.
Director, Mental Health Services, Stephenson Cancer Center; and Assistant Professor, University of Oklahoma College of Medicine, Department of Psychiatry and Behavioral Sciences, Oklahoma City, Oklahoma

Marilyn Price, M.D.
Assistant Professor of Psychiatry, Harvard Medical School; Member, Law and Psychiatry Service, Massachusetts General Hospital, Boston, Massachusetts

Divy Ravindranath, M.D., M.S., FACLP
Clinical Associate Professor (Affiliated), Department of Psychiatry and Behavioral Sciences, Stanford University School of Medicine, Stanford; Assistant Director of Inpatient Mental Health, Palo Alto Veterans Affairs Health Care System, Palo Alto, California

Patricia R. Recupero, J.D., M.D.
Clinical Professor of Psychiatry, Warren Alpert Medical School of Brown University; and Senior Vice President for Education and Training, Care New England Health System, Providence, Rhode Island

Phillip Resnick, M.D.
Professor of Psychiatry, Case Western Reserve University, Cleveland, Ohio

Elspeth Cameron Ritchie, M.D., M.P.H.
Chair of Psychiatry, Medstar Washington Hospital Center; Professor of Psychiatry, Uniformed Services University of the Health Sciences, Bethesda, Maryland; Vice Chair of Psychiatry, Georgetown University School of Medicine; and Clinical Professor of Psychiatry, George Washington University School of Medicine, Washington, DC

Ayal Schaffer, M.D.
Associate Professor, Department of Psychiatry, University of Toronto; and Head, Mood and Anxiety Disorders Program, Sunnybrook Health Sciences Centre, Toronto, Ontario

Lindsey Schrimpf, M.D.
Assistant Professor of Clinical Psychiatry, Department of Psychiatry, University of Missouri, Columbia, Missouri

Charles L. Scott, M.D.
Professor of Clinical Psychiatry, University of California, Davis, Sacramento, California

Andreea L. Seritan, M.D.
Professor of Clinical Psychiatry, University of California, San Francisco, San Francisco, California

Ruth Shim, M.D., M.P.H.
Luke and Grace Kim Professor in Cultural Psychiatry and Associate Professor of Clinical Psychiatry, Department of Psychiatry and Behavioral Sciences, University of California, Davis, Sacramento, California

Navneet Sidhu, M.D.
Teaching Faculty, St. Elizabeth's Hospital Forensic Psychiatry Fellowship Program, Washington, DC

Barbara Stanley, Ph.D.
New York State Psychiatric Institute and Vagelos College of Physicians and Surgeons, Columbia University, New York, New York

Katherine A. Straznickas, Ph.D.
Volunteer Associate Clinical Professor, University of California, San Francisco, San Francisco, California

Trisha Suppes, M.D., Ph.D.
Professor, Department of Psychiatry and Behavioral Sciences, Stanford University School of Medicine, Stanford; and Director, Bipolar and Depression Research Program, Veterans Health Administration Palo Alto Healthcare System, Palo Alto, California

Robert L. Trestman Ph.D., M.D.
Professor and Chair of Psychiatry and Behavioral Medicine, Virginia Tech/Carilion School of Medicine and Carilion Clinic, Roanoke, Virginia

Robert J. Ursano, M.D.
Professor of Psychiatry and Neuroscience, and Director, Center for the Study of Traumatic Stress, Department of Psychiatry, Uniformed Services University School of Medicine, Bethesda, Maryland

Donna Vanderpool, M.B.A., J.D.
Vice President, Risk Management, Professional Risk Management Services, Inc. (PRMS), Arlington, Virginia

Amy Wenzel, Ph.D., ABPP
Director, Main Line Center for Evidence-Based Psychotherapy, Bryn Mawr, Pennsylvania

James C. West, M.D.
Associate Professor of Psychiatry, and Scientist, Center for the Study of Traumatic Stress, Department of Psychiatry, Uniformed Services University School of Medicine, Bethesda, Maryland

Cheryl D. Wills, M.D.
Director, Child and Adolescent Forensic Psychiatric Services, Department of Psychiatry, University Hospitals of Cleveland, Case Western Reserve University, Cleveland, Ohio

Hal S. Wortzel, M.D.
Director, Neuropsychiatric Consultation Services, Rocky Mountain MIRECC; Michael K. Cooper Professor of Neurocognitive Disease, and Associate Professor of Psychiatry, Neurology, and Physical Medicine and Rehabilitation, University of Colorado School of Medicine, Aurora, Colorado

Brian W. Writer, D.O.
Staff Inpatient Psychiatrist, Audie L. Murphy Veterans Affairs Medical Center; and Adjunct Assistant Professor, Department of Psychiatry, University of Texas Health Science Center, San Antonio, Texas

Peter Yellowlees, M.B.B.S., M.D.
Chief Wellness Officer, UC Davis Health; Professor of Psychiatry and Vice Chair for Faculty Development, Department of Psychiatry, University of California, Davis, Sacramento, California

Disclosure of Interests

The following contributors to this book have indicated a financial interest in or other affiliation with a commercial supporter, a manufacturer of a commercial product, a provider of a commercial service, a nongovernmental organization, and/or a government agency, as listed below:

Peter Ash, M.D.   *Consultant:* Provides forensic psychiatric consultation to attorneys and courts on a variety of issues, including cases of malpractice arising from a completed suicide.

Antonio Fernando, M.D., ABPN   *Speaker:* Paid speaker for Teva Pharmaceuticals in a CME on Hypersomnia in Melbourne, Australia.

Pamela Howard, M.D., M.B.A.   President and majority shareholder, World Health Information Network (WHIN), a telehealth platform company. *Grants:* WHIN was recently awarded two Department of Health and Human Services/National Institutes of Health grants to detect and prevent suicidal behavior, ideation, and self-harm in youth who are in contact with the juvenile justice system and to develop applied research toward zero-suicide health care systems.

Ashley Blackmon Jones, M.D.   *Study/Research support:* Alpha Genomix Laboratories. Principal investigator studying use of pharmacogenomic testing to guide treatment for anxiety and depression.

The following contributors to this book indicated that they have no competing interests or affiliations to declare:

Richard Balon, M.D.; Michele Berk, Ph.D.; Susan Hatters Friedman, M.D.; Richard L. Frierson, M.D.; Rachel Funk-Lawler, Ph.D.; Glen O. Gabbard, M.D.; Michael Gitlin, M.D.; Liza H. Gold, M.D.; Annette Hanson, M.D.; Lindsay M. Hayes, M.S.; Kaustubh G. Joshi, M.D.; Dexter Louie, M.D.; Jeffrey L. Metzner, M.D.; Britta Klara Ostermeyer, M.D., M.B.A., FAPA; Rebecca A. Payne, M.D.; Jedidiah Perdue, M.D., M.P.H.; Marilyn Price, M.D.; Patricia R. Recupero, J.D., M.D.; Elspeth Cameron Ritchie, M.D., M.P.H.; Andreea L. Seritan, M.D.; Navneet Sidhu, M.D.; Katherine A. Straznickas, Ph.D.; Trisha Suppes, M.D., Ph.D.; Robert L. Trestman Ph.D., M.D.; Donna Vanderpool, M.B.A., J.D.; Cheryl D. Wills, M.D.; Brian W. Writer, D.O.; Peter Yellowlees, M.B.B.S., M.D.

Introduction

Liza H. Gold, M.D.
Richard L. Frierson, M.D.

Education of mental health professionals and non–mental health physicians is a critical component in addressing the serious public health problem of suicide in the United States. We are pleased to offer this third edition of the *American Psychiatric Association Publishing Textbook of Suicide Risk Assessment and Management* in the interest of improving the ability to address the problem of suicide and contributing to the education of psychiatrists as well as other mental and medical health professionals.

Mental health treatment can decrease rates of death from suicide and suicide attempts by recognizing and treating suicide risk factors and associated mental illness. When physicians identify patients at risk of death from suicide by asking about evidence-based risk factors, such as mental illness and substance use, suicide mortality decreases (Mann et al. 2005; Parra-Uribe et al. 2017). To date, all comprehensive approaches to suicide prevention demonstrated to reduce suicide rates include the training of health professionals as a critical component of their strategies (Mann et al. 2005; Schmitz et al. 2012).

Suicide risk assessment and management is a core competency (Jacobs et al. 2003; Rudd 2014; Simon 2012) for psychiatrists (Accreditation Council for Graduate Medical Education 2019) and psychologists (Cramer et al. 2013). Suicide risk assessment (SRA) training can enhance clinicians' knowledge, practical skills, and attitudes (Jacobson et al. 2012; McNiel et al. 2008; Pisani et al. 2011; Schmitz et al. 2012). Nevertheless, regardless of specialty, mental health professionals often lack basic skills and adequate training in SRA and do not regularly and systematically assess suicide risk (Cramer et al. 2013; Jacobson et al. 2012; Schmitz et al. 2012; Silverman 2014).

Primary care physicians also play a significant role in identifying and providing care for potentially suicidal patients (Luoma et al. 2002). Nevertheless, depression and other psychiatric disorders are underrecognized and undertreated in the primary care setting (Mann et al. 2005). Even when seeing patients with depressive symptoms, primary care physicians do not consistently inquire about suicidal ideation or plans (Graham et al. 2011). These findings have led to recommendations for increased training of primary care physicians in the recognition and management of suicide risk (Mann et al. 2005).

Suicide and Public Health

The need to improve training and skills in suicide risk assessment and management is imperative. Suicide is the tenth leading cause of death in the United States, the second leading cause of death for persons aged 10–34, and the fourth leading cause of death for those aged 35–54. Since 2009, the number of suicide deaths per year in the United States has surpassed the yearly total of deaths due to motor vehicle accidents (Centers for Disease Control and Prevention 2017a). In 2017, 47,173 people died from suicide. Of these, almost 2,500 were between the ages of 15 and 19; an additional 11,700 were between the ages of 20 and 34 (Centers for Disease Control and Prevention 2017b).

Even more disturbing is the fact that the age-adjusted U.S. suicide rate has increased 33%, from 10.5 per 100,000 in 1999 to 14.0 in 2017 (Hedegaard et al. 2018). Among U.S. women, the rate of deaths from suicide increased from 4.0 per 100,000 in 1999 to 6.1 in 2017 and the rate for U.S. men increased from 17.8 to 22.4. Compared with rates in 1999, U.S. suicide rates in 2017 were higher for males and females in all age groups from 10 to 74 years. This rise in U.S. suicide rates stands in sharp contrast to the significant decline in global suicide rates. Globally, age-standardized suicide rates decreased by 32.7% between 1990 and 2016 (Naghavi 2019). However, the average annual percentage increase in suicide death rates in the United States accelerated from approximately 1% per year from 1999 through 2006 to 2% per year from 2006 through 2017 (Hedegaard et al. 2018).

Stigmatization and Misconceptions

Many people find suicide difficult to discuss due to centuries of stigma associated with this subject. People who have suicidal thoughts or histories of suicidal behavior often are embarrassed or ashamed to discuss these experiences, fearing that others will think worse of them. Individuals with suicidal thoughts may report plans to make a suicide attempt appear to be an unintentional death in order to reduce a sense of embarrassment among surviving loved ones. Similarly, people who are concerned about others often are hesitant or fearful of directly asking about suicidal thoughts or plans. Many people fear that if they ask, they will be "suggesting" suicide or are concerned that the person will be insulted, offended, or humiliated.

Decreasing the negative social stigma attached to suicide is imperative. This requires that we recognize that suicide is not a "disease" or "psychiatric disorder." Suicide attempts and deaths can be the outcome of multiple medical and psychiatric disorders as well as the outcome of chronic and acute psychosocial stressors. "Respiratory failure" may be the ultimate cause of death in a variety of diseases and can be recognized as a cause of death even without knowing the underlying diagnosis. Similarly, suicidal thinking or behavior may be recognized by preceding signs and symptoms, even if the underlying cause has not been specifically identified.

Thus, addressing the stigma of suicide also requires that we change how we discuss this important subject with our patients and in our social discourse. The Centers for Disease Control and Prevention (CDC) National Center for Injury Prevention and

TABLE–1. **Centers for Disease Control and Prevention National Center for Injury Control and Prevention suggested terminology for suicide and self-directed injury**

Unacceptable term	Suggested replacement
Completed suicide or successful suicide	Suicide
Failed attempt or failed suicide	Suicide attempt or suicidal self-directed violence
Nonfatal suicide	Suicide attempt
Suicidality	Suicidal thoughts and suicidal behavior
Suicide gesture, manipulative act, or suicide threat	Nonsuicidal self-directed violence or suicidal self-directed violence

Source. Crosby et al. 2011, p. 23.

TABLE–2. **Centers for Disease Control and Prevention suggestions for uniform terms and definitions**

Term	Definition
Suicidal ideation	Thoughts of engaging in suicide-related behavior
Suicidal intent	Evidence (explicit and/or implicit) indicates that at the time of injury the individual intended to kill him- or herself or wished to die and that the individual understood the probable consequences of his or her actions
Suicidal plan	A thought regarding a self-initiated action that facilitates self-harm behavior or a suicide attempt, often including an organized manner of engaging in suicidal behavior such as a description of a time frame and method
Suicide attempt	A nonfatal, self-directed, potentially injurious behavior with any intent to die as a result of the behavior; may or may not result in injury
Suicide	Death caused by self-directed injurious behavior with an intent to die as a result of the behavior

Source. Crosby et al. 2011, pp. 21, 23, 90

Control examined commonly used terms in regard to suicides. They deemed many of these, including *failed attempt, successful suicide, suicide gesture or threat,* and *suicidality* unacceptable because they convey negative social judgments, are contradictory, or are vague and imprecise (see Table 1; Crosby et al. 2011, p. 23).

The CDC reviewers have offered uniform language and definitions to improve communication and precision about the nature of an individual's problems with suicidal thoughts or behavior (see Table 2). We encourage adoption of the CDC's terminology and have endeavored throughout this volume to use similar nonjudgmental and precise terms so as to decrease stigmatization associated with suicide. The use of the word *suicide* as a verb or the constructions *committed suicide* or *death by suicide* are problematic. Terms such as *suicide death, death from suicide,* or *died from suicide* are more neutral, accurate, and facilitate rather than hinder frank discussion of this serious public health problem.

Efforts to improve education and public discourse and decrease stigmatization also require that we directly address and correct widely held misconceptions regarding suicide. For example, many mistakenly believe that people intent on dying from suicide will find a way to do so, even if a suicide death is averted on one given occasion. The fact is that although a history of a suicide attempt is a risk factor for future suicide, only about 10% of individuals who make a suicide attempt go on to die from suicide (Barber and Miller 2014). After a suicide attempt, people are more likely to come to the attention of others and receive mental health treatment, which mitigates risk of future suicidal thoughts and behavior (Mann et al. 2005). Therefore, engagement in appropriate treatment may constitute a lifesaving intervention.

Similarly, the mistaken belief that people considering suicidal behavior will not tell anyone about their thoughts or plans is common. In fact, contact with mental health and primary care providers prior to suicide is common (Ahmedani et al. 2014; Luoma et al. 2002). Thus, each patient contact with a medical or mental health treatment provider provides an opportunity to decrease suicide risk through appropriate assessment and intervention.

Assessment of Risk Versus Prediction

A major change in perspective in how to best address suicide is one of the most important developments over past years and is reflected in the chapters of this volume. Mental health professionals and researchers have shifted from a model of "suicide prediction" to a model that emphasizes assessment and management of suicide risk. Psychosocial stressors, cultural factors, and chance circumstances, as well as psychiatric illness and substance use, may play a significant role in an individual's suicide death. Clinicians cannot assess all the multiple and dynamic variables involved in a suicide death and therefore cannot reliably predict of who will or will not attempt or die from suicide.

Despite being the tenth leading cause of death in the United States, suicide is a statistically rare event, and therefore the "absolute risk" of suicide death is low. Statistical analysis demonstrates that efforts to predict rare events, such as whether patients will attempt suicide or engage in a violent act, result in a large number of false positives (Maris 2002; Swanson 2011). The vast majority of people, even those who express active suicidal thoughts, do not die from suicide. In contrast, the assessment of "relative risk" of suicide is based on the fact that people with mental illness are significantly more likely to commit suicide than people who do not have mental illness. Suicide prevention efforts require the assessment of relative risk of death from suicide based on identifiable suicide risk and protective factors.

SRA and management of suicide risk factors is therefore the key to identification of suicidal thoughts and behaviors and implementing appropriate treatment interventions. Thorough, systematic, and repeated SRA on a case-by-case basis allows mental health professionals to identify factors that can be modified to reduce risk, assess the efficacy of treatment interventions, and address the unique circumstances that may increase or decrease a patient's risk of death from suicide. Some patients may require immediate psychiatric treatment, such as hospitalization for safety and initiation of pharmacotherapy to treat psychiatric disorders. Some patients may benefit just as much or more from interventions that increase social supports or address nonmedical needs.

Notably, competent suicide risk assessment and management has also become increasingly recognized as one of the most significant elements in the legal assessment of whether adequate care has been rendered to patients who attempt or die from suicide. Although the rates of professional claims made against psychiatrists are among the lowest of any medical specialty, suicide attempts or deaths constitute between 15% and as many as 37% of psychiatric professional negligence claims (Vanderpool 2018). Evidence in these cases requires expert testimony regarding the "standard of care," which is generally defined as the degree of attentiveness, caution, and prudence that a reasonable physician would exercise under similar circumstances.

Historically, experts have differed on what constitutes the standard of care for assessing and responding to suicide risk. Nevertheless, after a review of professional negligence cases involving suicide, Obegi (2017) identified the following as probable "expectations of clinical care, as they pertain to SRA, based on the legal concept of the reasonably careful person" (p. 453).

1. Gathering information from the patient
2. Gathering data from other sources
3. Estimating suicide risk
4. Treatment planning
5. Documentation
6. Reassessing risk at significant clinical junctures, such as changes in the patient's circumstances, condition, or treatment

Although no models of performing SRAs have been formally adopted by any professional organization or training program, all SRA models that have been suggested as guides for clinicians encompass these six elements.

The Purpose of This Third Edition

This edition has incorporated new perspectives regarding suicide on a variety of levels. The medical and social use of destigmatizing and more precise language, for example, was discussed earlier. In addition, chapter authors have reviewed research identifying additional suicide risk factors, such as sleep disorders, and their clinical implications. Topics integral to current issues related to suicide are also reviewed, including nonfatal, self-injurious behavior; physician-assisted suicide; and teaching suicide risk assessment and management during psychiatric residency. This edition also examines the increased rates of suicide among specific populations, including children, adolescents, and college students, and makes recommendations regarding suicide risk management in these populations.

We believe that psychiatrists at all level of practice, but especially those in training, will find much information in this volume of use. The material reviewed in this text is essential for those in mental health and primary care training programs. The information reviewed here also will be of value to other mental health professionals, including psychologists, advance practice nurses, psychiatric nurse clinicians, social workers, licensed professional counselors, and primary care physicians. Most importantly, we hope this volume will provide information and assistance to practicing clinicians and suicide prevention programs working with those who struggle with suicidal thoughts and behaviors.

Acknowledgments

We would like to thank the chapter authors for their contributions to this volume. Without their diligence and expertise, this edition would not be possible. We also thank American Psychiatric Association Publishing for giving us the opportunity to edit this edition of this essential text and to contribute to education and training of mental health and medical professionals. We hope that focusing on suicide risk assessment and management will result in a decrease in the rates of death from suicide in the United States and reverse what has been a deeply disturbing trend.

L.H.G.: Thanks to my family for their patience and support. I also wish to acknowledge my deep gratitude to and respect for Richard Frierson, friend and colleague, for the hard work of coediting this volume. His collaboration made this challenging project more enjoyable as well as more manageable.

R.L.F.: Thanks to Liza Gold for her encouragement during this process, her excellent editing skills, and her understanding of my very busy year. Also, thanks to colleagues, past and present, who make my work enjoyable.

References

Accreditation Council for Graduate Medical Education: ACGME Program Requirements for Graduate Medical Education in Psychiatry. Chicago, IL, Accreditation Council for Graduate Medical Education, 2019. Available at: https://www.acgme.org/Portals/0/PFAssets/ProgramRequirements/400_Psychiatry_2019.pdf?ver=2019–06–19–091051–927. Accessed August 3, 2019.

Ahmedani BK, Simon GE, Stewart C, et al: Health care contacts in the year before suicide death. J Gen Intern Med 29(6):870–877, 2014 24567199

Barber CW, Miller MJ: Reducing a suicidal person's access to lethal means of suicide: a research agenda. Am J Prev Med 47(3 suppl 2):S264–S272, 2014 25145749

Centers for Disease Control and Prevention: Injuries (website). Atlanta, GA, Centers for Disease Control and Prevention, 2017a. Available at: https://www.cdc.gov/nchs/fastats/injuries.htm. Accessed August 3, 2019.

Centers for Disease Control and Prevention: Suicide (website). Atlanta, GA, Centers for Disease Control and Prevention, 2017b. Available at: https://www.nimh.nih.gov/health/statistics/suicide.shtml. Accessed August 3, 2019.

Cramer RJ, Johnson SM, McLaughlin J, et al: Suicide risk assessment training for psychology doctoral programs: core competencies and a framework for training. Train Educ Prof Psychol 7(1):1–11, 2013 24672588

Crosby AE, Ortega L, Melanson C: Self-Directed Violence Surveillance: Uniform Definitions and Recommended Data Elements, Version 1.0. Atlanta, GA, Centers for Disease Control and Prevention, National Center for Injury Prevention and Control, 2011

Graham RD, Rudd MD, Bryan CJ: Primary care providers' views regarding assessing and treating suicidal patients. Suicide Life Threat Behav 41(6):614–623, 2011 22145822

Hedegaard H, Curtin SC, Warner M: Suicide mortality in the United States, 1999–2017. NCHS Data Brief No 330. Hyattsville, MD, National Center for Health Statistics, 2018

Jacobs DG, Baldessarini RJ, Conwell Y, et al: Practice Guideline for the Assessment and Treatment of Patients with Suicidal Behaviors. Arlington, VA, American Psychiatric Association, 2003

Jacobson JD, Osteen P, Jones A, et al: Evaluation of the recognizing and responding to suicide risk training. Suicide Life Threat Behav 42(5):471–485, 2012 22924960

Luoma JB, Martin CE, Pearson JL: Contact with mental health and primary care providers before suicide: a review of the evidence. Am J Psychiatry 159(6):909–916, 2002 12042175

Mann JJ, Apter A, Bertolote J, et al: Suicide prevention strategies: a systematic review. JAMA 294(16):2064–2074, 2005 16249421

Maris RW: Suicide. Lancet 360(9329):319–326, 2002 12147388

McNiel DE, Fordwood SR, Weaver CM, et al: Effects of training on suicide risk assessment. Psychiatr Serv 59(12):1462–1465, 2008 19033175

Naghavi M: Global, regional, and national burden of suicide mortality 1990 to 2016: systemic analysis for the Global Burden of Disease Study 2016. BMJ 364:194, 2019

Obegi JH: Probable standards of care for suicide risk assessment. J Am Acad Psychiatry Law 45(4):452–459, 2017 29282236

Parra-Uribe I, Blasco-Fontecilla H, Garcia-Parés G, et al: Risk of re-attempts and suicide death after a suicide attempt: a survival analysis. BMC Psychiatry 17(1):163, 2017 28472923

Pisani AR, Cross WF, Gould M: The assessment and management of suicide risk: state of workshop education. Suicide Life Threat Behav 41(3):255–276, 2011 21477093

Rudd MD: Core competencies, warning signs, and a framework for suicide risk assessment in clinical practice, in The Oxford Handbook of Suicide and Self-Injury. Edited by Nock MK. New York, Oxford University Press, 2014, 323–336

Schmitz WM, Allen MH, Feldman BN, et al: Preventing suicide through improved training in suicide risk assessment and care: an American Association of Suicidology task force report addressing serious gaps in U.S. mental health training. Suicide Life Threat Behav 42(3):292–304, 2012 22494118

Silverman MM: Suicide risk assessment and suicide risk formulation: essential components of the therapeutic risk management model. J Psychiatr Pract 20(4):373–378, 2014 25226200

Simon RI: Suicide risk assessment: gateway to treatment and management, in Textbook of Suicide Assessment and Management, 2nd Edition. Edited by Simon RI, Hales RE. Washington, DC, American Psychiatric Publishing, 2012, pp 3–28

Swanson JW: Explaining rare acts of violence: the limits of evidence from population research. Psychiatr Serv 62(11):1369–1371, 2011 22211218

Vanderpool D: Professional liability in psychiatric practice, in Textbook of Forensic Psychiatry, 3rd Edition. Edited by Gold LH, Frierson RL. Washington, DC, American Psychiatric Association Publishing, 2018, pp 169–184

PART I

Suicide Risk Assessment
and Treatment

CHAPTER 1

Suicide Risk Assessment

Liza H. Gold, M.D.

Death from suicide is a significant public health issue strongly associated with psychiatric illness and substance use disorders. Assessing suicide risk is a necessary clinical skill in all mental health and primary care settings and a core competency in medical student education and psychiatric residency training. To date, all comprehensive approaches to suicide prevention have included the training of health professionals as a critical component of their strategies (Schmitz et al. 2012). Physician education in suicide risk assessment and management begins with training in suicide risk assessment (SRA). SRA is the gateway to mental health treatment, one of only two interventions empirically demonstrated to reduce suicide mortality (Mann et al. 2005).

SRA is a complex and challenging clinical task. Suicide is not a diagnosis but a consequence of behavior associated with multiple psychiatric diagnoses as well as nonpsychiatric psychosocial circumstance. Moreover, patients with similar diagnoses are at varying degrees of risk for death from suicide, and level of risk can change rapidly and often without notice. Nevertheless, SRA should be routinely conducted with all patients, not just those already identified as being at risk.

Case Example

Mr. Nelson, a 68-year-old white male, was referred to Dr. Smith, a psychiatrist, because he was refusing low-risk surgery for removal of a benign tumor, stating, "Why bother? It will all be over soon anyway." At intake, Mr. Nelson told Dr. Smith that his wife of 35 years had died 2 years prior. Since then, Mr. Nelson has had increasing financial problems. He was living alone in the home he had shared with his wife but had stopped doing routine household chores. Mr. Nelson had three adult children but reported that since his wife died, "I don't talk to them much." He also reported he was drinking alcohol every night "because I can't sleep."

Dr. Smith asked Mr. Nelson whether he had thoughts about suicide. Mr. Nelson acknowledged considering killing himself, stating that in the past few weeks, while drinking, he had been handling his gun, loading and unloading it multiple times. Mr. Nelson stated that he has not shot himself because "I know my wife would be mad." However, he stated that he does not feel that he has any reason to go on living, and he

3

had hoped his tumor meant he had cancer so he would have a "good reason to kill my-self—you know, a reason my wife and kids would understand."

Dr. Smith called Mr. Nelson's son, who reported that his father had become with-drawn and isolative and that his family was "very worried about him." The son asked Dr. Smith, "Do you think he's going to kill himself?" Dr. Smith candidly told Mr. Nelson's son that she could not predict whether Mr. Nelson would actually try to kill himself but that he was at high risk of death from suicide. Dr. Smith recommended inpatient hospitalization for Mr. Nelson's safety and to begin treatment. After discussing Dr. Smith's recommendation with his son, Mr. Nelson agreed to a voluntary admission.

Suicide Risk Assessment: Prevention, Not Prediction

Efforts to predict whether patients will attempt suicide result in a large number of false-positives and false-negatives (Simon 2012b; Swanson 2011). The "absolute risk" that any individual will die from suicide is low because the vast majority of people, even those who express active suicidal thoughts, do not die from suicide. Despite being the tenth leading cause of death in the United States, suicide is a statistically rare event. In 2017, the overall national rate of suicide was 14.5 deaths per 100,000 people (Centers for Disease Control and Prevention 2019). Suicide prevention therefore focuses on the assessment of "relative risk" of death from suicide based on consideration of known suicide risk and protective factors. In contrast to absolute risk, the assessment of relative risk is based on the fact that people with mental illness are significantly more likely to die from suicide than people who do not have mental illness (Swanson 2011).

Methodology

Some mental health professionals rely on the clinical interview alone to assess suicide risk. Others rely on structured or semistructured checklists or patient self-surveys. The use of any of these methods does not, of itself, constitute an adequate SRA. Unaided and unstructured clinical judgment is central in identifying and assigning weight to the risk and protective factors identified through systematic assessment, but it is highly subject to error when relied on as the sole SRA methodology (Berman and Silverman 2014; Simon 2012b). In addition, patients at risk of death from suicide, particularly individuals who are intent upon dying, may deny or conceal a history of suicidal thoughts or behavior (Nock et al. 2008; Rudd 2014). For example, patients who made suicide attempts within 60 days of a health care visit reported they denied suicidal ideation because of fear of stigma, "clinician's overreaction," or loss of autonomy (Richards et al. 2019).

Similarly, use of any checklist alone does not constitute an adequate SRA (Simon 2012a, 2012b). Many suicide risk factors are not simply present or absent but may vary in degrees of severity. Some factors may contribute to risk in some individuals but not in others or may be relevant only when they occur in combination with particular psychosocial stressors (Jacobs et al. 2003).

General Principles

Clinicians can only determine the level of relative risk of death from suicide, as Dr. Smith in the case example informed Mr. Nelson's son. SRA is a process of semistructured assessment that assigns a level of risk based on systematic identification and prioritization of evidence-based acute or short-term risk factors, chronic or long-term risk factors, and protective factors (Simon 2012b). Higher versus lower levels of perceived risk carry greater imperatives for aggressive treatment planning, triage, and intervention (Berman and Silverman 2014).

A *suicide risk factor* is defined as a factor empirically demonstrated to correlate with suicide, regardless of when it first becomes present. Short-term risk factors, such as panic attacks, agitated depression, and insomnia, are those found prospectively and are statistically significant within 1 year of assessment. Long-term risk factors, derived from association with deaths from suicide 2–10 years after assessment, include suicidal ideation, severe hopelessness, and prior attempts. The presence of chronic or long-term risk factors establishes lifetime vulnerability to suicide risk (Berman and Silverman 2014; Rudd 2014). Protective factors are those that decrease risk of suicide, such as close, supportive family relationships, and identification of these is also integral to a thorough SRA.

Clinicians may include warning signs as a separate category of risk factors. These may overlap to some degree with short-term risk factors but are distinct in that they provide observable markers consistent with potentially increased intent. The presence of one or more warning signs is indicative of increased suicide risk in the context of lifetime vulnerability and may be the earliest detectable indications of acute heightened risk for death from suicide (Berman and Silverman 2014; Rudd 2014). Additionally, clinicians are more likely to assign a high-risk designation once objective evidence of suicide intent is identified, such as preparation and rehearsal behaviors (Rudd 2014).

No single risk factor or warning sign is pathognomonic for suicide. In addition, a single suicide risk factor, or even combination of risk factors, does not have the statistical significance on which to base an overall risk assessment due to the infrequency (i.e., low absolute risk) of suicide (Jacobs et al. 2003; Simon 2012b). The assessment of overall suicide risk involves an understanding of how risk factors interact and contribute to a heightened or lowered risk of suicide (Berman and Silverman 2014).

Suicidal ideation and planning are significant risk factors for suicide. When assessing suicidal ideation, clinicians should consider specific content, intensity, duration, and prior episodes (Berman and Silverman 2014; Rudd 2014). Fleeting, nonspecific suicidal thoughts with no associated subjective or objective intent should be investigated because they may indicate acute distress that might need to be addressed. Nevertheless, isolated, nonspecific thoughts of suicide typically are not evidence of escalation of risk of death from suicide. Reduced duration of suicidal thoughts frequently translates to reduced specificity, less severity, and lower intent, along with lower overall risk (Rudd 2014).

However, the presence or absence of suicidal thinking is not a particularly good indicator of escalating suicide risk, especially in individuals who have made multiple attempts and in those with chronic suicidal ideation (Rudd 2014; Simon 2012b). Many suicide attempts demonstrate a strong component of impulsivity. Most studies of impulsivity and suicide have found an absence of proximal planning or abruptness of attempt in more than 50% of cases (Rimkeviciene et al. 2015). Seventy-five percent of suicide attempts occur within 3 hours or less from the time of initial suicidal ideation, planning, or the decision to make an attempt. The length of time between first thoughts and an attempt has been found to be as little as a few minutes to a few hours (Ilgen et al. 2008; Yip et al. 2012).

Mr. Nelson, in the case example, demonstrated risk factors that—when taken together—led Dr. Smith to conclude that he was at high risk of suicide. These included symptoms of depression, suicidal thoughts, a plan, access to highly lethal means (a gun), alcohol abuse, and insomnia, all with onset in the past 2 years since the loss of his wife. In addition, Mr. Nelson's reason for not killing himself was not rational, indicating the possibility of cognitive impairment or delusional thinking. Other risk factors included financial problems and social withdrawal. Mr. Nelson's demographic risk factors included his sex (male), his ethnicity (white), and his age (over 65). Dr. Smith could not identify any significant protective factors. Finally, Dr. Smith noted Mr. Nelson's warning signs of preparation and rehearsal with his gun.

Suicide Risk Assessment and Treatment

Systematic risk assessment requires clinicians to gather essential information from multiple sources and not just rely on information based on patients' self-report. Collateral information may be a key element in SRA, particularly when a patient denies ideation, intent, or plans. Family members should be consulted if possible, as Dr. Smith did in Mr. Nelson's case, because family may be aware of changes in behavior or warning signs that the patient does not report (Simon 2012b). Additional collateral information may be obtained from medical records, the patient's medical and mental health providers, friends, and possibly other sources, such as police records (Silverman and Berman 2014; Simon 2012b; Table 1–1).

Clinicians typically use a dimensional scale of low, moderate, or high to describe suicide risk (Berman and Silverman 2014; Rudd 2014; Simon 2012b). As a general rule, as symptom severity and complexity increase, so does suicide risk, particularly if distinct warning signs also are present. Low risk is characterized by mild psychiatric symptoms with no associated suicidal intent or features. Moderate risk emerges as symptoms escalate, warning signs start to emerge, and evidence of subjective intent is identified. Dr. Smith's assessment of Mr. Nelson identified four essential elements that characterize high risk, including serious psychiatric symptoms and alcohol use, the presence of active intent (subjective or objective), the presence of warning signs, and limited protective factors (Rudd 2014).

Importantly, SRA should be an ongoing process, not a singular event. Suicide intent can increase with the accumulation of stressors or decrease as effective interventions are implemented. The accuracy of any SRA therefore decreases over time as circumstances and clinical risk factors change. Consequently, SRA needs to be repeated according to the clinical needs of the patient, particularly when a treatment decision that changes levels of safety or structure, such as discharge from inpatient treatment, is considered (Jacobs et al. 2003; Silverman and Berman 2014; Simon 2012b).

Treatment: Static and Dynamic Risk Factors

Systematic SRA is critical to clinical decision making, including safety planning and management; triage decisions; treatment planning, especially regarding voluntary or involuntary hospitalization; and overall risk management (Silverman and Berman 2014; Simon 2012b). Higher versus lower levels of perceived risk carry greater imperatives for aggressive treatment planning, triage, and intervention (Berman and Silverman 2014). Dr. Smith's assessment of Mr. Nelson's high risk indicated that inpatient treatment was needed both for his safety and to initiate treatment.

TABLE 1–1.   **Suicide risk assessment: approach to initial data gathering**

1. Identify distinctive individual suicide risk factors
2. Identify acute suicide risk factors
3. Identify protective factors
4. Evaluate medical history, including laboratory data if available
5. Obtain information from other clinical care providers such as primary care providers
6. Interview patient's significant others
7. Speak with current or prior mental health treatment providers, including treatment team if inpatient
8. Review patient's current and prior hospital records

Source.   Simon 2012a.

Decisions regarding specific treatment interventions rely on recognition of dynamic as opposed to static risk factors. *Static risk factors* are those that cannot be modified. Although static factors such as demographic characteristics, family history, or history of suicide attempts are important to identify, they cannot be the focus of clinical intervention. Mr. Nelson's static risk factors include his age, sex, and ethnicity. Awareness of the risk associated with these may lead clinicians to weigh other risk factors more heavily, but static risk factors themselves cannot be changed.

In contrast, *dynamic risk factors* are those that can be modified and thus should be identified as early as possible and treated aggressively. For example, anxiety, depression, insomnia, and psychosis may respond rapidly to medications as well as psychosocial interventions. In the case example, after admission to an inpatient unit, Mr. Nelson was prescribed an antidepressant that mitigated many of his depressive symptoms, including insomnia. Mr. Nelson also began attending Alcoholics Anonymous meetings, which he found helpful and which provided significant social support.

Clinicians should also identify and enhance, when possible, protective factors. For instance, psychosocial interventions can help a patient mobilize available social supports (Jacobs et al. 2003; Rudd 2014; Simon 2012b). In the case of Mr. Nelson, treatment providers were able to help him reconnect with his children, who became his most significant source of social support.

Structured Assessment of Suicide Risk Factors

Each patient contact is an opportunity to decrease suicide risk through appropriate assessment and intervention. Unfortunately, formal, systematic training of most mental health professionals in the assessment and management of suicidal patients is limited. Many mental health professionals appear to lack the requisite training and skills to appropriately assess for suicide risk (Jacobson et al. 2012; Schmitz et al. 2012). The lack of formal training is in part due to the fact that no guideline, methodology, or standard assessment tool has been formally endorsed for conducting SRAs (see Chapter 31, "Teaching Suicide Risk Assessment in Psychiatric Residency Training").

Nevertheless, suggested frameworks for SRA are generally consistent in their recommended methodology and typically combine semistructured tools, self-report surveys, and the clinical interview. Semistructured screening instruments, such as the

Columbia Suicide Severity Rating Scale (C-SSRS; Interian et al. 2018; Youngstrom et al. 2015), the Suicide Tracking Scale, and the Sheehan Suicidality Tracking Scale (Youngstrom et al. 2015) complement and improve routine clinical assessments and can provide support and corroboration for a well-conducted clinical SRA (Silverman and Berman 2014; Simon 2012b). They also increase opportunities for capturing significant information. For example, use of self-report measures, such as the Beck Depression Inventory (Green et al. 2015), in addition to a structured clinical interview, provides patients who have difficulty verbalizing suicidal ideation with another option to report this information (Silverman and Berman 2014).

SRAs should include inquiries about and review of demographic, short-term, and long-term risk factors as well as the individual patient's unique risk and protective factors (Simon 2012b). Clinicians should routinely obtain information regarding previous suicidal behavior, current suicidal thoughts or plans, life stressors and adverse events, the presence of psychiatric symptoms, substance use, access to highly lethal methods such as firearms, and protective factors. One SRA model (Rudd 2014) identifies seven categories of risk factors, or domains, with 24 different individual risk factors, as well as a domain for suicide warning signs and a domain for protective factors (Table 1–2).

Nevertheless, semistructured checklists alone also are not effective SRA methodologies (Jacobs et al. 2003; Simon 2012b). Checklists are overly sensitive, lack specificity, and cannot encompass all the relevant risk or protective factors for a given patient. None have been tested for reliability and validity (Silverman and Berman 2014; Simon 2012b). The key to SRA is conducting a comprehensive systematic assessment; the model presented here and other similar models should be considered an aid or guide to systematic assessment.

Suicide Risk Factors: An Overview

A detailed discussion of all risk and protective factors and the strength of the empirical evidence behind them is beyond the scope of this discussion. Psychiatric illness and substance use are the strongest risk factors for death from suicide (Ilgen et al. 2008; Nock et al. 2008). The following is a brief discussion of these and other highly significant risk factors. The association of death from suicide with specific diagnoses is discussed in subsequent chapters.

Psychiatric Disorders

As many as 90%–95% of suicide victims have a diagnosable psychiatric disorder at the time of death, and those who die from suicide are more likely to meet criteria for more than one psychiatric diagnosis (Arsenault-Lapierre et al. 2004; Nock et al. 2008). Analysis of the National Comorbidity Study data found that 82% of individuals who reported suicidal ideation, 95% of individuals who reported making suicide plans, and 88% of individuals who reported making suicide attempts met criteria for one or more DSM disorders (Kessler et al. 2005). Affective, substance-related, personality, and psychotic disorders account for most of the diagnoses among individuals who die from suicide. Of these, mood disorders, particularly depression, present high risk, followed closely by alcohol use disorders, with highest risk in those with both affective disorders and alcohol use disorders (Arsenault-Lapierre et al. 2004).

TABLE 1–2.   **Sample suicide risk assessment checklist**

Sample checklist: domain	Suicide risk assessment factors: specific risk
1. Predisposition to suicidal behavior	History of psychiatric diagnoses (including substance abuse): higher risk with recurrent disorders, comorbidity, chronicity
	History of suicidal behavior: higher risk with previous attempts, high lethality; considered chronic risk if two or more attempts have been made
	Recent discharge from inpatient psychiatric treatment; high risk in first year after discharge, higher in first month after discharge, highest risk during first week after discharge
	Demographic considerations: age, sex, ethnicity
	History of sexual, physical, or emotional abuse
2. Identifiable precipitants or stressors (most perceived as a loss)	Financial
	Interpersonal relationship(s) and relationship instability (loss of social support)
	Nursing home placement
	Professional identity, retirement
	Acute or chronic health problems (can encompass loss of independence, autonomy, or function)
3. Symptomatic presentation	Depressive symptoms: highest risk associated with comorbid anxiety and substance abuse symptoms
	In elderly, depression may present as misuse of medications, unexplained accidents, or intentional decreased intake
	Bipolar disorder: highest risk early in course of disorder
	Anxiety, especially acute agitation
	Schizophrenia, especially in time periods following active phases
	Borderline and antisocial personality features
4. Hopelessness	Severity
	Duration
5. Nature of suicidal thinking and behaviors	Current ideation: frequency, intensity, and duration
	Presence of suicidal plan, increased risk with specificity
	Availability of means (consider multiple methods)
	Access to (not just ownership of) firearms
	Lethality of means including both medical and perceived lethality
	Active suicidal behaviors including preparation and rehearsal behaviors
	Suicide intent with subjective and objective markers (warning signs)

TABLE 1–2.   **Sample suicide risk assessment checklist (continued)**

Sample checklist: domain	Suicide risk assessment factors: specific risk
6. Previous suicide attempts (and nonsuicidal self-injury)	Frequency
	Perceived lethality and outcome
	Opportunity for rescue and help seeking
	Preparatory behaviors (including rehearsals)
	Reaction to previous attempts (feelings about survival and lessons learned)
7. Impulsivity and self-control	Subjective self-control
	Objective control (e.g., substance abuse, impulsive behaviors, aggression)
8. Presence of suicide warning signs	Active suicidal thinking
	Preparation and rehearsal behavior
	Anger
	Recklessness, impulsivity, dramatic mood changes
	Anxiety and agitation
	Feeling trapped
	No reasons for living, no purpose in life
	Increased alcohol or substance abuse
9. Protective factors	Presence and accessibility of social support
	Problem-solving skills
	Active participation in treatment
	Presence of hopefulness
	Children/Grandchildren present in the home
	Religious commitment
	Life satisfaction
	Intact reality testing
	Fear of social disapproval
	Fear of suicide or death

Source. Adapted from Rudd 2014.

Alcohol and Drug Use

Suicide is one of the leading types of injury mortality linked with alcohol consumption (Conner et al. 2014). Individuals with a moderate to severe alcohol use disorder who come to clinical attention are at approximately nine times higher risk of death from suicide compared with the general population. Use of alcohol in the hours preceding suicidal behavior, regardless of the presence of an alcohol use disorder, is also highly prevalent and is a powerful independent risk factor beyond the risk conferred by chronic alcohol use (Kaplan et al. 2013). An analysis of the National Violent Death Reporting System data found that alcohol was present at the time of death in one-third of suicides by firearms, hangings, and poisonings, which constitute more than 90% of deaths from suicide in the United States. Moreover, the mean blood alcohol concentration levels in those who died from suicide exceeded 80 mg/dL, the legal limit for intoxication (Conner et al. 2014).

The association between other substance use disorders and suicidal behavior is as compelling as the association between alcohol use disorder and suicide. One meta-analysis (Poorolajal et al. 2016) found that individuals who abuse drugs had increased risk of suicidal ideation, suicide attempts, and suicide as compared to drug nonusers. Data from the 2014 National Survey of Drug Use and Health (Ashrafioun et al. 2017) indicated that prescription opioid misuse was significantly associated with suicidal ideation, suicide planning, and suicide attempts in those who misuse opioids, regardless of frequency of misuse.

Individuals with substance use disorders often enter treatment with depressive symptoms and a number of severe stressors, such as relationship loss, job loss, and health and financial problems. These may be the precipitants for seeking treatment, but these circumstances also put them at higher risk for suicidal behavior. Approximately 40% of patients seeking treatment in substance abuse programs for moderate to severe opiate use disorder and cocaine use disorder report a history of suicide attempts (Yuodelis-Flores and Ries 2015). In one study, 58% of those with polysubstance dependence (DSM-IV; American Psychiatric Association 1994) seeking treatment reported lifetime suicide attempts compared to 38% of those who were only alcohol dependent (Landheim et al. 2006).

Co-occurring psychiatric disorders and substance use disorders appear to have the strongest association with increased risk of suicide. In one study, the comorbidity of major depressive disorder and alcohol use disorder (severe) increased the risk of suicide by 4.5-fold in persons aged 20 years and 83-fold in those age 50 years (Conner et al. 2003). Higher rates of suicidal thinking and behavior have also been found in individuals with substance use disorders and comorbid schizophrenia, posttraumatic stress disorder, and borderline personality disorder (Yuodelis-Flores and Ries 2015).

Suicidal Ideation, Behavior, and Attempts

Suicidal ideation and related behaviors, including warning signs and intent, are also some of the most significant suicide risk factors. In the National Comorbidity Survey, Kessler et al. (1999) found that approximately 90% of unplanned suicide attempts and 60% of planned first attempts occurred within 1 year of the onset of suicidal ideation. The probability of transitioning from suicidal ideation to suicidal plan was 34%; the probability of transition from a plan to an attempt was 72%. A cross-national study (Nock et al. 2008) found that the lifetime prevalences of suicidal ideation, suicide plans, and suicide attempts were 9.2%, 3.1%, and 2.7%, respectively.

A history of having made a previous suicide attempt is also widely recognized as a risk factor for death from suicide. Studies of rates of death from suicide associated with a history of suicide attempt may significantly underestimate the strength of this association (Bostwick et al. 2016). Nevertheless, as many as 20%–25% of individuals who died from suicide had made attempts in the year prior to death, with risk significantly higher for men than for women (Cooper et al. 2005). Parra-Uribe et al. (2017) found that within 1 year of a first-time suicide attempt, 20.1% of individuals attempted suicide at least once more and 1.2% died from suicide. Younger age, the presence of a personality disorder, and alcohol use disorder were risk factors for reattempting; alcohol use and older age were risk factors for death from suicide.

Adverse Life Events

Major interpersonal stressful life events may increase suicide risk, particularly among adults with alcohol use disorders, other compromised coping skills, and psychiatric or psychological vulnerabilities (Nock et al. 2008). In vulnerable individuals, an adverse event may lead to a suicide attempt within a relatively short period of time. One meta-analysis (Liu and Miller 2014) found evidence for a consistent association between negative life events and suicidal ideation and behavior. Specifically, support for an association with life stressors was most consistent for death from suicide, followed by suicide attempts and, finally, suicidal ideation. Owens et al. (2003) found that half of all suicide decedents had experienced at least one adverse life event in their final month of life, most commonly concerning relationships, money, and work.

Exposure to a wide range of past and current adverse life events increases an individual's vulnerability to suicidal behavior (Pompili et al. 2011). A history of stressful life events, such as parental or family discord, impaired or neglectful parenting, and physical or sexual abuse during childhood have all been linked to suicide attempts and deaths from suicide. Examples of current life stressors that may precipitate suicidal thoughts and behavior in vulnerable individuals include loss of a significant relationship, interpersonal conflicts, financial or occupational problems, involvement in legal or disciplinary problems, or perceived public shame or humiliation.

Transient personal crises can create considerable emotional distress with intense negative emotions, such as anger, rage, shame, and guilt. These may arise quickly and in a crisis situation can lead to an unplanned suicide attempt (Rimkeviciene et al. 2015), particularly in individuals with a history of chronic, intermittent suicidal ideation and after recent alcohol consumption (Powell et al. 2001). Suicidal ideation among impulsive attempters may be more fleeting and temporary than that experienced by persons with chronic depression. Often, as the acute phase of a crisis passes, the urge to die from suicide decreases (Miller et al. 2012; Yip et al. 2012).

Protective Factors

Although less research is available identifying factors that protect individuals from suicide compared to research regarding suicide risk factors, protective factors are critically important in decreasing the probability of a fatal outcome. Like risk factors, protective factors vary with the distinctive clinical presentation of the individual patient (Simon 2012b). Arguably, the most important protective factor is accessible and available family or other social supports. The ability to engage in treatment is also a strong protective factor. Additional protective factors include feelings of responsibility to family, child-related concerns, strong religious beliefs, and cultural sanctions against suicide (Nock et al. 2008; Simon 2012b). Nevertheless, in any individual, a delicate balance may exist between suicide risk and protective factors, and acute high suicide risk may nullify protective factors (Berman and Silverman 2014; Simon 2012b).

The case example of Mr. Nelson demonstrated some of the most serious risk factors for suicide. Fortunately, a thorough assessment and timely treatment interventions were able to significantly decrease his short-term risk of suicide. Mr. Nelson benefited from inpatient admission to maintain his safety and initiate treatment with medication. Equally important, Mr. Nelson's treatment added and enhanced protective factors, which hopefully would continue to keep Mr. Nelson's future risk of death from suicide low. These included continuing outpatient treatment with medication and regular SRA; alcohol abstinence and increased social support through referral to Alcoholics Anonymous; and closer and more supportive relationships with his adult children and their families.

Conclusion

Mental health treatment has been demonstrated to decrease suicide mortality; SRA is the access point to mental health treatment. Thorough SRAs, repeated over time and at critical points in patients' treatment, will inform decisions regarding treatment and safety interventions. Each patient has unique risk and protective factors that must be considered in assessing an overall level of risk of death from suicide. Clinicians are less likely to overlook important factors that increase or decrease the risk of suicide if they conduct a systematic assessment that utilizes the clinical interview, patient self-report, a structured or semistructured instrument that can be adapted to each patient's circumstances, and information gathered from multiple sources.

Key Points

- Clinicians cannot predict death from suicide; only the risk of death from suicide can be assessed.

- Clinicians cannot rely on patient self-report or clinical judgment alone to determine suicide risk. Patients may not report suicidal ideation or behavior, and clinical judgment is highly subject to error.

- Suicide risk assessments (SRAs) require the use of a combination of semistructured instruments, clinical interview, and patient report.

- Data collection for SRAs should include collateral sources, medical records, and psychiatric history.

- Clinicians should consider aggressive clinical intervention in patients who present with high risk for suicide, particularly patients with combinations of risk factors highly associated with death from suicide.

- Psychiatric disorders, substance use, and a history of suicidal ideation, behavior, or attempts are some of the strongest risk factors for death from suicide.

- Treatment should address dynamic risk factors; the higher the level of risk assessed, the more imperative the need for treatment and, possibly, the need for inpatient hospitalization to maintain patient safety.

References

American Psychiatric Association: Diagnostic and Statistical Manual of Mental Disorders, 4th Edition. Washington, DC, American Psychiatric Association, 1994

Arsenault-Lapierre G, Kim C, Turecki G: Psychiatric diagnoses in 3275 suicides: a meta-analysis. BMC Psychiatry 4:37, 2004 15527502

Ashrafioun L, Bishop TM, Conner KR, et al: Frequency of prescription opioid misuse and suicidal ideation, planning, and attempts. J Psychiatr Res 92:1–7, 2017 28364579

Berman AL, Silverman MM: Suicide risk assessment and risk formulation, part II: suicide risk formulation and the determination of levels of risk. Suicide Life Threat Behav 44(4):432–443, 2014 24286521

Bostwick JM, Pabbati C, Geske JR, et al: Suicide attempt as a risk factor for completed suicide: even more lethal than we knew. Am J Psychiatry 173(11):1094–1100, 2016 27523496

Centers for Disease Control and Prevention: Injury Prevention and Control: Data and Statistics 2019. Atlanta, GA, Centers for Disease Control and Prevention, 2019. Available at: https://www.cdc.gov/injury/wisqars/index.html. Accessed April 19, 2019.

Conner KR, Beautrais AL, Conwell Y: Moderators of the relationship between alcohol dependence and suicide and medically serious suicide attempts: analyses of Canterbury Suicide Project data. Alcohol Clin Exp Res 27(7):1156–1161, 2003 12878922

Conner KR, Huguet N, Caetano R, et al: Acute use of alcohol and methods of suicide in a US national sample. Am J Public Health 104(1):171–178, 2014 23678938

Cooper J, Kapur N, Webb R, et al: Suicide after deliberate self-harm: a 4-year cohort study. Am J Psychiatry 162(2):297–303, 2005 15677594

Green KL, Brown GK, Jager-Hyman S, et al: The predictive validity of the Beck Depression Inventory suicide item. J Clin Psychiatry 76(12):1683–1686, 2015 26717528

Ilgen MA, Zivin K, McCammon RJ, et al: Mental illness, previous suicidality, and access to guns in the United States. Psychiatr Serv 59(2):198–200, 2008 18245165

Interian A, Chesin M, Kline A, et al: Use of the Columbia-Suicide Severity Rating Scale (C-SSRS) to classify suicidal behaviors. Arch Suicide Res 22(2):278–294, 2018 28598723

Jacobs DG, Baldessarini RJ, Conwell Y, et al: Practice Guideline for the Assessment and Treatment of Patients With Suicidal Behaviors. Arlington, VA, American Psychiatric Association, 2003. Available at: https://psychiatryonline.org/pb/assets/raw/sitewide/practice_guidelines/guidelines/suicide.pdf. Accessed April 22, 2019.

Jacobson JM, Osteen P, Jones A, et al: Evaluation of the recognizing and responding to suicide risk training. Suicide Life Threat Behav 42(5):471–485, 2012 22924960

Kaplan MS, McFarland BH, Huguet N, et al: Acute alcohol intoxication and suicide: a gender-stratified analysis of the National Violent Death Reporting System. Inj Prev 19(1):38–43, 2013 22627777

Kessler RC, Berglund P, Borges G, et al: Trends in suicide ideation, plans, gestures, and attempts in the United States, 1990–1992 to 2001–2003. JAMA 293(20):2487–2495, 2005 15914749

Kessler RC, Borges G, Walters EE: Prevalence of and risk factors for lifetime suicide attempts in the National Comorbidity Survey. Arch Gen Psychiatry 56(7):617–626, 1999 10401507

Landheim AS, Bakken K, Vaglum P: What characterizes substance abusers who commit suicide attempts? Factors related to Axis I disorders and patterns of substance use disorders. A study of treatment-seeking substance abusers in Norway. Eur Addict Res 12(2):102–108, 2006 16543746

Liu RT, Miller I: Life events and suicidal ideation and behavior: a systematic review. Clin Psychol Rev 34(3):181–192, 2014 24534642

Mann JJ, Apter A, Bertolote J, et al: Suicide prevention strategies: a systematic review. JAMA 294(16):2064–2074, 2005 16249421

Miller M, Azrael D, Barber C: Suicide mortality in the United States: the importance of attending to method in understanding population-level disparities in the burden of suicide. Annu Rev Public Health 33:393–408, 2012 22224886

Nock MK, Borges G, Bromet EJ, et al: Cross-national prevalence and risk factors for suicidal ideation, plans and attempts. Br J Psychiatry 192(2):98–105, 2008 18245022

Owens C, Booth N, Briscoe M, et al: Suicide outside the care of mental health services: a case-controlled psychological autopsy study. Crisis 24(3):113–121, 2003 14518644

Parra-Uribe I, Blasco-Fontecilla H, Garcia-Parés G, et al: Risk of re-attempts and suicide death after a suicide attempt: a survival analysis. BMC Psychiatry 17(1):163, 2017 28472923

Pompili M, Innamorati M, Szanto K, et al: Life events as precipitants of suicide attempts among first-time suicide attempters, repeaters, and non-attempters. Psychiatry Res 186(2-3):300–305, 2011 20889216

Poorolajal J, Haghtalab T, Farhadi M, et al: Substance use disorder and risk of suicidal ideation, suicide attempt and suicide death: a meta-analysis. J Public Health (Oxf) 38(3):e282–e291, 2016 26503486

Powell KE, Kresnow MJ, Mercy JA, et al: Alcohol consumption and nearly lethal suicide attempts. Suicide Life Threat Behav 32(1 suppl):30–41, 2001 11924693

Richards JE, Whiteside U, Ludman EJ, et al: Understanding why patients may not report suicidal ideation at a health care visit prior to a suicide attempt: a qualitative study. Psychiatr Serv 70(1):40–45, 2019 30453860

Rimkeviciene J, O'Gorman J, De Leo D: Impulsive suicide attempts: a systematic literature review of definitions, characteristics and risk factors. J Affect Disord 171:93–104, 2015 25299440

Rudd MD: Core competencies, warning signs, and a framework for suicide risk assessment in clinical practice, in The Oxford Handbook of Suicide and Self-Injury. Edited by Nock MK. New York, Oxford University Press, 2014, pp 323–336

Schmitz WM Jr, Allen MH, Feldman BN, et al: Preventing suicide through improved training in suicide risk assessment and care: an American Association of Suicidology Task Force report addressing serious gaps in U.S. mental health training. Suicide Life Threat Behav 42(3):292–304, 2012 22494118

Silverman MM, Berman AL: Suicide risk assessment and risk formulation. Part I: a focus on suicide ideation in assessing suicide risk. Suicide Life Threat Behav 44(4):420–431, 2014 25250407

Simon RI: Patient safety and freedom of movement: coping with uncertainty, in American Psychiatric Publishing Textbook of Suicide Assessment and Management, 2nd Edition. Edited by Simon RI, Hales RE. Washington, DC, American Psychiatric Publishing, 2012a, pp 331–346

Simon RI: Suicide risk assessment: gateway to treatment and management, in American Psychiatric Publishing Textbook of Suicide Assessment and Management, 2nd Edition. Edited by Simon RI, Hales RE. Washington, DC, American Psychiatric Publishing, 2012b, pp 3–28

Swanson JW: Explaining rare acts of violence: the limits of evidence from population research. Psychiatr Serv 62(11):1369–1371, 2011 22211218

Yip PS, Caine E, Yousuf S, et al: Means restriction for suicide prevention. Lancet 379(9834):2393–2399, 2012 22726520

Youngstrom EA, Hameed A, Mitchell MA, et al: Direct comparison of the psychometric properties of multiple interview and patient-rated assessments of suicidal ideation and behavior in an adult psychiatric inpatient sample. J Clin Psychiatry 76(12):1676–1682, 2015 26613136

Yuodelis-Flores C, Ries RK: Addiction and suicide: a review. Am J Addict 24(2):98–104, 2015 25644860

CHAPTER 2

Psychopharmacology and Neuromodulation

Robert L. Trestman, Ph.D., M.D.
Anita S. Kablinger, M.D., CPI, FAAP, FAPA, FACRP

As described in detail throughout this textbook, the characteristics of suicidal thoughts and behaviors and suicide are complex. Similarly, interventions that directly impact the functioning of the brain have complex effects. At times, distinguishing whether suicidal thoughts and behaviors are a manifestation of the underlying illness or of the treatment can be challenging. The interventions may also be misused: suicide by overdose with a therapeutic medication is an intrinsic risk that clinicians must weigh in treatment planning. In this chapter, we review the data regarding the effectiveness and risks of the different classes of psychopharmacological agents and address the risks and benefits of the rapidly evolving field of neuromodulation.

Psychopharmacology

Virtually any psychopharmacological agent, when taken in combination or at high enough dosage, can lead to death. This challenge is at the core of managing psychiatric illnesses, most of which increase the risk of death from suicide. Many mediators and moderators of risk exist, including underlying diagnosis, age and sex, cultural and social supports, past personal and family history, hopelessness, and psychosis. It is important to provide context as well to the relative lethality of prescription medications themselves commonly used in psychiatry (Giurca 2018).

The authors wish to acknowledge Brian Saway, B.A., currently a third-year medical student at Virginia Tech/Carilion School of Medicine, for his enthusiastic input, extensive neuromodulation literature search, and ideas concerning its use in suicidal thoughts and behaviors.

As may be seen in Table 2–1, when we provide a prescription to a patient for a month's supply of medication (maximum approved dosages are used in these examples), the potential for lethal overdose varies across two orders of magnitude by the medication chosen. These estimates do not take into consideration the person's biological state (e.g., whether someone is already malnourished or dehydrated) or whether multiple medications may be ingested.

Polypharmacy is a significant suicide risk factor: one recent study found use of antipsychotic drugs or polypharmacy with four or more medications were predictors of suicide death (Takeuchi et al. 2017). The type of medication used in an overdose attempt is also subject to what is available to the patient. Over the latter half of the twentieth century, use of tricyclic antidepressants (TCAs) in overdose was not an uncommon method of suicide; use of selective serotonin reuptake inhibitor (SSRI) antidepressants in overdose attempts is increasing, consistent with the transition in use from TCAs to SSRIs in the treatment of depression (Löfman et al. 2017).

Suicide risk is increased in individuals with mental illness, particularly depression. Treatment of depression reduces the risk of suicide, whether through pharmacological means, psychotherapy, or both (Weitz et al. 2014). The presence of suicidal ideation and behaviors at baseline may also be a predictor of treatment outcome in some populations (Bingham et al. 2017). Using the most appropriate rating scale in assessing measures of suicidal ideation remains an important factor as research in this area continues.

Antidepressants

The potential for increased risk of suicidal ideation linked to antidepressant use led to a black box warning for antidepressant use in 2004 in children, adolescents, and young adults. Most pharmacoepidemiological studies show a protective effect of antidepressants on suicidal ideation and behavior, though others find inconclusive or mixed results. A recent analysis of suicide deaths in Sweden of young women (ages 15–24 years between 1999 and 2013) found a trend for increased incidence of suicide death as antidepressant prescriptions increased in parallel (Larsson 2017). A large French dataset of outpatients newly prescribed antidepressants found that 9% of patients developed suicidal ideation *de novo* after drug initiation, with 1.7% attempting suicide (Courtet et al. 2014).

In addition to initial depressive manifestations and an association with suicidal ideation and behavior, lack of mood disorder improvement or worsening of symptoms also increased new thoughts or behaviors of suicide (Courtet et al. 2014). Analysis of the Northern Finland Birth Cohort of 1966 found that suicidal ideation was associated with the use of all antidepressants (without any significant difference between classes or types of antidepressants), but this association was no longer present when other symptoms of depression and anxiety were considered. Furthermore, insomnia itself was a predictor of suicidal ideation occurrence for depressed patients taking antidepressants (Rissanen et al. 2014). A focused review (Brent 2016) on antidepressants and suicidal thoughts and behaviors in young people found that 4–11 times more depressed young people benefit from antidepressants compared to experiencing a suicidal event, reflecting the need to not withhold antidepressants from patients and the potential benefits of careful treatment.

Treatment-emergent suicidal ideation in older depressed adults participating in a clinical trial was transient, early on in pharmacological exposure, and more likely due

TABLE 2–1. **Maximum daily dosage, LD50, and relative risk of death from overdose of selected common psychotropic medications**

Drug class and name	Maximum daily dosage, *mg*	LD50, *mg/kg*	Relative lethality
Selective serotonin reuptake inhibitors			
Escitalopram	20	980	1.0
Fluoxetine	80	452	8.9
Serotonin-norepinephrine reuptake inhibitors			
Desvenlafaxine	50	700	3.6
Duloxetine	120	279	21.5
Tricyclic antidepressants			
Protriptyline	60	299	10.0
Desipramine	300	320	46.9
Doxepin	300	147	102.0
Other antidepressants			
Mirtazapine	45	490	4.6
Trazodone	600	690	43.5
Mood stabilizers			
Topiramate	400	3,745	5.3
Lamotrigine	400	205	97.6
Lithium	1,800	525	171.4
Valproic acid	3,600	670	268.7
Antipsychotics			
Aripiprazole	30	953	1.6
Quetiapine	800	2,000	20.0
Clozapine	900	251	179.3
Chlorpromazine	800	145	275.9
Anxiolytics			
Alprazolam	4	3,100	0.1
Clonazepam	20	4,000	0.3

Note. LD50 is the lethal dose 50% of the time in animal models. The relative risk is based on a 30-day prescription at the maximum dosage to a 60-kg adult.

Source. Adapted from Giurca 2018.

to the depressive disorder itself rather than an adverse effect of medication (Cristancho et al. 2017). A very large Danish cohort study analyzing antidepressant prescriptions over a 10-year period showed an age-dependent decline in suicide rate in both antidepressant-treated men and women, with an opposite trend demonstrated in those not treated (Erlangsen and Conwell 2014). Alternatively, those initiated on antidepressants after age 75 seem to be more prone to suicidal behaviors, particularly if antidepressants are concomitantly used with anxiolytics and hypnotics (Hedna et al. 2018).

In sum, evidence reflects that adherence to antidepressant treatment of depression reduces suicide risk. Some evidence indicates that SSRIs decrease suicidal thoughts more than norepinephrine-dopamine reuptake inhibitors or serotonin-norepinephrine reuptake inhibitors during treatment (Henein et al. 2016). Other studies do not find a difference in the rates of suicidal ideation, behavior, or self-harm among classes of antidepressants (Valuck et al. 2016).

Another complicating factor related to experimental design is the general exclusion of patients at high risk of self-harm from clinical trials investigating potential antidepressant compounds, which has limited the assessment of suicidal ideation and behavior as markers of depression. This paradigm has been challenged with demonstrated transience of suicidal ideation in contrast to the durability of other depressive symptoms and can safely be investigated in the context of close monitoring. Additionally, the risk that suicidal thoughts may recur during a subsequent antidepressant or therapy trial after initial trial failure warrants continued close assessment (Perlis et al. 2012).

Antipsychotics

Antipsychotic medications are used to treat a wide range of psychiatric disorders and in the full age range of people with, for example, schizophrenia, bipolar disorder, and major depression. The efficacy of antipsychotic medications for treating psychosis and mania is well established, with less data generally available as to antisuicidal properties. The one major exception is clozapine. Clozapine-treated individuals with schizophrenia demonstrate reduction in rehospitalizations, better adherence to prescription refills, and a significantly lower risk of attempted suicide compared to other antipsychotic medications (Ringbäck Weitoft et al. 2014).

Clozapine's mechanism of action in reducing suicide behaviors, and by extension that of other second-generation antipsychotics, is postulated to be due to serotonergic involvement or to improved adherence from fewer side effects as compared to first-generation antipsychotics. Although akathisia, a recognized side effect of many pharmacotherapies, has been noted to increase the risk of suicide, in most studies this risk in inconsistent. This finding is hypothesized to be due to the countervailing benefit of treatment adherence versus lack of treatment in providing a net therapeutic benefit (Reutfors et al. 2016).

The use of first- and second-generation antipsychotics for treating patients with bipolar disorder is common. The effects of antipsychotics on suicidal ideation and behaviors in patients with bipolar disorder have not been clearly determined. Tondo and Baldessarini (2016) reviewed long-term treatment options for patients with bipolar disorder and the prevention of suicidal behavior, finding inconsistent benefit. Clozapine's antisuicidal benefits have been studied primarily in those with schizophrenia or schizoaffective disorder and not in those with bipolar disorder.

Mood Stabilizers

Mood-stabilizing agents have long been used in the treatment of a range of disorders, most notably bipolar disorder. Early recognition of illness and active treatment engagement are recognized as critical to long-term outcome and reduction of suicide risk in these patients. Longer duration of untreated bipolar illness and elevated risk of suicide attempts as well as increased frequency of suicide attempts emphasize the importance of early recognition and aggressive treatment of bipolar disorder (Tsai et al. 2016).

Lithium

The utility of lithium in reducing suicidal thoughts and behaviors is well established; along with clozapine, it has earned the U.S. Food and Drug Administration (FDA)'s indication for reducing these. The specific mechanism of action is unknown. A recent meta-review concluded that the evidence in support of lithium as effective in reducing suicide risk (across diagnosis, duration, and illness phase) is unambiguously positive and that lithium is underutilized in this regard (Smith and Cipriani 2017). Indeed, higher lithium levels in public drinking water have been associated with reduced suicide rates, particularly in men (Liaugaudaite et al. 2017). Proposed mechanisms include direct modulation of inositol monophosphatase or glycogen synthase kinase-3 (GSK-3) and indirect modulation of neurotrophic factors, neurotransmitters, and circadian rhythms (Can et al. 2014). Toffol et al. (2015) found that high-risk patients with bipolar disorder had a lower risk of suicide and all-cause mortality when treated with maintenance lithium therapy.

Antiepileptic Drugs

The FDA issued a warning regarding suicidal thoughts and behaviors and antiepileptic drugs in 2008 based on meta-analyses involving 11 antiepileptics, 199 studies, and more than 43,000 participants. Overall, antiepileptic drugs were associated with increased risk of suicidal thoughts and behaviors relative to placebo (Britton and Shih 2010). Clinical populations in this review included those with epilepsy, psychiatric disorders, and other conditions such as pain or agitation.

Consistent with these findings, Schuerch et al. (2016) recently reviewed retrospective cohort studies involving two large databases from the United Kingdom and Denmark to evaluate the relationship between selected antiepileptics (carbamazepine, gabapentin, lamotrigine, phenytoin, pregabalin, topiramate, and valproate) and suicidal thoughts and behaviors. Adjusted hazard ratios for suicide/suicidal behaviors ranged from 1.3 for lamotrigine and 2.7 for phenytoin in the United Kingdom and between 0.9 for valproate and 1.8 for phenytoin in Denmark. This study suggests a clinically significant association between some specific antiepileptic drugs and increased risk of suicide, although definitions and outcomes varied and emphasize the need for international standardization of terms.

Studies have also evaluated the relationship between antiepileptic drugs and specific populations. Patients with untreated bipolar disorder were at significantly greater risk of making suicide attempts and dying from suicide than those complying with treatment with antiepileptics and lithium (Caley et al. 2018). Furthermore, suicide risk appears to gradually decrease with continuing antiepileptic treatment, suggesting that the relationship between antiepileptics and suicidal behavior is confounded by multiple factors (Raju Sagiraju et al. 2018). In summary, although some studies suggest increased suicidal behavior in those treated with antiepileptic drugs, the balance of data reflects that antiepileptics are typically prescribed to patients with illnesses that predispose to death from suicide and that these drugs actually result in an overall reduction in the risk of suicide in these patients.

Ketamine and Other Glutamatergic Drugs

Ketamine is an *N*-methyl-D-aspartate (NMDA) receptor antagonist that has evidence for rapid antidepressant action and potential specific effectiveness in reducing suicidal thoughts and behaviors. Data suggest that ketamine may reduce suicidal ideation within 40 minutes of administration, with the beneficial effect lasting up to 1 week (Wilkinson et al. 2018). Although they are postulated to occur through NMDA-receptor antagonism mechanisms, ketamine's antisuicidal actions may manifest through anti-inflammatory pathways, γ-aminobutyric acid (GABA), or α-amino-3-

hydroxy-5-methyl-4-isoxazolepropionic acid (AMPA) receptors (Strasburger et al. 2017). Recent studies have examined the effects of esketamine, an intranasal formulation of the S enantiomer of ketamine, on depression and suicidal thoughts and behaviors (Canuso et al. 2018). Esketamine, in comparison to placebo and in addition to standard antidepressant treatment, appears to lead to rapid reduction in depression and some aspects of suicidal behavior in those at high risk for suicide.

Other Psychotropic Drugs

Smoking and smoking cessation have been associated with depression and suicide, with existing data suggesting that varenicline may increase the risk of suicidal thoughts and behaviors. Although this has led to a black box warning by the FDA, a recent meta-analysis of randomized trials suggests that varenicline does not magnify risk of suicide (Thomas et al. 2015).

A randomized, placebo-controlled trial using low-dosage buprenorphine, a partial μ-opioid agonist, for 4 weeks decreased suicidal ideation in 40 significantly suicidal patients without substance use disorders. Neither the use of concurrent antidepressants nor the diagnosis of borderline personality disorder affected the response to buprenorphine (Yovell et al. 2016). Tianeptine, a selective serotonin reuptake enhancer with μ-opioid receptor agonist properties, is an antidepressant in use in several countries but not approved by the FDA for use in the United States. One study has demonstrated a reduced risk of suicidal ideation associated with tianeptine compared with other antidepressants over the first 6 weeks of treatment of depressed outpatients (Nobile et al. 2018).

Neuromodulation

Research continues to illuminate the biological mechanisms that lead to psychiatric illness. Neuromodulation (also referred to as "interventional psychiatry") has become an area of rapidly expanding options. *Neuromodulation* involves both invasive and noninvasive procedures that influence the brain's neural activity and circuitry to alter behavior, cognition, or emotions. Research into neuromodulatory procedures and their roles in treating suicidal thoughts and behaviors has been sparse but is growing. Currently available interventions that have reached clinical practice include electroconvulsive therapy (ECT), transcranial magnetic stimulation (TMS), deep brain stimulation (DBS), and vagus nerve stimulation (VNS).

Electroconvulsive Therapy

We now have more than a half century of experience with ECT. The advancements in the technology used to administer ECT and in biometric telemetry have allowed for more precise control of the electrical stimulus while simultaneously monitoring the patient's electroencephalogram and vital signs. ECT has been shown to be effective in treating severe major depressive disorder (MDD) with or without psychotic features, manic or mixed episodes of bipolar disorder (Fink et al. 2014), and acute episodes of schizoaffective disorder or schizophrenia (Pompili et al. 2013). Several studies have shown promising short-term results with ECT leading to rapid improvement in suicidal thoughts and behaviors (Kellner et al. 2005), thought to be the result of the rapid reduction of severe depression, mania, and psychosis.

Furthermore, continuation treatment with a combination of nortriptyline and lithium after ECT has been demonstrated to be more effective in preventing suicidal ideation and behaviors than treatment with ECT alone (Kellner et al. 2005). Research examining the effect of ECT on suicidal ideation and behaviors 1 year after initial treatment has demonstrated that patients with MDD or bipolar disorder initially treated with ECT and continued on maintenance ECT and medication demonstrated significantly less suicidal behavior and fewer relapses compared to those treated with medication alone (Nordenskjöld et al. 2013).

With strong research backing the effectiveness of treating suicidal thoughts and behaviors with ECT (Fink et al. 2014), many researchers are now examining how the electrode placement, frequency of treatment, and concomitant treatment with pharmaceuticals can be altered to further improve ECT's effects. The safety and efficacy of ECT treatment and the findings indicating its direct or indirect effects on suicidal thoughts and behaviors support promptly assessing patients with significant suicidal preoccupation for suitability for ECT treatment, especially those admitted to the hospital and on suicide precautions. ECT may also be considered for pregnant (Spodniaková et al. 2015) and elderly (Geduldig and Kellner 2016) patients expressing acute suicidal ideation for whom pharmaceutical treatment may be contraindicated or who might have higher risk from pharmacotherapy than ECT.

Transcranial Magnetic Stimulation

TMS is a noninvasive procedure that uses electromagnetic induction to generate an electric current across the scalp and skull, altering the firing rates of targeted neurons in the brain. In 2008, the FDA approved TMS for the treatment of adults with MDD who have not experienced improvement from at least one prior treatment with an antidepressant at the standard treatment dosage and duration. TMS has some advantages over ECT as a treatment modality because it does not require anesthesia, induction of a seizure, or surgical intervention and has fewer side effects than ECT (McClintock et al. 2018).

Research has only recently begun to examine whether TMS can directly influence suicidal thoughts and behaviors. One study found that suicidal patients treated with repetitive TMS over 4–6 weeks had a significant decrease in suicidal thoughts and behaviors, with a rapid reduction in suicidal ideation occurring within the first day of treatment (George et al. 2014). Another study with depressed teenagers found that TMS treatment that resulted in measurable changes in long-interval intracortical inhibition (a measure of $GABA_B$-mediated inhibition) correlated significantly with a reduction in suicidal ideation (Lewis et al. 2019). The TMS procedure used may also be critical to treatment: bilateral, but not unilateral, TMS of the dorsolateral prefrontal cortex significantly reduced suicidal ideation in depressed patients who had failed at least two previous medication trials (Weissman et al. 2018). In an earlier retrospective study of 100 consecutive patients with treatment-resistant MDD (average of 3.4 previous failed medication trials) who were treated with TMS over a 6-month duration, 41% met criteria for response and 35% met criteria for remission. There were no suicide attempts in the entire cohort (Connolly et al. 2012). Substantial research is yet needed to refine TMS technology to more accurately target specific neural circuits and to explore TMS's potential to decrease suicidal ideation and behaviors in patients.

Deep Brain Stimulation

DBS is a neuromodulation procedure that involves the surgical implantation of a neurostimulating device into the brain. Through precise placement of the DBS device, electrical impulses can be administered to specific targets. Currently, the FDA has only approved DBS for the treatment of obsessive-compulsive disorder, advanced Parkinson's disease, chronic dystonia, and essential tremor. However, researchers are exploring the efficacy of this procedure in various other psychiatric disorders.

Studies examining whether DBS is an effective treatment for treatment-resistant depression have shown promising results. Several areas of the brain have been targeted for electrode placement in the treatment of depression, including the nucleus accumbens, ventral capsule/ventral striatum, and the posterior gyrus rectus. Bilateral electrode placement in the subcallosal cingulate gyrus has been the area most frequently targeted in recent studies of DBS and depression (Accolla et al. 2016). One study has found that use of high-resolution magnetic resonance imagery and tractography can further pinpoint the best area for electrode placement and provide an individualized surgical approach to DBS placement in patients with treatment-resistant depression. This study found that individualized placement increased treatment efficacy to 73% response at 6 months and 82% at 1 year (Riva-Posse et al. 2018).

However, suicide in patients receiving DBS is a concern. One study found that of 20 patients with treatment-resistant depression treated with DBS, 2 had died from suicide and 2 others had attempted suicide after a 3.5-year follow-up period (Kennedy et al. 2011). Although this is likely a reflection of the illness severity of individuals who receive DBS, it nevertheless reflects a need for ongoing clinical awareness of the persisting risk of suicide. In a 15-month study of 25 patients with a primary diagnosis of treatment-resistant depression, DBS (targeting the nucleus accumbens and ventral anterior limb of the internal capsule) significantly reduced depressive symptoms in 10 (40%) individuals. Suicide attempts or suicidal ideation occurred in six DBS patients, all nonresponders to treatment (Bergfeld et al. 2016). The indication for DBS (e.g., Parkinson's disease, epilepsy, depression), a previous history of suicidal thoughts and behaviors, and electrode placement (e.g., the subthalamic nucleus) may each contribute to postsurgery suicidal thoughts and behaviors (Voon et al. 2008). More research may clarify this complex issue.

Vagus Nerve Stimulation

VNS is another surgical procedure showing promising results in the treatment of suicidal thoughts and behaviors. This neuromodulatory intervention involves the surgical implantation of a pulse stimulator in the superficial anterior chest that transmits electrical pulses via an electrode to the left vagus nerve. The stimulation of the left vagus nerve leads to downstream impulses that affect various mood centers in the brain.

VNS has been FDA approved since 2005 as an adjunctive treatment of treatment-resistant depression in adult patients who have not had adequate response to at least four antidepressant medication trials. Relatively few well-designed randomized clinical trials exist, but data from two systematic reviews suggest a significant long-term reduction in depressive symptoms overall (Berry et al. 2013; Cimpianu et al. 2017). Researchers are now specifically investigating VNS's capability to treat suicidal thoughts and behaviors in this patient population. For example, a 5-year observational study of patients with treatment-resistant depression treated with VNS (*N*=795) found that subjects treated with VNS showed a significantly greater reduction in their suicidal thoughts and behaviors profile compared with subjects receiving standard psychopharmacological treatment (Aaronson et al. 2017). This trial supports the need for further research to determine the mediators and moderators of VNS in the successful treatment of suicidal thoughts and behaviors.

Conclusion

Patients with medical, neurological, and neuropsychiatric illnesses have a higher risk for suicidal behavior. The difficulty in assessing whether psychotropic drugs may also independently increase the risk of suicide adds to the complexity of caring for this vulnerable population. Ultimately, treating those at high risk for suicide remains an important area of clinical concern and calls for increasing access to quality care and increasing public education to reduce the rates of suicide in the United States.

Key Points

- Appropriately selected and monitored medications and neuromodulation techniques may be very helpful in the treatment of patients with suicidal ideation and behavior.

- Psychopharmacological interventions that may indirectly decrease suicidal ideation are those that effectively treat the underlying psychiatric disorders of mood and psychotic disorders.

- Certain psychopharmacological agents may directly reduce suicidal thoughts and behaviors. Antidepressant agents, mood stabilizers including anticonvulsants, and glutamatergic drugs may be effective in decreasing suicidal risk.

- Each psychopharmacological agent, or combination of them, carries different risks of potential use in overdose attempts.

- More controlled studies are needed to assess the efficacy of novel neuromodulation approaches in the treatment of psychiatric disorders and suicide.

References

Aaronson ST, Sears P, Ruvuna F, et al: A 5-year observational study of patients with treatment-resistant depression treated with vagus nerve stimulation or treatment as usual: comparison of response, remission, and suicidality. Am J Psychiatry 174(7):640–648, 2017 28359201
Accolla EA, Aust S, Merkl A, et al: Deep brain stimulation of the posterior gyrus rectus region for treatment resistant depression. J Affect Disord 194:33–37, 2016 26802505
Bergfeld IO, Mantione M, Hoogendoorn MLC, et al: Deep brain stimulation of the ventral anterior limb of the internal capsule for treatment-resistant depression: a randomized clinical trial. JAMA Psychiatry 73(5):456–464, 2016 27049915

Berry SM, Broglio K, Bunker M, et al: A patient-level meta-analysis of studies evaluating vagus nerve stimulation therapy for treatment-resistant depression. Med Devices (Auckl) 6:17–35, 2013 23482508

Bingham KS, Rothschild AJ, Mulsant BH, et al: The association of baseline suicidality with treatment outcome in psychotic depression. J Clin Psychiatry 78(8):1149–1154, 2017 28445632

Brent DA: Antidepressants and suicidality. Psychiatr Clin North Am 39(3):503–512, 2016 27514302

Britton JW, Shih JJ: Antiepileptic drugs and suicidality. Drug Healthc Patient Saf 2:181–189, 2010 21701630

Caley CF, Perriello E, Golden J: Antiepileptic drugs and suicide-related outcomes in bipolar disorder: a descriptive review of published data. Ment Health Clin 8(3):138–147, 2018 29955559

Can A, Schulze TG, Gould TD: Molecular actions and clinical pharmacogenetics of lithium therapy. Pharmacol Biochem Behav 123:3–16, 2014 24534415

Canuso CM, Singh JB, Fedgchin M, et al: Efficacy and safety of intranasal esketamine for the rapid reduction of symptoms of depression and suicidality in patients at imminent risk for suicide: results of a double-blind, randomized, placebo-controlled study. Am J Psychiatry 175(7):620–630, 2018 29656663

Cimpianu CL, Strube W, Falkai P, et al: Vagus nerve stimulation in psychiatry: a systematic review of the available evidence. J Neural Transm (Vienna) 124(1):145–158, 2017 27848034

Connolly KR, Helmer A, Cristancho MA, et al: Effectiveness of transcranial magnetic stimulation in clinical practice post-FDA approval in the United States: results observed with the first 100 consecutive cases of depression at an academic medical center. J Clin Psychiatry 73(4):e567–e573, 2012 22579164

Courtet P, Jaussent I, Lopez-Castroman J, et al: Poor response to antidepressants predicts new suicidal ideas and behavior in depressed outpatients. Eur Neuropsychopharmacol 24(10):1650–1658, 2014 25112546

Cristancho P, O'Connor B, Lenze EJ, et al: Treatment emergent suicidal ideation in depressed older adults. Int J Geriatr Psychiatry 32(6):596–604, 2017 27162147

Erlangsen A, Conwell Y: Age-related response to redeemed antidepressants measured by completed suicide in older adults: a nationwide cohort study. Am J Geriatr Psychiatry 22(1):25–33, 2014 23567434

Fink M, Kellner CH, McCall WV: The role of ECT in suicide prevention. J ECT 30(1):5–9, 2014 24091903

Geduldig ET, Kellner CH: Electroconvulsive therapy in the elderly: new findings in geriatric depression. Curr Psychiatry Rep 18(4):40, 2016 26909702

George MS, Raman R, Benedek DM, et al: A two-site pilot randomized 3 day trial of high dose left prefrontal repetitive transcranial magnetic stimulation (rTMS) for suicidal inpatients. Brain Stimul 7(3):421–431, 2014 24731434

Giurca D: Decreasing suicide risk with math. Curr Psychiatr 17(2):57–59, 2018

Hedna K, Andersson Sundell K, Hamidi A, et al: Antidepressants and suicidal behaviour in late life: a prospective population-based study of use patterns in new users aged 75 and above. Eur J Clin Pharmacol 74(2):201–208, 2018 29103090

Henein F, Prabhakar D, Peterson EL, et al: A prospective study of antidepressant adherence and suicidal ideation among adults. Prim Care Companion CNS Disord 18(6):1–4, 2016 27907275

Kellner CH, Fink M, Knapp R, et al: Relief of expressed suicidal intent by ECT: a consortium for research in ECT study. Am J Psychiatry 162(5):977–982, 2005 15863801

Kennedy SH, Giacobbe P, Rizvi SJ, et al: Deep brain stimulation for treatment-resistant depression: follow-up after 3 to 6 years. Am J Psychiatry 168(5):502–510, 2011 21285143

Larsson J: Antidepressants and suicide among young women in Sweden 1999–2013. Int J Risk Saf Med 29(1-2):101–106, 2017 28885220

Lewis CP, Camsari DD, Sonmez AI, et al: Preliminary evidence of an association between increased cortical inhibition and reduced suicidal ideation in adolescents treated for major depression. J Affect Disord 244:21–24, 2019 30292987

Liaugaudaite V, Mickuviene N, Raskauskiene N, et al: Lithium levels in the public drinking water supply and risk of suicide: a pilot study. J Trace Elem Med Biol 43:197–201, 2017 28385387

Löfman S, Hakko H, Mainio A, et al: Affective disorders and completed suicide by self-poisoning, trend of using antidepressants as a method of self-poisoning. Psychiatry Res 255:360–366, 2017 28628870

McClintock SM, Reti IM, Carpenter LL, et al: Consensus recommendations for the clinical application of repetitive transcranial magnetic stimulation (rTMS) in the treatment of depression. J Clin Psychiatry 79:16cs10905, 2018 28541649

Nobile B, Jaussent I, Gorwood P, et al: Tianeptine is associated with lower risk of suicidal ideation worsening during the first weeks of treatment onset compared with other antidepressants: a naturalistic study. J Psychiatr Res 96:167–170, 2018 29073492

Nordenskjöld A, von Knorring L, Ljung T, et al: Continuation electroconvulsive therapy with pharmacotherapy versus pharmacotherapy alone for prevention of relapse of depression: a randomized controlled trial. J ECT 29(2):86–92, 2013 23303421

Perlis RH, Uher R, Perroud N, et al: Do suicidal thoughts or behaviors recur during a second antidepressant treatment trial? J Clin Psychiatry 73(11):1439–1442, 2012 23059018

Pompili M, Lester D, Dominici G, et al: Indications for electroconvulsive treatment in schizophrenia: a systematic review. Schizophr Res 146(1-3):1–9, 2013 23499244

Raju Sagiraju HK, Wang CP, Amuan ME, et al: Antiepileptic drugs and suicide-related behavior: is it the drug or comorbidity? Neurol Clin Pract 8(4):331–339, 2018 30140585

Reutfors J, Clapham E, Bahmanyar S, et al: Suicide risk and antipsychotic side effects in schizophrenia: nested case-control study. Hum Psychopharmacol 31(4):341–345, 2016 27108775

Ringbäck Weitoft G, Berglund M, Lindström EA, et al: Mortality, attempted suicide, rehospitalisation and prescription refill for clozapine and other antipsychotics in Sweden—a register-based study. Pharmacoepidemiol Drug Saf 23(3):290–298, 2014 24435842

Rissanen I, Jääskeläinen E, Isohanni M, et al: Antipsychotics and antidepressants and their associations with suicidal ideation—the northern Finland birth cohort 1966. Schizophr Res 153(suppl 1):S359, 2014

Riva-Posse P, Choi KS, Holtzheimer PE, et al: A connectomic approach for subcallosal cingulate deep brain stimulation surgery: prospective targeting in treatment-resistant depression. Mol Psychiatry 23(4):843–849, 2018 28397839

Schuerch M, Gasse C, Robinson NJ, et al: Impact of varying outcomes and definitions of suicidality on the associations of antiepileptic drugs and suicidality: comparisons from UK Clinical Practice Research Datalink (CPRD) and Danish national registries (DNR). Pharmacoepidemiol Drug Saf 25(suppl 1):142–155, 2016 27038360

Smith KA, Cipriani A: Lithium and suicide in mood disorders: updated meta-review of the scientific literature. Bipolar Disord 19(7):575–586, 2017 28895269

Spodniaková B, Halmo M, Nosálová P: Electroconvulsive therapy in pregnancy: a review. J Obstet Gynaecol 35(7):659–662, 2015 25526509

Strasburger SE, Bhimani PM, Kaabe JH, et al: What is the mechanism of ketamine's rapid-onset antidepressant effect? A concise overview of the surprisingly large number of possibilities. J Clin Pharm Ther 42(2):147–154, 2017 28111761

Takeuchi T, Takenoshita S, Taka F, et al: The relationship between psychotropic drug use and suicidal behavior in Japan: Japanese adverse drug event report. Pharmacopsychiatry 50(2):69–73, 2017 27595297

Thomas KH, Martin RM, Knipe DW, et al: Risk of neuropsychiatric adverse events associated with varenicline: systematic review and meta-analysis. BMJ 350:h1109, 2015 25767129

Toffol E, Hätönen T, Tanskanen A, et al: Lithium is associated with decrease in all-cause and suicide mortality in high-risk bipolar patients: a nationwide registry-based prospective cohort study. J Affect Disord 183:159–165, 2015 26005778

Tondo L, Baldessarini RJ: Suicidal behavior in mood disorders: response to pharmacological treatment. Curr Psychiatry Rep 18(9):88, 2016 27542851

Tsai CJ, Cheng C, Chou PH, et al: The rapid suicide protection of mood stabilizers on patients with bipolar disorder: a nationwide observational cohort study in Taiwan. J Affect Disord 196:71–77, 2016 26919054

Valuck RJ, Libby AM, Anderson HD, et al: Comparison of antidepressant classes and the risk and time course of suicide attempts in adults: propensity matched, retrospective cohort study. Br J Psychiatry 208(3):271–279, 2016 26635328

Voon V, Krack P, Lang AE, et al: A multicentre study on suicide outcomes following subthalamic stimulation for Parkinson's disease. Brain 131(Pt 10):2720–2728, 2008 18941146

Weissman CR, Blumberger DM, Brown PE, et al: Bilateral repetitive transcranial magnetic stimulation decreases suicidal ideation in depression. J Clin Psychiatry 79(3):e11692, 2018 29701939

Weitz E, Hollon SD, Kerkhof A, et al: Do depression treatments reduce suicidal ideation? The effects of CBT, IPT, pharmacotherapy, and placebo on suicidality. J Affect Disord 167:98–103, 2014 24953481

Wilkinson ST, Ballard ED, Bloch MH, et al: The effect of a single dose of intravenous ketamine on suicidal ideation: a systematic review and individual participant data meta-analysis. Am J Psychiatry 175(2):150–158, 2018 28969441

Yovell Y, Bar G, Mashiah M, et al: Ultra-low-dose buprenorphine as a time-limited treatment for severe suicidal ideation: a randomized controlled trial. Am J Psychiatry 173(5):491–498, 2016 26684923

CHAPTER 3

Cognitive and Behavioral Therapy

Amy Wenzel, Ph.D., ABPP

Abby Adler, Ph.D.

Many variables that contribute to understanding and treating suicidal thoughts and behavior are psychological in nature. For example, increasing attention has focused on recognizing and heeding warning signs for suicidal behavior or indicators that an individual is entering into an acute suicidal crisis, much in the same way as, for example, arm pain and shortness of breath would be for a heart attack (Rudd 2008). Some of these warning signs, such as hopelessness, withdrawal, anger, and aggression, can be addressed through psychotherapeutic interventions as they are occurring, as well as in a preventive manner so that patients know how to manage them if they arise in the future. Cognitive-behavioral therapy (CBT), a short-term, time-sensitive psychotherapy approach, is one such acute psychological intervention that directly addresses such psychological variables to prevent suicide.

This chapter examines four specific CBT packages for the treatment of suicidal ideation and behavior: 1) cognitive therapy for suicide prevention (CT-SP; Wenzel et al. 2009) and its adaptations; 2) brief CBT for suicide prevention (BCBT; Rudd 2012) for active military populations; 3) dialectical behavior therapy (DBT; Linehan 1993) for emotion dysregulation and its adaptations; and 4) internet-delivered CBT (van Spijker et al. 2014). Notable aspects of each treatment approach and evidence of their efficacy are discussed. In addition, professional issues of which cognitive-behavioral therapists should be mindful when treating patients with suicidal thoughts and behaviors are reviewed.

The Cognitive-Behavioral Approach

CBT is characterized by several distinctive features. First, CBT is an active, problem-focused approach that is meant to have a clear endpoint so that patients can, eventually, implement tools and strategies in their lives without the aid of a therapist. To achieve this aim, patients receive psychoeducation about cognitive-behavioral principles, practice corresponding skills and strategies, and consider ways to generalize their learning to their lives outside of the therapy session. Second, CBT is a collaborative approach to treatment; the therapist and patient work together as a team to customize the intervention to meet the patient's individual needs, strengths, and learning style. This feature increases the likelihood that patients will take ownership over their role in treatment and fully engage in the treatment process. Collectively, these factors increase the likelihood that patients will make meaningful changes in their lives even after therapy has completed. Empirical research has determined that CBT is efficacious for countless clinical conditions (Butler et al. 2006) because cognitive and behavioral intervention strategies are versatile and have relevance to the thinking, emotional experiencing, and behaviors associated with most types of emotional distress and adjustment problems.

This approach to treatment is a strong match for work, specifically, with patients who report suicidal thoughts or behavior. Although some risk factors for suicidal thoughts and behavior are static (e.g., age, ethnicity), many risk factors are modifiable and can be targeted in psychotherapy to prevent a future suicidal crisis. These risk factors include (but are not limited to) suicidal ideation, chronic hopelessness, impulsivity, impulsive aggression, an overgeneral memory style (i.e., difficulty recalling specific memories about one's life), poor problem solving, low problem-solving self-efficacy, perfectionism, the frequent committal of cognitive distortions, and symptoms of many mental health disorders (e.g., Brown et al. 2000). CBT is an approach that helps patients address many of these modifiable risk factors, and strategies targeting these factors are routinely delivered in clinical practice.

Empirical research is accumulating in support of CBT as an evidence-based treatment for suicidal ideation and behavior. For example, one meta-analysis examined the efficacy of the broad family of cognitive-behaviorally based psychotherapeutic approaches in the reduction of suicidal and nonsuicidal self-injurious behavior (Tarrier et al. 2008). Most of the active cognitive-behaviorally based interventions included in the analyses were variations of CT-SP, DBT, and an older form of problem-solving therapy (Salkovskis et al. 1990) and were compared to a usual-care condition (i.e., treatment received in the community that could include medication, supportive counseling, a combination of treatments, or no treatment at all). In this meta-analysis, CBT outperformed usual care on many outcome measures, including suicidal ideation, suicidal behavior, and hopelessness.

Another review summarized outcomes for five cognitive-behavioral approaches that primarily targeted suicidal cognitions (Mewton and Andrews 2016). The authors of this review concluded that these treatment approaches were highly efficacious in reducing suicidal ideation and both suicidal and nonsuicidal self-injurious behavior. Interestingly, studies evaluating the efficacy of these CBT interventions found that effects were observed primarily on variables directly relevant to suicidal thoughts and behaviors rather than secondary outcome measures (e.g., depression). This pattern of results suggests that CBT focused specifically on suicide prevention in a targeted, transdiagnostic manner achieves its primary aim.

Denchev et al. (2018) examined the cost-effectiveness and the societal impact of suicide-prevention interventions initiated in emergency departments. They determined that for patients who present to emergency departments with suicidal risk, connecting patients with a suicide-focused CBT program improves outcomes (e.g., prevents suicide deaths and reattempts) with an incremental cost of $18,800 USD per life-year, which is significantly less than an estimated societal willingness to pay to reduce mortality of $50,000 USD per life-year. In the next sections, we describe four specific cognitive-behavioral approaches to suicide prevention.

Cognitive Therapy for Suicide Prevention

CT-SP is modeled in the spirit of traditional "Beckian" cognitive therapy as originally conceived by the "father" of CBT, Dr. Aaron T. Beck (1967). CT-SP was developed in the late 1990s as a response to prevailing clinical practices in which patients with suicidal thoughts and behaviors were generally treated for depression (combined with high-risk management), rather than for suicide risk itself. Dr. Beck and his colleagues observed that not all patients with suicidal thoughts and behaviors are depressed and, moreover, that tailoring treatment to a diagnosis rather than to suicidal behavior itself had the potential to miss essential targets of treatment that could ultimately prevent suicide (Wenzel et al. 2009).

Thus, CT-SP was developed as a transdiagnostic treatment approach that could be delivered as an adjunct to other psychiatric treatments (e.g., pharmacotherapy, substance abuse treatment), facilitating a holistic treatment-team approach. Although the term "cognitive therapy" is used to designate this protocol, most scholars and practitioners use the terms "cognitive therapy" and "CBT" interchangeably. Indeed, CT-SP focuses on cognitive change and behavior change equally, which is relevant to reducing suicide risk.

CT-SP is divided into three phases: an early phase, a middle phase, and a late phase. The early phase of treatment has numerous goals, which are addressed in approximately the first three sessions. Throughout the entire early phase of treatment, the cognitive therapist takes great measures to engage the patient in treatment because research shows that a large proportion of patients at risk for suicide who are referred for treatment do not follow through (Lizardi and Stanley 2010).

First, cognitive-behavioral therapists obtain informed consent for treatment. Informed consent is important upon the commencement of any course of mental health intervention. However, informed consent, particularly confidentiality limitations, are important to address systematically with patients with suicidal thoughts and behaviors at the outset of treatment because these patients are at an increased likelihood, relative to other general psychiatric patients, to be in a position in which it is necessitated that confidentiality be broken. Therefore, cognitive-behavioral therapists carefully explain the limits of confidentiality and exactly what will happen if confidentiality is compromised. At the same time, during the informed consent process, cognitive-behavioral therapists have an opportunity to educate patients about the treatment approach, its structure, and what it can offer as a means of instilling hope so that patients have a sense that their lives can be different.

After obtaining informed consent, cognitive-behavioral therapists conduct a thorough suicide risk assessment to determine the appropriate frequency of sessions and the need for referrals to other services as well as to begin the development of a case formulation of their patient's clinical presentation. In addition, therapists develop a collaborative safety plan for patients to consult in between sessions when they experience or become aware of an impending suicidal crisis. The safety plan is a written summary of warning signs for suicidal crises; coping skills that patients can use on their own; people to whom they can reach out for general support and connection, or specifically for help; and contact information for professionals who can help. Although the safety plan was originally developed as part of this treatment protocol, it has since been extended into a stand-alone intervention that is used with individuals with a suicide-related concern who present to emergency departments for acute services (Stanley et al. 2018).

In the middle sessions of treatment, cognitive-behavioral therapists deliver standard and adapted cognitive and behavioral strategies targeted toward the relevant psychological factors in effect during the patient's most recent suicidal crisis (e.g., narrowed attention on suicide as the sole solution to problems). Therapists also address modifiable factors that put patients at risk for future suicidal crises (e.g., perfectionism). Standard cognitive therapy interventions typically used in CT-SP include cognitive restructuring (i.e., the identification, evaluation, and modification of unhelpful thinking); behavioral activation (i.e., the promotion of active engagement in meaningful and pleasurable activities); and social problem solving (i.e., the solving of "real-life," often interpersonal, stressors that the patient is facing).

For patients who report interpersonal strife with family members, conjoint sessions are often indicated. Family sessions are particularly applicable in CT-SP with adolescent patients so that parents can help teens use their CBT strategies when needed. For patients who report difficulty accessing health care services or complying with other treatments, cognitive therapists provide coaching in making phone calls to schedule appointments, communicating with other health care professionals, and developing organizational skills to take medications as indicated and attend appointments.

Above all, the middle sessions of CT-SP are devoted to the identification and cultivation of reasons for living because research shows that an absence of reasons for living, combined with many reasons for dying, is associated with an increased risk of suicidal behavior (Jobes and Mann 1999). Having reasons for living combats an array of suicide-relevant beliefs that are activated during suicidal crises. These include the belief that the future is hopeless, that continued existence is unbearable, that the individual does not belong to a larger group, and that the individual is a burden on others (Rudd 2000). Although reasons for living can be discussed in session and written down for patients to consult outside of session, the most innovative method of gathering reminders of reasons for living is to construct a "hope box." In its original form, the hope box was a shoebox in which patients placed tangible reminders for living (e.g., photographs of loved others, verses from religious texts). At present, many patients use mobile phone applications to remind them of reasons for living, such as the Virtual Hope Box, which can be downloaded for free from the "app store" on a mobile phone device.

The final phase of treatment focuses on relapse prevention, or steps that can be put in place to reduce the likelihood of a future suicidal crisis. The key activity in this phase of treatment is a *relapse prevention task*, which involves patients imagining in vivid detail the suicidal crisis that brought them to treatment and rehearsing ways in which the cognitive-behavioral tools acquired in treatment would be useful for managing distress. Patients also have the opportunity to imagine a potential crisis that could be encountered in the future and describe the future application of cognitive-behavioral tools to avert suicidal ideation and behavior. Throughout the late phase of treatment, patients consolidate their learning by summarizing what skills they have learned and how they can use them in the future as well as prepare for the ending of treatment or the continuation of treatment focused on goals other than the reduction of risk for suicidal behavior.

In the landmark study evaluating the efficacy of CT-SP, Brown et al. (2005) randomized 120 patients who were seen in an emergency department within 48 hours after a suicide attempt to CT-SP plus usual care or usual care only. Across an 18-month period following baseline, patients randomized to the CT-SP condition had a lower suicide reattempt rate than patients randomized to the usual-care condition. In addition, relative to patients receiving usual care, patients receiving CT-SP reported a lower level of depression on a standard self-report inventory at the 6-, 12-, and 18-month reassessments and a lower level of hopelessness at the 6-month reassessment. Results from this study show that CT-SP can reduce the rate of suicide reattempts by as much as 50%.

Although the Brown et al. (2005) study is the only published clinical trial evaluating the efficacy of this protocol (Wenzel et al. 2009), CT-SP has had widespread influence upon many applications of the cognitive-behavioral approach to reducing suicide risk in specific populations. For example, CT-SP has been modified into a brief format (six 60- to 90-minute individual sessions) to be delivered to patients on an inpatient unit while hospitalized after a suicidal crisis, with preliminary results indicating that it outperforms usual care in reducing depression, hopelessness, suicidal ideation, and posttraumatic stress symptoms (Ghahramanlou-Holloway et al. 2018).

In addition, CBT served as the model for the psychotherapy intervention used in the Treatment of Adolescent Suicide Attempters study (Brent et al. 2009), a clinical trial that was originally intended to compare psychotherapy, medication, or combined treatment but was ultimately modified to allow families to choose their preferred treatment. The vast majority of participants in this study received either psychotherapy alone or in combination with medication, and results indicated that the reattempt rate was lower than in comparable samples. Finally, CT-SP has been adapted for older men who are at risk for suicidal behavior (but who often deny the presence of hopelessness and suicidal ideation), and results from a large clinical research trial applying the CT-SP protocol to this population are pending (Bhar and Brown 2012).

Brief Cognitive-Behavioral Therapy

BCBT (Rudd 2012) incorporates many elements of CT-SP as well as the extensive program of research by its developers and specifically targets active-duty members of the military. The basis of this treatment is the developer's observation of six common elements across a range of CBTs for suicide prevention used in clinical trials: 1) an easy-to-understand model of suicidal behavior; 2) a focus on treatment compliance; 3) the identification of skills to be targeted in treatment; 4) an emphasis on the patient's personal responsibility for treatment; 5) easy access to crisis and emergency services; and 6) an easy-to-understand written treatment plan.

Like CT-SP, BCBT is divided into three phases, labeled in this protocol as phase I: orientation; phase II: skill focus; and phase III: relapse prevention. Although many aspects of this protocol are similar to CT-SP, one notable evolution from the Brown et al. (2005) protocol is its early emphasis on the identification of reasons for living and the development of a hope box (or "survival kit") and a reasons for living coping card in phase I of treatment to decrease suicidal intent and instill hope. Moreover, four specific skill sets are targeted in phase II, including problem solving, mindfulness, cognitive appraisal (much like cognitive restructuring), and relaxation (Rudd 2012).

In a large-scale evaluation of BCBT (Rudd et al. 2015), active-duty army soldiers at Fort Carson, Colorado, were randomly assigned to BCBT ($n=76$) or usual care ($n=76$). Results replicated and extended the impressive findings reported in the Brown et al. (2005) study, with only 13.8% of patients receiving BCBT making at least one suicide attempt in the 24-month follow-up period compared with 40.2% of patients receiving usual care. Group differences in suicide attempts emerged at the 6-month follow-up reassessment and widened throughout the remaining 18 months of follow-up. However, no group differences emerged for secondary outcome variables, including depression, hopelessness, anxiety, and posttraumatic stress. Interestingly, a near-statistically significant trend was noted, with fewer patients in the BCBT condition retired for medical reasons, relative to patients in the usual-care condition (26.8% vs. 41.8%). Results from this study provide evidence that BCBT can reduce suicide attempt rates by 60%, suggesting that it optimized the efficacious features of CT-SP.

Dialectical Behavior Therapy

DBT is a cognitive-behaviorally based psychotherapeutic approach that garnered attention in the mid-1990s for treatment of patients with borderline personality disorder who engage in chronic self-harm behavior with both suicidal and nonsuicidal intent (Linehan 1993). DBT is a multifaceted treatment approach that involves five main components (described later). All patients have an individual therapist who takes a dialectical approach of balancing opposing ideas to address the problematic behaviors that put patients at risk for harm and exacerbate symptoms. For the therapist, this includes striving for a balance between providing validation of emotional pain and facilitating behavior change within each session. Furthermore, therapists encourage patients to work toward balancing acceptance and change within themselves and throughout their daily lives.

Targets of treatment during the individual therapy component of DBT include 1) reduction in suicidal and nonsuicidal self-injurious behaviors; 2) reduction in therapy-interfering behaviors; 3) reduction in symptoms associated with previous trauma; 4) reduction in behaviors that detract from quality of life; and 5) increase in behaviors that make life worth living. In addition, patients participating in DBT enroll in a concurrent skills training group where they participate in four modules geared toward developing skills in mindfulness, interpersonal effectiveness, emotion regulation, and distress tolerance. Patients are coached by their individual therapist in the application of these skills to their daily lives, often via telephone coaching sessions that occur in between individual therapy appointments. The final two features of DBT programs include case management and peer consultation for therapists.

Dialectical behavioral therapists apply many strategies to help patients reduce suicidal and nonsuicidal self-harm behavior. When patients report self-harm behavior, dialectical behavior therapists conduct a *chain analysis* to identify the antecedents and consequences of the behavior so patients can identify points leading up to the behavior at which they could apply their learned coping skills. Throughout the course of treatment, patients are coached in the application of emotion regulation skills to decrease the likelihood of crises leading to self-harm behavior and distress tolerance skills to help them "survive" moments of intense emotional distress without doing something to hurt themselves. As dialectical behavioral therapists deliver these interventions, they simultaneously communicate a stance of acceptance and validation of the emotional pain that patients have been enduring and of the notion that patients are coping with this pain as best they can.

DBT's efficacy has been evaluated in 21 randomized controlled trials and 15 uncontrolled trials examining its usefulness for patients with borderline personality disorder who engage in self-harm behavior as well as patients with comorbid conditions such as substance use disorders, posttraumatic stress disorder, and eating disorders (Granato et al., in press). In the first landmark study evaluating its efficacy, Linehan et al. (1991) randomized 22 patients to DBT and 22 patients to usual care and examined rates of parasuicide (defined as acts with both suicidal and nonsuicidal intent) as the main outcome variable. Results indicated that 95.5% of the usual-care patients had engaged in a parasuicidal act during the year of treatment relative to 63.6% of the DBT patients, a difference that is considered large and significant. In addition, relative to patients in usual care, those who received DBT had fewer medically severe parasuicidal incidents, were more likely to be retained in treatment, and had fewer inpatient psychiatric days.

In a second landmark study, Linehan et al. (2006) randomized 52 patients to DBT and 49 patients to nonbehavioral psychotherapy delivered by skilled clinicians, the latter representing the highest-quality treatment patients could receive in the community. Results indicated that 23.1% of patients receiving DBT attempted suicide during the 2-year study period, relative to 46% of patients treated by community expert psychotherapists. In addition, the medical risk of parasuicidal acts (with and without suicidal intent) was lower for DBT patients than for patients treated by community experts, as were the rates of crisis services use and treatment dropout. Results from this study were particularly striking because they demonstrated that DBT is associated with a specific suicide-prevention effect that goes above and beyond that achieved by some of the highest-quality psychotherapy offered in the community.

Internet-Delivered Cognitive-Behavioral Therapy

CBT has been listed as an evidence-based approach to prevent suicide by the Substance Abuse and Mental Health Services Administration. However, one major challenge facing the greater CBT field is the accessibility to patients of therapists who are adequately trained to deliver this intervention at a level of acceptable competency. CBT is not taught in all training programs, and many clinicians do not receive adequate training in suicide risk assessment, management, or treatment. As a result, scholar-practitioners have worked to identify innovative ways to bring CBT to those who might benefit from this treatment, especially people who live in underserved and remote locations. One way to achieve wider availability of CBT is through the use of a CBT protocol that patients can access via the internet.

Recently, CBT for suicide prevention has been translated to an internet-delivery intervention for people with mild-to-moderate depression who report suicidal ideation (van Spijker et al. 2014). In this study, 236 people were randomized to the cognitive-behavioral intervention (*n*=116) or to a waitlist control condition (*n*=120). The intervention integrated components of Beckian cognitive therapy, DBT, problem-solving therapy, and mindfulness-based cognitive therapy. The program consisted of six weekly sessions that targeted cognitive restructuring, emotion regulation, and relapse prevention. Results indicated that people who completed the intervention reported significant reductions in suicidal ideation and worry relative to people who were assigned to a waitlist control condition. Per participants' self-report, four people in the intervention condition attempted suicide during the study period, relative to seven people in the waitlist control condition. No participant in either condition died from suicide during the study.

A logical concern about an internet-based intervention for suicide prevention is the safety of participants who are at higher risk to engage in suicidal behavior than the typical psychiatric patient. A safeguard was included in the van Spijker et al. (2014) study in which participants deemed to be at elevated risk for suicidal behavior through their responses to self-report measures of depression and suicidal ideation were contacted by a study staff member and completed a risk assessment. Participants' general practitioners were contacted if participants were identified as being at elevated risk after the risk assessment or if the participant could not be contacted. Thus, although safety concerns must be paramount as innovative interventions are developed, these preliminary results suggest that internet-based cognitive-behavioral interventions are feasible and can serve as a valuable resource in suicide prevention efforts to assist in reaching a broader population.

Working With Suicidal Patients

Cognitive-behavioral therapists aim to be mindful of "practicing what they preach," such that they strive to apply cognitive and behavioral principles and strategies in their own lives to manage stress, engage in appropriate self-care, and make use of positive social support (Wenzel et al. 2009). Although these practices are important for all mental health providers, they are imperative for providers who work with patients with suicidal thoughts and behaviors who may require crisis management and extra sessions and who may experience sudden changes in clinical and suicide risk status. Cognitive-behavioral therapists are encouraged to use cognitive restructuring techniques to manage hopeless or catastrophic cognitions about their clinical work; they should use interpersonal effectiveness techniques to communicate with patients, their family members, and other care providers; and they are encouraged to use behavioral strategies to manage their mood and stress level, such as by getting proper sleep, nutrition, and exercise.

Of particular note, cognitive-behavioral therapists are advised to make use of consultation with peers and mentors when working with suicidal patients (Linehan 1993; Wenzel et al. 2009). When possible, they advocate for a "treatment team" approach so that multiple health care providers are available to provide input and share responsibility for the patient's well-being. In DBT, for example, peer consultation is worked into the treatment model so that therapists working with patients with suicidal thoughts and behaviors can obtain regular support (Linehan 1993).

Conclusion

Suicide and suicidal behavior are a significant public health problem for which effective intervention is essential. Although great strides have been made in understanding the phenomenology and epidemiology of and risk factors for suicidal behavior, recent data show that suicide rates in the United States have increased since 1999 despite the attention that this problem has received in scholarly and clinical arenas (Hedegaard et al. 2018). Thus, continued work is clearly needed to optimize and further disseminate efficacious interventions for individuals with suicidal thoughts and people at risk for suicidal behavior.

Nevertheless, CBT for suicide prevention is a treatment of choice for patients with suicidal thoughts and behaviors because of its active problem-solving focus and its structure, both of which allow patients to acquire tangible skills for managing and preventing emotional distress. Two well-established CBT packages, CT-SP and DBT, have demonstrated efficacy in reducing suicide attempts during treatment and follow-up periods, and a related approach, BCBT, has also demonstrated efficacy in reducing suicide attempts specifically among active-duty military personnel.

CBT for suicide prevention is now being adapted for the needs of special populations, including adolescents, older adults, inpatients, and people with substance use disorders, as well as in special formats, such as an internet-based program. Across these treatment packages, research findings support the use of CBT strategies to directly target the factors contributing to suicidal thoughts and behaviors, regardless of diagnosis, in order to prevent suicide. Furthermore, regardless of the particular CBT protocol adopted, cognitive-behavioral therapists strive to apply the principles and strategies of CBT in their own lives as they work with patients at high risk of suicide in order to maintain a balanced and adaptive mindset, engage in healthy self-care, and obtain positive social support.

Key Points

- Cognitive-behavioral therapy (CBT) is a transdiagnostic psychotherapeutic approach that focuses on suicide-relevant thoughts, behaviors, risk factors, and warning signs rather than on one specific mental health diagnosis.

- Cognitive therapy for suicide prevention (CT-SP) is a brief, adjunctive treatment in which patients develop a safety plan to deal with suicidal crises, develop coping skills, cultivate reasons for living, and test their acquired skills in an innovative relapse prevention task.

- CT-SP has been adapted for many distinct clinical populations, including inpatients who have been hospitalized after a suicide attempt, adolescents who attempt suicide, older men with suicidal thoughts and behaviors, and active-duty military service people.

- Landmark studies have shown that CBT reduces the rate of suicide attempts by approximately 50%–60%.

- Dialectical behavior therapy (DBT) is a multifaceted treatment aimed at reducing self-harm behavior with and without suicidal intent, composed of individual therapy, skills training group, telephone coaching, case management, and peer consultation for therapists.

- Randomized controlled trials have demonstrated that DBT reduces self-harm behavior with and without suicidal intent, the medical lethality of self-harm behavior, and the usage of crisis services relative to usual care and treatment delivered by experts in the community.

- The delivery of CBT has been extended to internet-based approaches, which can address a pressing need for evidence-based treatment to reach underserved populations in rural and remote areas.

- Cognitive-behavioral therapists strive to apply the principles and strategies of treatment to themselves to practice stress management, self-care, and the appropriate solicitation of support in working with often challenging patients at high risk for death from suicide.

References

Beck AT: Depression: Causes and Treatment. Philadelphia, University of Pennsylvania Press, 1967

Bhar SS, Brown GK: Treatment of depression and suicide in older adults. Cogn Behav Pract 19(1):116–125, 2012

Brent D, Greenhill L, Compton S, et al: The Treatment of Adolescent Suicide Attempters study (TASA): predictors of suicidal events in an open treatment trial. J Am Acad Child Adolesc Psychiatry 48(10):987–996, 2009 19730274

Brown GK, Beck AT, Steer RA, et al: Risk factors for suicide in psychiatric outpatients: a 20-year prospective study. J Consult Clin Psychol 68(3):371–377, 2000 10883553

Brown GK, Ten Have T, Henriques GR, et al: Cognitive therapy for the prevention of suicide attempts: a randomized controlled trial. JAMA 294(5):563–570, 2005 16077050

Butler AC, Chapman JE, Forman EM, et al: The empirical status of cognitive-behavioral therapy: a review of meta-analyses. Clin Psychol Rev 26(1):17–31, 2006 16199119

Denchev P, Pearson JL, Allen MH, et al: Modeling the cost-effectiveness of interventions to reduce suicide risk among hospital emergency department patients. Psychiatr Serv 69(1):23–31, 2018 28945181

Ghahramanlou-Holloway M, LaCroix JM, Perera KU, et al: Inpatient psychiatric care following a suicide-related hospitalization: a pilot trial of post-admission cognitive therapy in a military medical center. Gen Hosp Psychiatry 2018 Epub ahead of print

Granato HF, Sewart AR, Vinograd M, et al: Dialectical behavior therapy, in American Psychological Association Handbook of Cognitive Behavioral Therapy. Edited by Wenzel A. Washington, DC, American Psychological Association, in press

Hedegaard H, Curtin SC, Warner M: Suicide rates in the United States continue to increase. NCHS Data Brief 309(309):1–8, 2018 30312151

Jobes DA, Mann RE: Reasons for living versus reasons for dying: examining the internal debate of suicide. Suicide Life Threat Behav 29(2):97–104, 1999 10407963

Linehan MM: Cognitive-Behavioral Treatment of Borderline Personality Disorder. New York, Guilford, 1993

Linehan MM, Armstrong HE, Suarez A, et al: Cognitive-behavioral treatment of chronically parasuicidal borderline patients. Arch Gen Psychiatry 48(12):1060–1064, 1991 1845222

Linehan MM, Comtois KA, Murray AM, et al: Two-year randomized controlled trial and follow-up of dialectical behavior therapy vs therapy by experts for suicidal behaviors and borderline personality disorder. Arch Gen Psychiatry 63(7):757–766, 2006 16818865

Lizardi D, Stanley B: Treatment engagement: a neglected aspect in the psychiatric care of suicidal patients. Psychiatr Serv 61(12):1183–1191, 2010 21123401

Mewton L, Andrews G: Cognitive behavioral therapy for suicidal behaviors: improving patient outcomes. Psychol Res Behav Manag 9:21–29, 2016 27042148

Rudd MD: The suicidal mode: a cognitive-behavioral model of suicidality. Suicide Life Threat Behav 30(1):18–33, 2000 10782716

Rudd MD: Suicide warning signs in clinical practice. Curr Psychiatry Rep 10(1):87–90, 2008 18269900

Rudd MD: Brief cognitive behavioral therapy (BCBT) for suicidality in military populations. Mil Psychol 24(6):592–603, 2012

Rudd MD, Bryan CJ, Wertenberger EG, et al: Brief cognitive-behavioral therapy effects on post-treatment suicide attempts in a military sample: results of a randomized clinical trial with 2-year follow-up. Am J Psychiatry 172(5):441–449, 2015 25677353

Salkovskis PM, Atha C, Storer D: Cognitive-behavioural problem solving in the treatment of patients who repeatedly attempt suicide: a controlled trial. Br J Psychiatry 157:871–876, 1990 2289097

Stanley B, Brown GK, Brenner LA, et al: Comparison of the safety planning intervention with follow-up vs usual care of suicidal patients treated in the emergency department. JAMA Psychiatry 75(9):894–900, 2018 29998307

Tarrier N, Taylor K, Gooding P: Cognitive-behavioral interventions to reduce suicide behavior: a systematic review and meta-analysis. Behav Modif 32(1):77–108, 2008 18096973

van Spijker BAJ, van Straten A, Kerkhof AJFM: Effectiveness of online self-help for suicidal thoughts: results of a randomised controlled trial. PLoS One 9(2):e90118, 2014 24587233

Wenzel A, Brown GK, Beck AT: Cognitive Therapy for Suicidal Patients: Scientific and Clinical Applications. Washington, DC, American Psychological Association, 2009

CHAPTER 4

Psychodynamic Treatment

Andreea L. Seritan, M.D.
Katherine A. Straznickas, Ph.D.
Glen O. Gabbard, M.D.

Treatment of the suicidal patient may be likened to negotiating the perils of a minefield—with each step, one is terrifyingly aware of the potential lethality underfoot. Most, if not all, psychiatrists will eventually find themselves attempting to guide a patient through this terrain fraught with risk and uncertainty. A psychodynamically informed road map may be helpful to both strengthen the clinician's footing and identify hazards on the path to recovery.

Psychodynamic treatment refers not only to psychotherapy but also to a broader approach to treatment in general. Clinicians can use this conceptual model to determine the most appropriate interventions designed to alter the patient's fundamental wish to die. The patient-specific psychodynamic treatment strategy is largely derived from the clinician's exploration of the patient's internal world, including unconscious conflicts, deficits and distortions of intrapsychic structures, and internal object relations (Gabbard 2014). This understanding must, of course, be integrated with contemporary findings from the neurosciences and psychopharmacology.

Psychodynamic psychiatry is shaped by a number of theoretical models, including ego psychology, with its central notion of unconscious conflict; object relations theory; self psychology; and attachment theory. From the outset of each therapeutic relationship, the psychiatrist undertakes a dynamic assessment of the patient's needs and uses the findings to construct a coherent conceptual framework from which all future interventions are prescribed. The dynamic psychiatrist employs a wide range of treatment modalities, including pharmacotherapy, risk factor assessment and modification, mobilization of social support, and psychotherapy. Regardless of whether the patient's plan of care includes dynamic psychotherapy, the treatment is, by definition, *dynamically informed*.

A set of time-honored principles guides the dynamic psychiatrist's approach to the treatment of the suicidal patient. These ideological cornerstones include the belief that suicidal thoughts and behaviors may have unconscious meanings, that the past repeats itself in the present, that unconscious motivations may lead to patient resistance, that transference to the clinician may have a major impact on the treatment, and that the treater's countertransference responses to the patient must be taken into account to avoid potential errors.

Literature Review

Efficacy

Evidence for the efficacy of dynamic therapy in the treatment of suicidal patients has been building over the past several decades. Guthrie et al. (2001) randomly assigned 119 patients who presented to the emergency department after deliberate self-poisoning to receive either brief psychodynamic interpersonal therapy or treatment as usual (outpatient follow-up with a general practitioner). Those who received therapy had a significantly greater reduction in suicidal ideation and were less likely to report repeat self-harm attempts at 6-month follow-up. Petersen et al. (2008) examined the outcomes of 38 patients enrolled in a 5-month-long day treatment program combining psychodynamic and cognitive-behavioral therapy in group and individual settings. The intervention group showed a significant reduction in hospitalizations and suicide attempts and improved social functioning. Chiesa et al. (2009) explored the effectiveness of a community-based psychodynamic therapy program by prospectively following for 2 years a group of 68 patients with severe personality disorders. Patients in the psychodynamic therapy group improved to a significantly greater degree with regard to three clinical outcome measures—hospital admissions, self-mutilation, and suicide attempts—and had significantly lower early dropout rates.

Dynamic therapy has shown promise in the care of suicidal patients with borderline personality disorder (BPD). Research involving the treatment of BPD using a randomized controlled trial of psychodynamically based partial hospitalization (in which dynamic individual therapy and group therapy were the foundation of the program) demonstrated dramatic reductions in suicidal thoughts and behaviors (Bateman and Fonagy 2001). Although 95% of the sample of 38 patients with BPD had attempted suicide in the 6 months prior to the study, at 18-month follow-up there had been only 4 attempts in the treatment group compared to 28 in the control group (Bateman and Fonagy 2001). In a randomized clinical trial of 104 women with BPD treated for 1 year with either transference-focused psychotherapy (TFP) or by experienced community therapists, significantly fewer patients in the TFP group attempted suicide, although self-harm behavior was not reduced in either group (Doering et al. 2010).

Psychodynamic Themes

Further studies have sought to delineate the psychodynamic themes relevant to suicidal patients. Preexisting psychological variables may increase the likelihood of acting on suicidal thoughts. Projective tests allow expression of intrapsychic conflicts and object relations schemas, even though individuals may not consciously acknowledge them, and have been used by researchers to explore unconscious representations in suicidal patients (de Kernier 2012). Instruments such as the Implicit Association Test (IAT;

available at https://implicit.harvard.edu/implicit), a brief computer-administered test, can reveal unconsciously held beliefs. The IAT uses the subject's reaction times when classifying semantic stimuli to measure automatic mental associations on various topics. In a study of 157 patients seeking treatment at a psychiatric emergency department, the implicit association of death/suicide with self was significantly stronger in individuals who presented after suicide attempts than in those seen for other reasons. Moreover, patients who held implicit associations of death with self had a sixfold higher risk of attempting suicide in the next 6 months (Nock et al. 2010).

Psychodynamic clinicians have developed a substantial literature that provides useful exploration of the varying meanings of the wish to die as well as the formidable obstacles that may be encountered as one attempts to treat the suicidal patient. Operating under the assumption that the ego could kill itself only by treating itself as an object, Freud (1917/1963) postulated that suicide results from displaced murderous impulses—destructive wishes toward an internalized object that are instead directed against the self. After the development of the structural model (Freud 1923/1961), Freud redefined suicide as the victimization of the ego by a sadistic superego.

Karl Menninger's (1933) conceptualization was more complex, with a view of the suicidal act as consisting of at least three wishes—the wish to kill, the wish to be killed, and the wish to die. In other cases, aggression plays less of a role, and the patient's motivation is instead fulfillment of a wish to reunite with a lost loved one or with a loving superego figure. Lindner (2010) also identified a conflict between fusion and separation wishes. When an individual's self-esteem and self-integrity depend on attachment to a lost object, suicide may seem to be the only way to restore self-cohesion.

The pursuit of perfectionism or an idealized view of the self that is rigidly held to despite repeated disappointments may also lead to the belief that suicide is the only way out (Gabbard 2014). Empirical studies (Beevers and Miller 2004; Hamilton and Schweitzer 2000) have consistently linked high levels of perfectionism with suicidal thoughts and behaviors. In fact, one study (Beevers and Miller 2004) demonstrated the impact of perfectionism to be both independent of and equal in significance to hopelessness, a factor commonly regarded as the best cognitive predictor of suicidal ideation. Pennel et al. (2018) also found that patients with higher neuroticism and an anxious attachment style had a fourfold-higher risk of repeat suicide attempts, as compared to patients without these traits, in study of 60 patients who were seen in emergency departments after a suicide attempt.

Many theorists have emphasized the role of intolerable affective states ("mental pain" or "psychache") in precipitating suicide, particularly in people with limited capacity to modulate emotions. Hendin et al. (2007) surveyed the therapists of 36 patients who had died from suicide while in treatment (mostly dynamic therapy). They explored the frequency with which patients had expressed nine intense affects in the period just before their suicides and found that seven—desperation, hopelessness, feelings of abandonment, self-hatred, rage, anxiety, and loneliness—were significantly more frequent among the patients who had died from suicide than among age-matched, severely depressed, nonsuicidal patients. Maltsberger (2004) described four progressive stages that culminated in suicide: "affective flooding, desperate maneuvering to counter the resulting mental emergency, loss of control as the self begins to disintegrate, and grandiose magical scheming for mental survival as the self-representation splits up and body jettison becomes plausible" (p. 653). He viewed these phenomena as manifestations of sev-

TABLE 4–1.	Psychodynamic factors that may contribute to suicide attempts

Conflict between fusion and separation wishes

Unconscious association of self with death/suicide

Excessively high self-expectations

Overcontrol of affect, particularly aggression

Inability to regulate intense affect (affect flooding)

Wish to destroy the part of self that responds to idealized parental expectations (in adolescents)

Negative self-schema/fragmentation

Loss of ego integrity

Loss of reality testing

Source.   Adapted from de Kernier 2012; Lindner 2010; Maltsberger 2004; Nock et al. 2010.

eral dysfunctional processes: failed affect regulation, ego helplessness, narcissistic surrender, breakdown of the representational world, and loss of reality testing (Maltsberger 2004). Table 4–1 summarizes psychodynamic factors that may contribute to suicide attempts.

Countertransference Pitfalls

Psychodynamic clinicians (Gabbard and Wilkinson 2000; Perry et al. 2013) have also stressed the countertransference pitfalls associated with treatment of suicidal patients, particularly patients with significant characterological pathology. Hate, rescue fantasies, and narcissistic vulnerability are among the most prominent responses. Intensive psychotherapy of suicidal patients can stir sadistic and murderous wishes in the therapist, a reaction noted to be opposite the fervent wish to rescue the patient. When the therapist assumes the role of savior or omnipotent rescuer who will go to all forms of self-sacrifice to save the patient, countertransference hate and resentment are often unfortunate by-products. This may lead to aversion, provoking the therapist to abandon the patient in subtle ways (forgetting appointments, withdrawing emotionally) or malice, filling the therapist with impulses to respond to the patient in overtly hostile or sarcastic ways. Therapists may fear that a patient's suicide will make them look bad to their colleagues, and this recognition of the patient's power over them may breed resentment. In addition, borderline patients often realize that the therapist's narcissism is on the line when a patient is contemplating suicide. They may exploit this vulnerability by enjoying the sadistic power they wield over the therapist.

Patients who have experienced severe child abuse and neglect will approach psychotherapy with the expectation that they deserve to be compensated for their tragic past by extraordinarily special treatment on the part of the therapist. The ordinary professional boundaries of therapeutic work are felt as depriving and even sadistic. Therapists may feel coerced into desperate efforts to demonstrate that they are completely different from the abusive object from the past, an approach that has been termed "disidentification with the aggressor" (Gabbard 2003). One reason this strategy fails is that the patient is searching for a "bad enough object" (Gabbard 2000). In other words, such patients desperately need the therapist to take on characteristics of the abusive internal object that they carry within themselves, because abusive object relations are both predictable and familiar to these patients. If therapists do not allow

TABLE 4–2.	Countertransference reactions in psychodynamic therapy with suicidal patients

Anxiety regarding death and suicide

Anger, hatred

Fear of hopelessness

Fear of failure

Narcissistic vulnerability

Overly active stance, to fight off projective identifications of helplessness

Rescue fantasies

Source. Adapted from Gabbard and Wilkinson 2000; Orbach 2001; Perry et al. 2013.

themselves to be transformed into the bad object role, the patient will continue to escalate the demands until they finally provoke the therapist into exasperation.

The most useful principle for managing these countertransference pitfalls is prevention. By refusing to take the role of the patient's rescuer, the therapist can avoid the resentment and hatred often accompanying that role. Monitoring one's responses and the defensive postures assumed to deal with such hateful feelings are essential measures in managing countertransference. Perry et al. (2013) showed that avoiding therapist errors that stem from negative countertransference and helping patients process their negative reactions to treatment leads to faster decrease in suicidal thoughts and behaviors.

Therapists should also examine their own anxiety surrounding death and fear of hopelessness, which, if not adequately addressed, may contribute to suicidal acting out by patients (Orbach 2001). Carefully balancing the empathic validation of the patients' wish to die with relentless confrontation of their self-destructive impulses is key in psychodynamic therapy with suicidal patients. In addition, dynamic therapists who treat suicidal patients with severe, terminal medical illnesses have to constantly monitor their feelings of helplessness. Countertransference enactments may include making special accommodations for patients (above and beyond those dictated by the patients' physical limitations) and becoming overly active in treatment, taking on most of the work of therapy, in an attempt to fight off projective identifications of helplessness. This overly active stance may backfire, leading to the patient's withdrawal in a passive mode, thus compounding their feelings of ineffectiveness in dealing with their severe medical illness or other stressors. Table 4–2 illustrates common countertransference reactions that may occur in the psychodynamic treatment of suicidal patients.

Treatment Steps

Navigating the perilous landscape of psychodynamic treatment of suicidal patients is best embarked upon in a series of deliberate, carefully placed steps (Table 4–3).

First and foremost, a solid therapeutic alliance between the patient and clinician must be established to ensure honest communication of any suicidal threat. Second, differentiating between the *fantasy of suicide* as a means of escape and the intent to carry out the *act of suicide* is of the utmost importance. Clarifying these states may be important in determining whether the psychodynamic treatment will be conducted on

TABLE 4–3.	Steps in the psychodynamic treatment of suicidal patients

Establish a therapeutic alliance

Differentiate between the fantasy and the act of suicide

Discuss the limits of treatment

Investigate precipitating events

Explore fantasies of the interpersonal impact of suicide

Establish level of suicidal thoughts and behaviors present at baseline

Monitor transference and countertransference

an outpatient basis or on an inpatient psychiatric unit (see Chapters 15, "Outpatient Treatment of the Suicidal Patient," and 16, "Inpatient Treatment"). Third, the clinician and patient must have a frank discussion about the limits of treatment. Therapists should clearly indicate that they cannot stop patients from dying from suicide. Moreover, the therapist's responsibilities and the patient's responsibilities within the context of the therapeutic alliance must be clearly differentiated. Fourth, the therapist must investigate precipitating events that may have triggered the patient's suicidal thoughts and behaviors. These stressors may provide hints about the relevant dynamic themes that inform the meaning of the suicide. Exploring the patient's fantasy about the specific interpersonal impact of suicide may also be productive. In the chronically suicidal patient, a baseline level must be established so that a descent into an acute risk state can be detected. Finally, as treatment progresses, the therapist must carefully monitor both transference and countertransference.

Hendin et al. (2006) interviewed therapists for 36 patients who died from suicide while receiving open-ended therapy and medication. Six potential problem areas were identified: poor communication with another provider involved in the case, permitting patients or relatives to control the therapy, avoidance of issues related to sexuality, ineffective or coercive actions resulting from the therapist's anxieties about a patient's potential suicide, not recognizing the meaning of the patient's communications, and untreated or undertreated symptoms. Paying close attention to these critical areas can optimize treatment and decrease the risk of suicide while recognizing that tragic outcomes cannot entirely be prevented.

Case Example 1: Acute Suicidal Ideation and Behaviors

Ms. A, a 34-year-old single female with no previous history of suicide attempts, was in twice-weekly psychotherapy for longstanding difficulties in romantic relationships. She came to a session one day in considerable distress. She said that the man she was dating had told her on their second date that he was not ready to commit to a relationship so soon after his recent divorce. She said he had been very considerate to her and had behaved "like a gentleman." She found herself deeply wounded by his wish to end their budding relationship. She said that she no longer wanted to date and felt hopeless about ever finding the right man. She looked at Dr. B, her therapist, and asked poignantly, "Do you think any man is ever going to want me?"

Her therapist, knowing that he was on potentially perilous ground, tried his best to respond in a helpful way: "Well, it's a hard question for me to answer with any certainty, but I definitely don't think it's hopeless like you do. You've had some very positive relationships."

Ms. A replied, "Yeah, but they never go anywhere."

Dr. B attempted to reassure Ms. A. "But most relationships don't result in marriage. It doesn't mean that there aren't positive things about them."

After a pause, Ms. A made a hesitant admission: "When I was lying awake last night, I kept thinking about committing suicide. I couldn't get it out of my mind."

Dr. B was taken aback by this revelation. Unable to suppress his surprise, he expressed his frank amazement (somewhat unempathetically): "I don't understand. You've known this man for a few weeks and been on two dates with him. Is he worth committing suicide over?"

Ms. A responded, "I know it makes no sense. I can't understand why I'm reacting this intensely."

Dr. B asked what it was about her date that made the loss so unbearable. Ms. A thought for a moment. "He just seemed like a great catch—caring, thoughtful, and financially well off. He's worldly, too. He's been everywhere, has a kind of class about him, and he's older and wiser than most of the men I've dated."

The therapist knew that Ms. A had lost her father when she was 10, leading him to formulate the possibility that the current loss had reawakened the pain and longing from the childhood loss. He posed a tentative interpretive understanding in the form of a simple observation: "Old enough to be your father."

Ms. A hesitated. "Yeah, but he's different than my father—at least the way I remember him."

"Yes, of course he's not exactly like your dad," Dr. B responded. "But sometimes one loss reawakens feelings about an earlier loss."

Ms. A became reflective. "There must be something like that going on. It just doesn't make sense that I'd feel this much pain. I didn't even know him that well."

The therapy then continued to explore the meaning of the precipitating event: the linkage—previously unconscious, now more conscious—between the much older romantic partner and Ms. A's father. Recognizing that the patient's hopelessness and suicidal thoughts and behaviors were serious, Dr. B engaged the patient in further discussion to assess suicide risk. Although Ms. A admitted to fantasizing about suicide, she denied any specific plan or intent to carry out the act. Dr. B decided that outpatient care with frequent follow-up was most appropriate and, after discussion with the patient, recommended Ms. A begin an antidepressant medication.

This case of acute suicidal thoughts and behaviors in a woman who had never considered suicide before supports the findings that parental death before age 18 is associated with an increased long-term risk of suicide (Guldin et al. 2015). The therapist explored the meaning of the triggering event and helped the patient understand how a previous loss was amplifying the impact of the current loss.

Case Example 2: Chronic Suicidal Thoughts and Behaviors in Borderline Personality Disorder

Ms. G was a 23-year-old patient with BPD who was admitted to a psychiatric inpatient unit after the latest in an extensive history of suicide attempts, this time by overdose. She was then referred to Dr. H for psychotherapy. She met with Dr. H while still hospitalized. Dr. H asked Ms. G if she wanted to work on the reasons for her chronic suicidal thoughts and behaviors. Ms. G said that she really did not want to work on it; she just wanted to die. Dr. H asked why she was intent on dying. Ms. G told her that it was impossible for her to live up to her parents' expectations. Her parents, both academics, had raised her to follow in their footsteps. Throughout her childhood, they had gone over homework assignments with her, corrected her grammar on English papers, and helped her memorize material for examinations. She said she knew they loved her, but she could not measure up to their expectations. She contrasted herself to her brother, a Ph.D. candidate at a prestigious university. Ms. G had graduated from college with a good grade point average but had been denied admission to the highly competitive program to which she had applied. Hence, she had started graduate school in comparative literature at what she regarded as a "mediocre university." She explained that her chronic level of suicidal thoughts and behaviors had become worse when she received a B on her first essay in a graduate course in an area of great interest to her.

Dr. H made a simple observation: "A B is a pretty decent grade."

"No it isn't," Ms. G replied. "In grad school you really have to get As or you'll never get a job."

Dr. H argued a bit with her. "But it's only your first paper. Most professors grade a little lower at first and expect improvement in the course of the semester."

"My professor hates me. There is no way she will ever give me an A. My parents would be so upset if they knew I was getting Bs," Ms. G insisted.

Noting Ms. G's combination of intense perfectionism and her borderline tendency to see "bad objects" everywhere, Dr. H asked, "Do you think your parents hate you, too?"

Ms. G thought for a moment. "Well, I know they think I'm a failure and a brat for giving up and trying to kill myself. I hate them for what they've done to me."

"Well, suicide is one way to get back at them," Dr. H observed quietly. "They must be terribly worried about you right now."

Ms. G's face became twisted with scorn. "I think they'd be glad if I died because I'm such a pain in the ass for them."

Dr. H asked, "Is it possible that they might think differently than you imagine?"

Ms. G was puzzled. "What do you mean?"

"Well, you said earlier that you knew they loved you when they tried to help you with your homework as a child. I'm sure that no matter how much of a pain in the ass you have been recently, they still have feelings of love for you."

"How do you know that?" Ms. G asked.

"I don't know for sure," replied Dr. H. "But in my experience, parents rarely stop loving their kids. Has it occurred to you that they might be devastated if you killed yourself and might never get over it?"

Dr. H continued to stress this approach of helping the patient see that her parents' reaction to her suicide might be quite different than what she may have imagined. Ultimately, with the help of meetings with her parents and the social worker on the inpatient unit, she realized that she had misread her parents' attitude toward her. She told Dr. H, "I realize now that if I killed myself, I wouldn't be eliminating my pain. I'd simply be passing it on to them." Dr. H also helped her realize that she had internalized her parents' expectations so that now her perfectionism reflected her own internal expectations of what she should do. Her parents made it clear to her that they would love her "even if she was a ditchdigger."

After helping her own her perfectionism and her need to berate herself for never achieving her excessively high self-expectations, the therapy then focused on the need to mourn this tormenting and idealized view of herself and settle for more reasonable goals. Ms. G gradually began to accept that she could be a worthwhile person despite having flaws. At the same time, she could see that she could achieve excellence in her writing while still being less than perfect.

The case of Ms. G illustrates a number of key principles in the psychodynamic treatment of suicidal patients. First, one must differentiate acute suicidal thoughts and behaviors from the chronic baseline of suicide risk in patients with BPD. Second, as with many borderline patients, Ms. G's ability to mentalize was impaired (Bateman and Fonagy 2004). *Mentalization* refers to the capacity to understand that one's own and others' thinking is representational in nature and that one's own and others' behavior is motivated by internal states, such as thoughts and feelings. Ms. G found it difficult to imagine how the mind of her parents might be different from her own mind. Dr. H worked in therapy to help her appreciate that the impact of her suicide on her parents would be much more devastating than she thought. Similarly, the therapist helped her see that one meaning of her wish to die was to seek revenge against her parents. She could make them suffer and get back at them for driving her to perform at a level that met their expectations. Dr. H also helped Ms. G see that her parents' perfectionistic expectations were now internalized as her own. She had to take responsibility for them and recognize that they were so unreasonable that they led to feelings of hopelessness and a wish to die. She had to mourn her fantasized achievements to ultimately lead a more realistic existence.

Conclusion

The psychodynamic treatment of suicidal patients is anchored by several fundamental elements, including a coherent biopsychosocial formulation to help ensure a good understanding of the underlying biological and psychosocial aspects, a thorough suicide risk assessment, and close monitoring of transference and countertransference processes. Clinicians should pay attention to countertransference pitfalls and recognize their limitations while navigating the perilous waters of psychodynamic therapy with suicidal patients.

Key Points

- Suicidal ideation and behaviors have meanings that vary from patient to patient. These meanings may be multiple and complicated; thus, they require careful exploration in the context of a strong therapeutic alliance.

- Suicidal patients may induce intense countertransference feelings ranging from anxiety to despair, hatred, and beyond. These feelings can lead to boundary violations as well as life-threatening treatment errors if they are not heeded and addressed.

- Thoughtful reflection on the transference/countertransference developments in psychotherapy often reveals the major interpersonal themes relevant to the patient's suicidal thoughts and behaviors.

- Patients who are suicidal must be cautioned that no one can save them from suicide. They are ultimately responsible for their own safety while working in psychotherapy to find ways to live with pain.

References

Bateman A, Fonagy P: Treatment of borderline personality disorder with psychoanalytically oriented partial hospitalization: an 18-month follow-up. Am J Psychiatry 158(1):36–42, 2001 11136631

Bateman AW, Fonagy P: Mentalization-based treatment of BPD. J Pers Disord 18(1):36–51, 2004 15061343

Beevers CG, Miller IW: Perfectionism, cognitive bias, and hopelessness as prospective predictors of suicidal ideation. Suicide Life Threat Behav 34(2):126–137, 2004 15191269

Chiesa M, Fonagy P, Gordon J: Community-based psychodynamic treatment program for severe personality disorders: clinical description and naturalistic evaluation. J Psychiatr Pract 15(1):12–24, 2009 19182561

de Kernier N: Suicide attempt during adolescence: a way of killing the "infans" and a quest for individuation-separation. Crisis 33(5):290–300, 2012 22562857

Doering S, Hörz S, Rentrop M, et al: Transference-focused psychotherapy v. treatment by community psychotherapists for borderline personality disorder: randomised controlled trial. Br J Psychiatry 196(5):389–395, 2010 20435966

Freud S: The ego and the id (1923), in The Standard Edition of the Complete Psychological Works of Sigmund Freud, Vol 19. Translated and edited by Strachey J. London, Hogarth, 1961, pp 1–66

Freud S: Mourning and melancholia (1917), in The Standard Edition of the Complete Psychological Works of Sigmund Freud, Vol 14. Translated and edited by Strachey J. London, Hogarth, 1963, pp 237–260

Gabbard GO: On gratitude and gratification. J Am Psychoanal Assoc 48(3):697–716, 2000 11059393

Gabbard GO: Miscarriages of psychoanalytic treatment with suicidal patients. Int J Psychoanal 84(pt 2):249–261, 2003 12856351

Gabbard GO: Cluster B personality disorders: borderline, in Psychodynamic Psychiatry in Clinical Practice, 5th Edition. Washington, DC, American Psychiatric Publishing, 2014, pp 427–479

Gabbard GO, Wilkinson SM: On victims, rescuers, and abusers, in Management of Countertransference With Borderline Patients. Northvale, NJ, Jason Aronson, 2000, pp 47–70

Guldin MB, Li J, Pedersen HS, et al: Incidence of suicide among persons who had a parent who died during their childhood: a population-based cohort study. JAMA Psychiatry 72(12):1227–1234, 2015 26558351

Guthrie E, Kapur N, Mackway-Jones K, et al: Randomised controlled trial of brief psychological intervention after deliberate self poisoning. BMJ 323(7305):135–138, 2001 11463679

Hamilton TK, Schweitzer RD: The cost of being perfect: perfectionism and suicide ideation in university students. Aust N Z J Psychiatry 34(5):829–835, 2000 11037370

Hendin H, Haas AP, Maltsberger JT, et al: Problems in psychotherapy with suicidal patients. Am J Psychiatry 163(1):67–72, 2006 16390891

Hendin H, Maltsberger JT, Szanto K: The role of intense affective states in signaling a suicide crisis. J Nerv Ment Dis 195(5):363–368, 2007 17502800

Lindner R: [Psychodynamic hypothesis about suicidality in elderly men]. Psychother Psychosom Med Psychol 60(8):290–297, 2010 19753510

Maltsberger JT: The descent into suicide. Int J Psychoanal 85(pt 3):653–667, 2004 15228702

Menninger KA: Psychoanalytic aspects of suicide. Int J Psychoanal 14:376–390, 1933

Nock MK, Park JM, Finn CT, et al: Measuring the suicidal mind: implicit cognition predicts suicidal behavior. Psychol Sci 21(4):511–517, 2010 20424092

Orbach I: Therapeutic empathy with the suicidal wish: principles of therapy with suicidal individuals. Am J Psychother 55(2):166–184, 2001 11467255

Pennel L, Quesada JL, Dematteis M: Neuroticism and anxious attachment as potential vulnerability factors for repeat suicide attempts. Psychiatry Res 264:46–53, 2018 29626831

Perry JC, Bond M, Presniak MD: Alliance, reactions to treatment, and counter-transference in the process of recovery from suicidal phenomena in long-term dynamic psychotherapy. Psychother Res 23(5):592–605, 2013 23937543

Petersen B, Toft J, Christensen NB, et al: Outcome of a psychotherapeutic programme for patients with severe personality disorders. Nord J Psychiatry 62(6):450–456, 2008 18836927

CHAPTER 5

Split Treatment

The Psychiatrist's Role

Richard Balon, M.D.

Split treatment arrangements in psychiatric patient care are increasingly common. Managing a suicidal patient in split treatment is challenging and may be made even more so when the roles and responsibilities of each provider are unclear. Although patients derive certain benefits from split treatment, they may also be at increased risk of adverse outcomes, including suicide. Split treatment has become more prevalent, so familiarity with the best arrangements for split treatment and the complex management of suicidal thoughts and behaviors in this setting is imperative.

Split Treatment Defined

Split treatment refers to a treatment setting in which a patient is seen by two mental health professionals, a therapist and a physician, usually a psychiatrist or a primary care physician. Depending on the level of collaboration between the two clinicians, split treatment could be also called *collaborative treatment* (Riba et al. 2018). In split or collaborative treatment, the physician prescribes medication (usually psychotropic agents) and the therapist provides psychotherapy as indicated, for example, cognitive-behavioral therapy in depressive disorders. In contrast, the term *integrated treatment* is commonly used to describe treatment in which psychiatrists provide both medication and psychotherapy. At times, the term *medication backup* has been used interchangeably for both split and collaborative treatment. In this chapter, the term *split treatment* is used because it better captures the fragmentation of the current system of care (Riba et al. 2018).

Split treatment has been widely practiced over the past few decades. This practice has developed for various reasons. First, the combination of pharmacotherapy and psychotherapy has been proven beneficial in many circumstances and frequently superior to the efficacy of either pharmacotherapy or psychotherapy alone. The two modalities could be delivered either simultaneously or sequentially. Second, psychiatrists and primary care physicians may not be able to provide both pharmacotherapy and psychotherapy, either due to lack of skills or lack of patient or system resources, including limitations imposed by insurers focused on cost containment.

Split Treatment Arrangement

Treating patients in a split treatment setting and effectively addressing their suicidal thoughts and behaviors depends on the type and setting of the psychiatrist's practice. In an inpatient setting, split treatment is the norm, but safety concerns are integrated into inpatient management (see Chapter 16, "Inpatient Treatment"). In addition, those participating in split treatment in inpatient settings are familiar with professional qualifications of hospital staff and typically have institutionally facilitated or defined means of communication and responsibilities (unless the psychiatrist is in a consultative role, as discussed later). Finally, issues regarding coverage of care during the absence of one provider usually are addressed systemically and rarely become problematic.

Managing split treatment safety issues in other settings, such as outpatient practices or partial hospitalization programs, presents additional challenges and raises a number of questions with significant clinical implications:

1. Is the setting a clinic in which several psychiatrists and therapists work together?
2. Is the setting a solo practice without any formal arrangement between the psychiatrist and therapist(s) in the community?
3. If there is no formal arrangement, have the psychiatrist and the therapist(s) worked together before, and if so, have issues or problems been identified previously?
4. Has the patient been referred to the psychiatrist by a therapist or was the patient self-referred?
5. If self-referred, is the patient already working with a therapist?

Before establishing the boundaries and role definitions of split treatment—that is, the roles and responsibilities of each provider—psychiatrists should consider areas such as therapist qualification, legal implications and risks, and ethical issues. For example, the American Psychiatric Association (APA)'s *Guidelines for Psychiatrists in Consultative, Supervisor, or Collaborative Relationships With Nonphysician Clinicians* (American Psychiatric Association 2009, pp. 1–2) states, "When psychiatrists extend their services to other health professionals in meaningful collaboration (which includes supervision of cases or participation in interdisciplinary teamwork), they are obliged to know about and to be willing to assume the established legal responsibilities involved."

Some physicians may have a good source of referral for therapy in the community or may work in an office (or hospital setting) with a number of therapists. However, some psychiatrists may not work in such settings. Similarly, many therapists practicing alone or in a group without access to a psychiatrist may have difficulties finding a psychiatrist for their patients when those patients might benefit from psychotropic medication. This situation is worse in areas with a greater shortage of psychiatrists, such as rural communities. In addition, patients may have insurance that limits the available pool of therapists, and the psychiatrist may not have a connection to a therapist in the pool. Increasingly, the treating psychiatrist does not personally know the therapist, which adds certain challenges to split treatment and the communication required for such treatment to be of maximum benefit. Patients may also prefer to see a therapist closer to their home yet not mind traveling farther for less frequent visits with a physician.

In a way, split treatment is, unfortunately, a minefield of possible clinical problems, including increased risk of suicidal thoughts and behaviors, and a lack of clarity regarding boundaries and responsibilities may cause various clinical problems during treatment. Finally, as new treatment "settings" (e.g., telepsychiatry) become increasingly utilized, further arrangements regarding split treatment should be considered but are likely to remain the same as those outlined here.

Clarification and Delineation of the Relationship Between Psychiatrist and Therapist

Clarification of the relationship between psychiatrist and therapist is very important because it delineates the roles and responsibilities. The APA guidelines (American Psychiatric Association 2009) describe three types of relationships between psychiatrists and therapists: consultative, supervisory, and collaborative. In a *consultative relationship*, psychiatrists do not assume responsibility for patient care. They evaluate the information provided and offer opinions, which the therapist may or may not accept. In a *supervisory relationship*, psychiatrists

> retain direct responsibility for patient care and give professional direction and active guidance to the nonphysician clinician….The psychiatrist remains ethically and medically responsible for the patient's care as long as the treatment continues under his or her supervision. The patient should be fully informed of the existence and nature of, and any changes in, the supervisory relationship. (American Psychiatric Association 2009, p. 2)

Finally, in a *collaborative* relationship, psychiatrists and therapists implicitly and mutually share

> responsibility for the patient's care in accordance with the qualifications and limitations of each nonphysician clinician's discipline. The patient must be informed of the respective responsibilities of each nonphysician clinician. In support of patient-centered services, a patient has the right and responsibility to seek his/her own healthcare. If a patient autonomously and independently seeks nonphysician services, the psychiatrist does not have supervisory responsibility over the nonphysician clinician. (American Psychiatric Association 2009, p. 2)

Interprofessional Considerations

Delineation of the roles in split treatment is related to considerations of licensure and training of both parties. Physicians must be licensed by the state where they practice (unless they practice in a federal facility, such as U.S. Department of Veterans Affairs [VA] facilities, where license in any state allows them to practice). Many physicians, including psychiatrists, are certified by their specialty board, such as the American Board of Psychiatry and Neurology for psychiatrists. However, not every therapist is properly trained and licensed. Psychologists, social workers, and substance abuse therapists are usually required to undergo formal and highly structured training through institutional programs, including a required number of supervised therapy hours, and typically must be licensed.

Nevertheless, psychiatrists are well advised to discuss the training, licensure, and liability insurance of the collaborating therapist with that therapist. Meyer (2012) noted that in many jurisdictions licensure is not required for psychotherapists. Physicians may start inquiries about therapists' backgrounds in a friendly, neutral manner by presenting a brief summary of their own qualifications and then asking about the therapist's qualifications and licensure. A significant amount of information can be found online, because many professionals post information about their services, backgrounds, board certifications (if any), and licensure.

Psychiatrists may also consider obtaining more specific information about future collaborating therapists:

1. Does the therapist have experience in handling certain conditions or disorders specific to the case(s)?
2. Does the therapist have any experience treating patients with co-occurring substance use disorders?
3. Does the therapist have additional training in certain types of therapies that may be useful for potentially suicidal patients, such as crisis intervention, cognitive-behavioral therapy, or dialectical behavioral therapy?

This information is best obtained through face-to-face or voice-to-voice communication. Personal communication may, at times, help to determine whether the psychiatrist and the therapist "click" with each other. Unfortunately, for a variety of reasons, psychiatrists sometimes neglect to obtain all this information. "Many split-treatment pairs of clinicians may know nothing of each other.... Split treatment 'teams' are often independent providers who are respectively ignorant of each other's professional training, experience, and clinical methods" (Meyer 2012, p. 265). This can result in significant treatment problems and, in the case of patients with suicidal ideation or behavior, may lead to a fatal outcome.

Emergency Situations, Urgent Access, and Coverage for Weekends, Holidays, and Vacations

The patient and providers should clearly understand which provider is responsible for what sort of care in emergency or urgent situations. This should be established with full agreement and understanding of all three parties: the psychiatrist, the therapist, and the patient. The nature of what constitutes an emergency or urgent situation should be discussed and determined. Whom the patient should contact in these situations can vary: it could be the therapist, who likely sees the patient more frequently than the psychiatrist; it could be agreed that the patient should contact both; or it may be agreed that in the case of emergence of suicidal thoughts and behaviors, the psychiatrist takes the primary treatment role.

Psychiatrists should also make sure that the patient has easy access to both treating professionals by phone, by e-mail (voice and e-mail may be connected so that voice messages could appear in one's e-mail), or through an answering service. The physician and the therapist should also be able to easily reach each other to discuss an emergency situation management. Use of social media for contact related to patient care and for any communication with or about patients is not advisable because social media is inherently insecure and not confidential.

Psychiatrists using voicemail should also consider their own and their collaborating therapists' systems. Many voicemail systems ask the caller to call 911 (or some other emergency service number) in case of "emergency" or instruct them to go to the nearest emergency department. Patients in a suicidal crisis find themselves in complex and complicated situations and may be extremely distressed; a phone message referring patients elsewhere may feel like rejection. Preferably, patients in crisis should understand how to reach the appropriate provider to be able to discuss their suicidal feelings and decide together what steps should be taken. If possible, the psychiatrist and the therapist should communicate with each other in such situations. However, if their suicidal thoughts and behaviors seem urgent, for example, if a patient has a clear suicidal plan, the contacted clinician should err on the side of caution and arrange for immediate in-person evaluation in the office or emergency department or for direct admission to a psychiatric inpatient setting.

Coverage for services when one provider is absent, for example, on vacation, is not a clear-cut affair in split treatment settings. Both clinicians should arrange for their own coverage. The covering psychiatrist or therapist should be informed about the split treatment arrangement and be given contact information for the other treating party. Therapists may ask the psychiatrist or primary care physician to cover for them during vacation or extended illness instead of having their own coverage. If the treating psychiatrist is agreeable with this arrangement, then it can be implemented. However, the reverse is usually not possible because nonmedical therapists may not be able to address all the medical needs of the patient, such as issues that arise regarding medication side effects. Arrangements similar to vacation coverage should be implemented for weekends and holidays, depending on all parties' preferences.

Termination Versus Abandonment

It may seem difficult or premature to discuss the issues of how, when, and why termination of split treatment should be instituted, yet, like other arrangements, this one should be clear to the psychiatrist and the therapist from the beginning of their relationship. The reasons that a split treatment arrangement might need to be terminated are numerous, for example, the psychiatrist may be physically leaving the area or may be unable to work with the specific therapist; the patient's insurance company may change terms of their financial coverage such that patients can no longer afford to consult either the psychiatrist or the therapist; or one treating party may disagree with the other regarding appropriate treatment, making it difficult to continue to work collaboratively.

Patients should never be abandoned during the process of termination of split treatment arrangements. In the case of suicidal patients, failure to consider appropriate termination can have disastrous outcomes. In addition to the damage that may be done to patients and families, clinicians may also expose themselves to significant liability. As Gutheil and Simon (2003) noted,

> a clinician may—from a legal perspective—choose not to treat, may cease treating, or may refuse to treat anyone at any time for any reason, with exceptions. The typical exceptions to this generalization represent the legal basis of abandonment: *The clinician may not cease treatment during a crisis or emergency and may not leave a patient in need of treatment completely without some recourse, such as referral or alternative care. To do either of these actions constitutes legal abandonment.* (p. 175)

Clinicians who work in settings in which they are required to accept some patients for treatment due to regional regulations should be careful to avoid violations of these as well.

Psychiatrists may leave split treatment patient care arrangements (if not in an emergency situation) but need to arrange for referrals to another physician or direct patients to their insurance companies for referrals if financial issues become problematic. Alternatively, psychiatrists may solicit referral recommendations from the treating therapists or direct the patient to do so (Gutheil and Simon 2003). Unless a patient clearly does not require medication but may still benefit from continuing therapy, the psychiatrist cannot pass all treatment responsibilities to a therapist only.

Even if medication is no longer required, psychiatrists should make certain that the patient and therapist understand whether they may reach out to the physician in the future if a crisis occurs or the need for pharmacotherapy arises again. If the psychiatrist cannot provide this assurance regarding future availability, patients should be given the name of another psychiatrist in case of future emergency. Finally, as Meyer and Simon (1999) recommended, the patient's best interest should guide what information is communicated to the patient about the decision to dissolve the split treatment arrangement or about any disagreements and misgivings between clinicians.

Initial Contact and Communication About a Specific Patient

Initial contact within an established office or clinic where both the psychiatrist and the therapist work is often straightforward. At times, the therapist may send an e-mail, place a call, or personally inform the psychiatrist that a therapy patient needs to be seen for medication management. Similarly, treating psychiatrists may communicate directly with therapists that they have a patient who would benefit from therapy and that they are making a referral. This should be followed by a review of the patient's chart and further discussion. The patient should always be informed that this communication is going to happen.

However, some mistakenly believe that the Health Insurance Portability and Accountability Act (HIPAA) requires patient consent for this type of communication. In fact, pertinent clinical information between a psychiatrist and a therapist can be disclosed without patient consent, whether clinicians work for the same entity or not. Sharing clinical information via electronic and other means of communication without patient consent is also possible, as long as this communication is properly secured. Information disclosure requires patient consent in two circumstances: transmission of the written psychotherapy notes if these are not part of the official medical record and substance abuse treatment records maintained by a licensed substance abuse program. Nevertheless, psychiatrists are advised to check that the regulations in their

TABLE 5–1.	The "eight Cs" of collaborative treatment
Clarity	Roles, boundaries, coverage, supervision, if any
Contract	Reflecting roles, boundaries, etc. (preferably written)
Communication	Contact information for both treating parties
Consent	By all parties to collaborative treatment arrangement
Contact	Routine, regular, when indicated or desired
Comprehensive view	Both treating parties
Credentialing	For both treating parties
Consultation	Disagreement between treating parties may signal need for consultation

own states are not more restrictive and whether any additional legal rules apply. Of note, communication with family members requires patient consent.

Communication Between Providers

Psychiatrists should be certain to establish clear boundaries and expectations between themselves and therapists. Routine contact is advisable, particularly for patients with a history of suicide attempts or suicidal ideation. For example, the therapist may see a patient on a weekly basis and agree to contact the medicating psychiatrist once a month at a minimum, even if only to leave a voicemail message regarding the patient's therapy status. Prescribing psychiatrists who evaluate patients in split treatment on a monthly basis or even less often may agree to contact the therapist—again, even if only to leave a voicemail message indicating no change in status—after a routine medication management appointment. The physician and the therapist should discuss the progress of treatment or lack of progress, possible side effects, emerging patient splitting, and similar issues. Certainly, physicians and therapists should agree and expect to communicate in the event of a problem or crisis.

Gutheil and Simon's (2003) eight Cs of collaborative treatment are a good summary of the elements of split or collaborative treatment arrangements (Table 5–1).

Rush and Thase (2018) outlined the essential patient–clinician collaborations in patient-centered medical management of depression. These can be adapted for split treatment as follows:

1. The decision making in the formulation of the treatment plan should be shared by all three parties.
2. Expectations as to the duration of treatment, critical decision points, and management of medication side effects should be shared and aligned by all.
3. Education, information, and action plans for managing suicidal ideation, side effects, substance abuse, and concurrent medical conditions should be provided to the patient and therapist.
4. The patient should be engaged in monitoring symptoms, functioning, side effects, and health activities and should share these with both psychiatrist and therapist.
5. New interventions to enhance adherence should be anticipated, discussed, and planned by both clinicians.
6. Psychiatrists and therapists should discuss, define, and counteract obstacles to full recovery.
7. Psychiatrists and therapists should develop a relapse prevention/amelioration plan.

Negative Aspects of Split Treatment With Possible Adverse Outcome

Negative aspects of split treatment may include problematic ethical issues involving supervision of and relationship with nonmedical professionals and interdisciplinary tension and politics as well as transference and countertransference issues within the triangular relationship (i.e., patient–psychiatrist–therapist) (Goldsmith et al. 1999). In addition, both psychiatrists and therapists may be subject to various misperceptions. Either treatment provider (or both) may overvalue psychotherapy, ignore the psychological meaning of medication, believe that psychiatrists should manage all questions related to medication, or think that the patient is too acutely symptomatic to treat through therapy. Therapists sometimes feel that the psychiatrist is undervaluing the role of therapy and pushing the therapist aside. They may incorrectly assume that the psychiatrist will provide coverage for the therapist if the therapist is away or temporarily unavailable or that the psychiatrist will take full responsibility for the patient's care if the patient's condition worsens. Psychiatrists may believe that the therapist should always agree and support the physician's decisions or that the therapist feels free to discuss disagreements. Psychiatrists may also have concerns about malpractice and liability issues.

Patients may also have misperceptions that should be communicated and addressed as they become identified. For example, patients may be confused about the roles of the treating parties, especially in the primary care setting, in addressing their mental health issues. Patients may believe that the psychiatrist is interested only in prescribing medications, that all uncomfortable feelings can be attributed to the side effects of medication, or that the physician may precipitously stop medication or force hospitalization. Additional pitfalls in split treatment may include issues related to confidentiality, such as one provider keeping secrets from the other or providers failing to communicate with each other effectively.

One issue that commonly arises in collaborative treatment is that of "patient splitting," in which the patient unconsciously may create an adversarial or conflicted situation between the psychiatrist and therapist. Collaborative treatment increases the risk of patient splitting. Such situations are particularly problematic in patients with a history of suicide attempts or suicidal ideation, because splitting may compromise patient safety.

Suicidal Ideation and Behaviors, Suicide, and Split Treatment

The treating parties in split treatment should be aware that many of these misperceptions, problematic situations, and pitfalls may lead directly to situations endangering the life of the patient or even a treatment team member. The issue of death from suicide and suicidal behavior in the split treatment setting has not been studied, and very little literature addressing this issue is available. Suicidal behavior itself is not a mental disorder. The treatment of suicidal ideation and behavior occurs within the framework of treating mental disorders in which these thoughts and actions may be part of a patient's symptomatology, or a patient's symptoms may be associated with an increased risk of death from suicide. The classification of suicidal thoughts and behaviors could change in the future; DSM-5 (American Psychiatric Association 2013) lists "suicidal behavior disorder" as one of several conditions for further study.

The psychiatric disorders associated with increased risk of death from suicide include mood disorders (including bipolar disorder, which clinicians do not always consider to be associated with increased risk of death from suicide), schizophrenia and other psychotic disorders, anxiety disorders, impulse-control disorders, substance use disorders, and some personality disorders, primarily borderline personality disorder. Physical illness can also be associated with increased risk of death from suicide, for example, AIDS, cancer (especially head and neck, gastrointestinal, and pulmonary), epilepsy, multiple sclerosis, renal failure on dialysis, and spinal cord injury (Maris et al. 2000). In the primary care setting, where the physician may prescribe an antidepressant for depression during these illnesses and refer the patient to a therapist, increased risk of death from suicide associated with physical illness should dictate routine suicide risk assessment. The risk of death from suicide is even higher in patients with a combination of disorders or diseases. One such area requiring increased attention is the complex relationship of pain, opioid use, opioid overdose, and death from suicide (Bohnert and Ilgen 2019).

Split treatment situations may at times increase the risk of death from suicide, particularly in the absence of clear boundaries, treatment roles, and communication. For example, the patient may be confused about the open lines of communication with both the psychiatrist and the therapist and may not fully reveal the degree of his or her suicidal thoughts and behaviors to either treatment provider. Alternatively, the therapist may believe that a patient's suicidal thoughts and behaviors are the psychiatrist's responsibility. This belief may arise from the therapist's misperception that they represent a severe problem that cannot be addressed effectively through therapy. The therapist may believe that suicidal thoughts and behaviors must be treated primarily through medication. Inexperienced therapists may send a patient with suicidal ideation or behavior to the treating psychiatrist immediately after finding that the patient is suicidal. This can create an even more complicated clinical situation that increases risk of death from suicide because the patient may feel rejected by the therapist.

On the other hand, the psychiatrist or primary care physician may not pay enough attention to the patient's reports of emerging suicidal ideation and behaviors, for example, as a result of the use of certain antidepressants or during stressful psychosocial situations. Psychiatrists may mistakenly believe that the therapist is "talking to the patient about feelings" and would either address the issue of suicide in therapy or contact the psychiatrist to discuss the issue if the therapist remains concerned. Primary care physicians are frequently limited in their discussions with patients due to time constraints and may not elicit suicidal ideation. Yet primary care is an ideal setting to identify suicide risk and suicidal thoughts and behaviors, especially in older patients, and to initiate some type of care (Raue et al. 2014). Primary care physicians are more likely than other types of physicians to see older adults, and older adults may be more likely to discuss various aspects of their mental health with their primary care physicians, especially if they have a long and trusting relationship with them.

Good communication between both clinicians, including consulting the other party, is critical to avoid various treatment challenges with patients at increased risk of death from suicide, particularly the risk associated with splitting. Splitting by the patient may also complicate patient reporting of suicidal thoughts and behaviors, including a suicidal plan. Splitting typically takes the form of the good guy/bad guy, a characterization that may change from moment to moment, which may make it difficult to recognize as it occurs (Goldsmith et al. 1999). Some patients with personality disorders, especially those diagnosed with borderline personality disorder, may try to play clinicians against each other. When unrecognized, this can further complicate or damage communication between clinicians and may divert attention from the patient's suicidal ideation and behaviors.

Ideological or interdisciplinary differences could also lead to lack of communication and compromise assessment of suicidal thoughts and behaviors in the shared patient. Physicians may believe that certain therapists lack appropriate training to treat patients and that only they have sufficient understanding of treatment issues. Similarly, therapists may believe that certain physicians are not attuned to psychological issues, are only interested in medication, and thus are unable to help therapists manage issues of suicidal thoughts and behaviors. At times, unfortunately, patients may recognize the lack of respect of one treating party for the other (or mutual lack of respect). That may lead to more desperation and a pessimistic view of treatment outcome.

Unclear arrangements regarding coverage also may increase risk of death from suicide. A patient with suicidal ideation who tries to reach a therapist who is unavailable may not be informed that the psychiatrist is providing covering services for the therapist. Similarly, the patient may be referred by a voice message to the emergency department or to an emergency number but nevertheless leaves a voicemail message that he or she "feels suicidal and would like to talk to you about it in a day or two." If the message remains unanswered, the patient may start to feel more desperate while waiting for a response.

Prevention and Management of Suicidal Ideation and Behaviors in Split Treatment Setting

Preventive measures or measures to decrease suicidal thoughts and behaviors and risk of death from suicide in split treatment include the proper split treatment arrangements outlined earlier and addressing the negative aspects of split treatment. Close collaboration between psychiatrist and therapist, monitoring adherence, and addressing nonadherence to treatment are also measures that may help to decrease suicidal thoughts and behaviors and risk of death from suicide. All these measures are based on best clinical practices in general rather than any specific research evidence because, as noted, research on this subject is not available.

Management begins with proper assessment of risk of death from suicide as discussed in Chapter 1 ("Suicide Risk Assessment") of this book. The timing of assessment depends on the character and acuity of the patient's suicidal thoughts and behaviors. Patients, especially those with mood disorders and substance use disorders, should be carefully assessed for suicidal ideation and risk of death from suicide by both the physician and the therapist at the outset of split treatment. Ideally, the assessment should be discussed between the psychiatrist and the therapist. However, unless the patient reports suicidal ideation to at least one of the two clinicians, this discussion may not take place (although suicidal ideation is not the only risk factor that increases risk of death from suicide). Patients may not necessarily report suicidal ideation to both treating parties in a split arrangement for various reasons.

Raue et al. (2006) recommended sequential assessment of suicide risk based on severity of suicidal ideation: from passive to active suicidal ideation to a specific detailed plan, including intention to harm oneself, reasons for living, and impulse control. They wrote, "While definitive data do not exist on when this evaluation should be conducted, we suggest that patients with passive suicidal ideation be evaluated within a week" (Raue et al. 2014, p. 466). They also recommended increased frequency of visits for patients with suicidal ideation or patients started on antidepressants. Finally, they stated that patients "endorsing active suicidal ideation even when lacking a specific plan or intention require immediate, same-day evaluation" (p. 466). In such situations, the treating clinician(s) should make every effort to conduct a same-day evaluation. However, if clinicians are unable to evaluate the patient themselves, the patient should be referred to the nearest emergency department (ideally a psychiatric one) or directly admitted to an inpatient psychiatric unit (preferably with the patient's family's help).

The evaluation and management of a suicidal patient in split treatment should be a joint effort of physician and therapist. Both clinicians should actively ask about suicidal ideation and conduct ongoing assessments of suicidal thoughts and behaviors. They should not rely on the other clinician to address this issue. In addition, each clinician should inform the other treatment provider whenever a patient reports suicidal ideation or a plan, and neither clinician should address the patient's suicidal ideation and behaviors without the other clinician's input. Both physician and therapist should be cautious about using so-called suicide prevention contracts. These contracts should not substitute for ongoing assessment of suicidal ideation, and no evidence is available that indicates that they mitigate the risk of death from suicide (Edwards and Sachmann 2010). Also, clinicians should remain aware that suicidal thoughts and behaviors are fluctuating phenomena, and as noted, patients may not always disclose them to either treating clinician.

Psychopharmacology and psychotherapy should not be the only modalities used in split treatment. Psychoeducation (of patients and families) should also be implemented. Families may play an important role in mitigating risk of death from suicide; however, both psychiatrist and therapist should be aware that involvement of family members may increase the possibility of splitting. As Rush and Thase (2018) pointed out, multiple factors affect outcomes with any therapy, such as patient care systems, clinicians, sociocultural factors, patient-clinician factors, and the patient's support system. These factors impact the outcome of suicidal thoughts and behaviors as well. They should be included in the discussion between the psychiatrist (or any other physician) and the therapist in split treatment.

Conclusion

Psychiatrists should be aware that management of the suicidal patient in a split treatment arrangement could be challenging and complicated. Definitive guidelines for the management of suicidal thoughts and behaviors in split treatment are not available. Proper arrangement of split treatment and established routes of communication between psychiatrist (or primary care physician) and therapist are necessary to minimize risks generally associated with split treatment, and the potential for increase in risk of death specifically from suicide. Proper collaboration, without interdisciplinary or ideological conflicts, and ongoing good communication between psychiatrist and therapist could help in early detection and management.

Key Points

- Split treatment is a complex treatment arrangement that replaces the traditional therapeutic dyad with a triad—a treatment relationship involving a psychiatrist or other physician, a therapist, and the patient.

- Psychiatrists and therapists in split treatment should make every effort to work as a team.

- Patients should be properly informed about the arrangements (e.g., coverage), roles, responsibilities, and rules and should be involved in decision discussions.

- Setting appropriate boundaries, defining roles, and establishing routines regarding communication at the outset of a split treatment arrangement are important not only for effective split treatment but also for assessment and management of suicidal thoughts and behaviors in this setting.

- Both the psychiatrist's and the therapist's expertise should be used in detecting, assessing, and managing suicidal thoughts and behaviors, without professional or ideological bias.

- Assessment of suicidal thoughts and behaviors in split treatment should be an ongoing process, and its results should be communicated between the treating parties.

References

American Psychiatric Association: Guidelines for Psychiatrists in Consultative, Supervisor, or Collaborative Relationships With Nonphysician Clinicians (Resource Document). Washington, DC, American Psychiatric Association, 2009. Available at: https://www.psychiatry.org/File%20Library/Psychiatrists/Directories/Library-and-Archive/resource_documents/rd2009_CollaborativeRelationships.pdf. Accessed January 20, 2019.

American Psychiatric Association: Diagnostic and Statistical Manual of Mental Disorders, 5th Edition. Arlington, VA, American Psychiatric Association, 2013

Bohnert ASB, Ilgen MA: Understanding links among opioid use, overdose, and suicide. N Engl J Med 380(1):71–79, 2019 30601750

Edwards SJ, Sachmann MD: No-suicide contracts, no-suicide agreements, and no-suicide assurances: a study of their nature, utilization, perceived effectiveness, and potential to cause harm. Crisis 31(6):290–302, 2010 21190927

Goldsmith RJ, Paris M, Riba MB: Negative aspects of collaborative treatment, in Psychopharmacology and Psychotherapy: A Collaborative Approach. Edited by Riba MB, Balon R. Washington, DC, American Psychiatric Press, 1999, pp 33–63

Gutheil TG, Simon RI: Abandonment of patients in split treatment. Harv Rev Psychiatry 11(4):175–179, 2003 12944125

Maris RW, Berman AL, Silverman MM, et al: Physical illness and suicide, in Comprehensive Textbook of Suicidology. Edited by Maris RW, Berman AL, Silverman MM. New York, Guilford, 2000, pp 342–356

Meyer DJ: Split treatment, in The American Psychiatric Publishing Textbook of Suicide Assessment and Management, 2nd Edition. Edited by Simon RI, Hales RE. Washington, DC, American Psychiatric Publishing, 2012, pp 263–282

Meyer DJ, Simon RI: Split treatment: clarity between psychiatrist and psychotherapist, part II. Psychiatr Ann 29(5):327–332, 1999

Raue PJ, Brown EL, Meyers BS, et al: Does every allusion to possible suicide require the same response? J Fam Pract 55(7):605–612, 2006 16822448

Raue PJ, Ghesquiere AR, Bruce ML: Suicide risk in primary care: identification and management in older adults. Curr Psychiatry Rep 16(9):466, 2014 25030971

Riba MB, Balon R, Roberts LW: Competency in Combining Pharmacotherapy and Psychotherapy: Integrated and Split Treatment, 2nd Edition. Washington, DC, American Psychiatric Association Publishing, 2018

Rush AJ, Thase ME: Improving depression outcome by patient-centered medical management. Am J Psychiatry 175(12):1187–1198, 2018 30220219

Cultural Humility and Structural Competence in Suicide Risk Assessment

Poh Choo How, M.D., Ph.D.

Christine Kho, M.D.

Ruth Shim, M.D., M.P.H.

Suicide rates among some racial and ethnic minority groups have steadily increased over the past two decades (Stone et al. 2018). For example, the suicide rate among Native American and Alaskan Native groups has recently surpassed that of non-Hispanic whites by at least 50% (Suicide Prevention Resource Center 2013). East Asian American women have the highest suicide rates among all American women over the age of 65 years (Li et al. 2018), and the rate of suicide among African American children younger than 13 years of age is twice that of white children of the same age group (Bridge et al. 2018). Overall, trends point to an increasing suicide rate in ethnic minority populations.

At the same time, suicide rates may be underestimated in racial and ethnic minority populations due to underrepresentation in research (Cha et al. 2018), misclassifications of causes of death (Rockett et al. 2010), and an underreporting of suicidal ideation (Anderson et al. 2015). Research on suicidal thoughts and behaviors has been predominantly conducted among white, non-Hispanic young adults and less frequently includes or reports on participants' race, ethnicity, veteran status, gender identification, or sexual orientation (Cha et al. 2018). This cultural bias has important clinical and research implications, and its recognition supports the need for broader, more inclusive, and equitable approaches to help us understand factors that contribute to suicide risk in racial, ethnic, sexual, and other minority groups.

Previous discussions on cultural competence in suicide risk assessment (SRA) have focused on how differences in culture, race, and ethnicity impact suicide rates.

This chapter departs from past attempts to categorize race and ethnicity into discrete groups in order to evaluate differences in suicide risk. We present an approach to SRA that allows for a multidimensional evaluation of risk factors through the lens of cultural humility and structural competence. This approach incorporates the consideration of upstream factors (e.g., social determinants of health), including adverse childhood experiences (ACEs), that contribute to the lifetime suicide risk of individuals from all population groups.

Role of Cultural Humility in Evaluating Suicide Risk

The concept of cultural competence arose to emphasize the clinical need to deliver care and services that effectively meet the social, cultural, and linguistic needs of diverse groups of patients. However, the term *cultural competence* implies that providers with majority backgrounds are the default "normal" and have a responsibility to educate themselves on the "different" and—possibly by implication—"abnormal" perspectives of patients of minority backgrounds who have varied cultural perspectives worthy of openness or understanding (Yeager and Bauer-Wu 2013). A cultural competence framework often oversimplifies culture by categorizing discrete racial and ethnic groups without fully considering the role played by intersectionality of multiple cultural identities held at an individual level (e.g., people of mixed-racial identities or the intersection of gender, subcultural, and other identities).

Furthermore, cultural competence is often presented in a decontextualized state, listing various traditions and ideals that minorities and immigrants may hold and applying them broadly to members of a group without regard for unique life experiences (e.g., racism and discrimination, ACEs, migration, and acculturation) (Yeager and Bauer-Wu 2013). This promotes stereotyping and bias and contributes to a two-dimensional, static view of the individual rather than an image of respect, flexibility, and fluidity. Ultimately, this perspective limits the comprehensiveness of an SRA as well as clinicians' overall understanding of the unique experiences of the individual patient to whom they are providing treatment.

In contrast, a culturally informed SRA calls for a multidimensional, dynamic consideration of the individual in relation to the environmental, historical, societal, and other factors with which they interact. This view can be achieved through the lens of *cultural humility*, a cultural framework that adopts a lifelong commitment to self-reflection and critique and calls for providers to approach clinical encounters with an attitude of curiosity, openness, and a willingness to learn from the patient (Tervalon and Murray-García 1998; Figure 6–1).

Cultural humility also emphasizes the awareness of the power differential between patient and provider, which has significant implications for SRAs. For example, studies have shown that some individuals from ethnic minority groups were more likely to hide suicidal ideation (Anderson et al. 2015) or omit answering questions about suicide (Cha et al. 2018). A culturally competent framework may explain this phenomenon as predominantly related to higher rates of stigma about mental illness and suicide among certain racial, ethnic, and religious minority groups. In contrast, a perspective through the lens of cultural humility would also consider that individuals may not reveal their suicidal ideation to providers because they know that providers

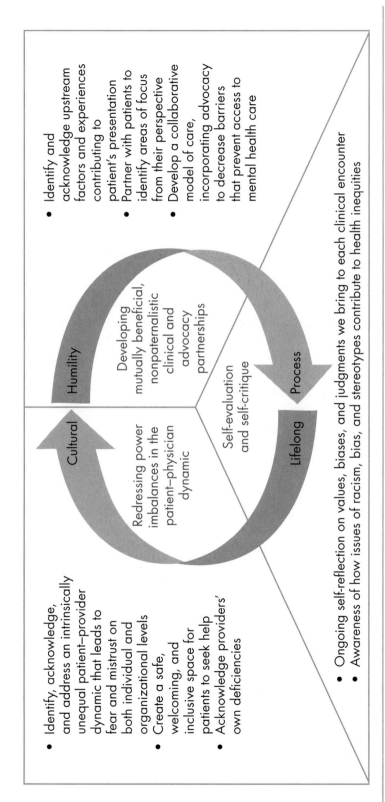

Figure 6–1.   Applying cultural humility in the clinical encounter and in the provider–patient relationship.

can take measures against a patient's will, such as involuntary hospitalization. Although decreasing stigma when conducting SRAs is important, a cultural humility approach's additional perspective calls for simultaneously addressing the power differential between the patient and provider in order to foster safety, collaboration, and partnership in suicide assessment and management.

Although most SRAs take place in one-on-one clinical encounters, many of the perspectives considering the influence of culture on mental health outcomes require taking a population health approach. The cultural humility framework allows us to shift from a view of SRA from the perspective of individual patient characteristics and the clinical encounter as a snapshot moment in time to the longitudinal, lifespan, generational, and societal influences as well as systemic factors that lead to disparities and inequities in suicide risk. Mitigation of suicide risk at both individual and population levels calls for providers to develop structural competence to address these disparities and inequities.

Structural Competence and the Suicide Risk Assessment

Structural competence is defined as the development of skills that empower physicians to act on systemic causes of health inequities while considering social determinants of health and mental health (Hansen et al. 2018). Inequities in mental health outcomes are evidenced in epidemiological studies that have found differences in incidence and prevalence of depression and rates of suicide across sex, age, race, and ethnicity (González et al. 2010). However, the causes of these inequities are not always clearly stated or understood. The World Health Organization (2008) stated that the social determinants of health are most responsible for the health inequities that exist in societies.

Addressing the differences in suicide rates among different groups requires that clinicians become able to recognize the structural causes of mental illness and suicidal thoughts and behaviors, rearticulate "cultural" formulations of this ideation and behavior in structural terms, and identify appropriate structural interventions. As an example, previous discussions about the disproportionately high rates of suicide in Native American/Alaskan Native communities examined factors such as tribal attitudes toward suicide and the prevalence of alcohol use. These discussions have shifted over the past decade to incorporate structural violence, lack of access to health care, inequitable social policies, loss of culture and cultural identity, historical trauma, and systemic oppression as upstream factors leading to inequities in health care and to higher suicide rates in this racial and ethnic group (Figure 6–2) (Browne et al. 2016; Suicide Prevention Resource Center 2013). Browne et al. (2016) proposed inequity-responsive, culturally safe, trauma- and violence-informed, and contextually tailored care to address these inequities.

Social Determinants of Mental Health and Suicide Risk

The main goal of the SRA is to consider those risk factors that contribute to a higher risk of completing suicide as well as protective factors that mitigate suicide risk.

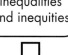

Historical influences on present-day inequalities and inequities

What historical influences have determined which communities are presently privileged versus underprivileged/oppressed?

For example
- Removal of Native Americans from ancestral lands (Removal Act, 1830)
- Slavery of African Americans
- Chinese Exclusion Act (1882)
- Internment of Japanese Americans (1942–1946)
- Racial segregation, Jim Crow laws, red-lining
- Criminalization of homosexual activity

Sociopolitical and cultural context and structural inequities

What current laws and policies determine which communities have access to economic and political opportunities, education, and health care?

For example
- Voting rights laws, immigration laws, health care laws
- Systemic racism (e.g., school-to-prison pipeline)
- War, violence, forced migration, fear of retribution (for refugees and asylum seekers)

Social determinants of health

What historical and current sociopolitical influences contribute to the social determinants of health for communities and individuals?

For example
- Socioeconomic status, access to or lack of social capital
- Access to health care, housing, education, employment opportunities
- Discrimination
- Adverse childhood experiences disproportionately affect historically, socially, politically, and economically disadvantaged individuals

Individual

What facets of identity (e.g., culture, gender, religion, nationality, ability, sexual orientation) influence individual life experiences and access to means of advancement?

Inequities upstream can lead to lack of basic services, including
- Education
- Health care

FIGURE 6–2. Upstream structural influences on mental health and suicide risk.

However, in considering the best points of intervention to prevent suicide, psychiatrists should understand that the social determinants of health are the upstream factors that lead to increased rates of suicide attempts and suicide within and between populations. These upstream factors include things such as ACEs, structural discrimination, social exclusion, income inequality, unemployment, and other determinants of health. Table 6–1 lists specific social determinants of health and cites examples of how they contribute to inequities in suicide rates (Office of Disease Prevention and Health Promotion 2018).

TABLE 6–1.   **Social determinants of health**

Domain	Definition	Example as it relates to suicide
Economic stability	Connection between a person's financial resources (e.g., income, cost of living, socioeconomic status) and health. Domain includes key issues such as poverty, employment, food security, and housing stability.	Lower socioeconomic status and low education levels are risk factors for suicide.
Health and health care	Reflects connection between a person's access to and understanding of health services and his/her health. Domain includes key issues such as access to health care, access to primary care, and health literacy.	Lack of access to mental health care increases the risk of suicide.
Neighborhood and built environment	Reflects connection between where a person lives (e.g., housing, neighborhood, and environment) and his/her health and well-being. Domain includes key issues such as access to healthy food, quality of housing, crime and violence, and environmental conditions.	Exposure to violence and living in neighborhoods with greater income disparities are risk factors for suicide.
Social and community context	Reflects connection between aspects of a person's social environment (e.g., social support, family circumstances, community engagement) and his/her health and well-being. Domain includes key issues such as social cohesion, civic participation, incarceration, and discrimination.	Racial and other forms of discrimination, decreased supportive networks, and social cohesion are risk factors for suicide. For example, not living in two-parent households increases suicide risks, especially for racial/ethnic minority populations.

Source.   Office of Disease Prevention and Health Promotion 2018.

The link between social determinants of health and increased rates of mental illness and suicide is not limited to the United States. For example, in South Korea (Lee et al. 2017), Brazil (Machado et al. 2015), and Europe (Das-Munshi and Thornicroft 2018), low socioeconomic status has been linked to increased suicide rates. Similarly, educational inequalities between Northern and Southern European countries are fueling differences in suicide rates between these regions (Das-Munshi and Thornicroft 2018) because lower education level limits opportunities for employment and access to resources.

Structural racism is defined as "macro-level systems, social forces, institutions, ideologies, and processes that interact with one another to generate and reinforce inequities among racial and ethnic groups" (Gee and Ford 2011, p. 117). This type of racism is a major contributor to increased risk of suicide among groups most commonly impacted by the detrimental effects of structural racism and discrimination (including African

Americans, Native Americans/Alaskan Natives, Latinx populations, women, immigrants, and LGBTQ populations) (Gee and Ford 2011). African American women have the highest rate of medically treated suicide attempts, defined as attempts with consequences severe enough to require medical intervention (Spicer and Miller 2000). Other studies identified racial discrimination as having both direct and mediated effects on suicide and morbid ideation in African American youth (see Chapter 18, "Children and Adolescents"; Walker et al. 2017) as well as among older Chinese Americans (Li et al. 2018).

When considering the intersectionality of cultural identities, risk factors accumulate and contribute to elevated suicide risk in those who identify with multiple cultural groups. One study suggests increased risk for suicidal ideation and behavior among African American women at the intersection of poverty, gender inequality, and racism (Perry et al. 2013). Another study found that African American and Latinx sexual minority youth have suicide rates two to seven times higher than heterosexual youth of similar racial/ethnic background, because these sexual minority youth disproportionately experience increased discrimination, school failure, familial rejection, violence, and mental health problems (see Chapter 23, "Suicide and Gender"; Craig and McInroy 2013).

An abundance of data associate ACEs with many negative health outcomes, including liver disease, cardiovascular disease, major depressive disorder, and early mortality. These associations are often seen in a graded fashion, in which the risk of poor outcomes increases with the number of ACEs one experiences. Suicide attempts follow this pattern, with the risk of suicide increasing significantly as it relates to the number of ACEs that one recalls from childhood (Dube et al. 2001). Although ACEs are universally problematic, those children at risk for high numbers of ACEs (more than seven) often are interacting early with the child welfare system and are often either in foster care or involved with the juvenile justice system. Recent studies have demonstrated that having one ACE in any category increases an individual's suicide risk by more than double while having an ACE score of six and above increases suicide risk by a factor of 24 (Merrick et al. 2017).

Case Example 1

Heidi is a 26-year-old Native American woman currently incarcerated at the county jail. She was observed crying and refusing meals for several days and endorses feelings of sadness and anxiety. This is the third year in a row that she is serving time for driving under the influence. She started to drink heavily 4 years ago and endorses one past suicide attempt by trying to jump off the fourth story of a building. She also endorses a previous experience of intimate partner violence. Currently, Heidi denies suicidal thoughts and states that she "just want[s] to get help" because "I don't want to get in trouble with custody."

How can we consider Heidi's suicide risk through the lens of cultural humility and with a structural competence approach? The standard approach for assessment and management of suicide risk would involve an inventory of the strongest risk and protective factors for suicidal ideation and behaviors and may include standardized screening tools. In this case, we would consider prior suicide attempts, depressed mood, hopelessness, substance use, impulsive behavior, and severe anxiety. The usual approach to SRA would direct clinicians to consider how suicide disproportionately affects Native American/Alaskan Native communities and that Native American/Alaskan Native women in this patient's age group have the highest rate of suicide (19 per 100,000) among women of all ethnic groups, more than three times the rate for white women (Suicide Prevention Resource Center 2013). Furthermore, a previous suicide attempt increases Heidi's lifetime risk of a repeat attempt; untreated alcohol use disorder further adds to her risk. Given Heidi's history of intimate partner violence, the contribution of an undiagnosed mental illness (major depressive disorder or posttraumatic stress disorder [PTSD]) to her overall risk for suicide must also be considered.

Looking through the lens of cultural humility, clinicians should consider the influence of the forensic context that is likely affecting the already imbalanced provider–patient dynamic. This model suggests that clinical assessment should consider whether further challenges to Heidi's safety and confidentiality may affect her readiness to reveal thoughts about suicide in this setting. Addressing stigma and misconceptions about the consequences of expressing suicidal ideation or receiving mental health treatment in a combined forensic and clinical setting may be useful, considering her expressed fear and uncertainty about the consequences of the evaluation/encounter on her custody.

> After reassuring Heidi that the mental health evaluation neither is punitive nor would it affect her time served, Heidi reveals that she thinks about suicide daily. Her previous attempt had been triggered by the removal of her children from her custody by Child Protective Services. This occurred in conjunction with being charged with child endangerment for exposing her children to her abusive partner. However, Heidi has not taken further steps to end her life because she desperately hopes to be reunited with her children one day. In the community, she turns to alcohol to help her control her suicidal ideation, depression, and anxiety.

Let us also consider the upstream factors, structural inequities, social determinants of health, and ACEs that have contributed to Heidi's current situation and suicide risk. Here, the social history portion of the psychiatric evaluation is the most informative.

> On further exploration, Heidi reveals that she grew up on a rural reservation in a single-parent home. Her father was often incarcerated. Her mother was also affected by intimate partner violence and worked far away to earn enough to support the family. Heidi expressed fondness for spending time with her grandparents and participating in sweat lodge ceremonies with them. When they died, Heidi no longer felt connected to the traditions and ceremonies of the Miwok tribe to which she belongs. Heidi left high school after the tenth grade and moved to a nearby town to start work. There, she began a relationship with the father of her children. She expressed that having come from a broken home, her family and children became very important to her. Sadly, her partner ended up abusing her. The nearest primary care clinic where she could obtain both medical and psychiatric care was 150 miles away. Heidi had made the 300-mile round trip journey once, but she had not been able to follow up because she could not afford the cost of fuel for subsequent appointments. When her children were separated from her, Heidi could not imagine living life without them, precipitating her attempt to end her life.

The historical oppression, structural violence, and inequitable social policies and practices (e.g., social exclusion, unjust land allotment, and forced acculturation) that disproportionately affect the Native American/Alaskan Native community have been well documented (Browne et al. 2016; Suicide Prevention Resource Center 2013).

These upstream factors contributed to decreased community cohesion. In addition, the forced resettlement of these communities to rural settings resulted in many members of this population living in areas where access to health and mental health care, education, and employment, among other things, were limited. As a result, Heidi's overall suicide risk is further elevated due to social determinants such as lower socio-economic status, lower level of education, lack of access to health care, exposure to violence, lack of social cohesion, and social exclusion. Heidi also has multiple ACEs (six total), which further adds to her suicide risk. The social significance and societal origins of Native American/Alaskan Native suicide underscore the linkages between shared risk factors, such as historical trauma, and personal risk factors, such as acculturation, discrimination, and even reluctance to seek mental health services (Suicide Prevention Resource Center 2013).

A structural formulation of this case identifies systemic barriers that exacerbate lack of access to care. Similarly, a structural competence approach to Heidi's care includes identification of interventions to address structural inequities, for example, by advocating for increased access to mental health treatment (e.g., through loan forgiveness programs for mental health practitioners in rural/tribal areas, providing mobile mental health services that travel to reservations, or use of telepsychiatry). Certainly, making treatment for alcohol use disorder more widely available or using a preventive health approach to diminish rates of alcohol abuse would have widespread positive outcomes.

Promoting and creating upstream changes can have significant positive downstream changes. For example, a Canadian study demonstrated that cultural continuity (defined as having infrastructure, such as the presence of cultural facilities, and sovereignty, such as self-government) not only is a protective factor for suicide but is also related to lower rates of depression and alcohol use disorders (Chandler and Lalonde 2008).

Mental Health Issues Associated With Migration and Immigration

The push and pull of modern-day migratory forces have led to an unprecedented number of 210 million migrants worldwide. Globalization, economic pressures, population demographic shifts, environmental threats, wars and conflicts, and human rights abuses are some of the reasons for this movement of people within and across countries (Nygren-Krug 2013). In June 2018, the United Nations High Commissioner for Refugees (2018) estimated there are a record 68.5 million forcibly displaced people worldwide, of whom 25.4 million are refugees, 3.1 million are asylum seekers, and the majority, 40 million, are internally displaced people. The process of migration is not a simple one, particularly for refugee and asylum seekers, and has significant implications on mental health and suicide risk. See Table 6–2 for definitions of terms used to describe different migrant populations.

Research on the mental health of refugee populations historically has focused on psychopathology as a posttraumatic reaction to the acute stressors of war; however, this life events model fails to take into account the multiple and varied stressors that accumulate premigration, perimigration, and postmigration (Priebe et al. 2016). Expo-

TABLE 6–2. **Definition of terms and implications for suicide risk among migrants**

Term	Definition	Factors contributing to increased suicide risk
Migrant	A person who changes his or her country of usual residence regardless of reason for departure.	Experience of discrimination/social exclusion, limited health care, lack of economic opportunity, housing insecurity, and other social determinants of mental health in host country
Refugee	A migrant who is outside of his or her country of origin due to "well-founded fear of being persecuted for reasons of race, religion, nationality, membership of a particular social group or political opinion" (United Nations General Assembly 1951, p. 152) and is protected from forced return to their homeland unless the situation that prompted their flight improves (under the United Nations Refugee Convention of 1951). Host countries are responsible for providing favorable conditions, including the right to work, freedom of movement, and public services.	Exposure to violence and trauma pre-, peri-, and postmigration; breakdown of family including parental separation, social identity, and community cohesion
Asylum seekers	Migrants who have sought international protection after entering another country on a temporary visa or without any documents of their own whose refugee status has not been determined.	Forced detention, uncertainty of delayed asylum processing, having variable access to freedom to travel, access to health care, and rights to public services depending on host country due to unprotected status in addition to other risk factors
Irregular migrants	Individuals who do not have a residence permit allowing regular stay in a host country.	

Source. Nygren-Krug 2013; Priebe et al. 2016; Silove et al. 2017.

sures to risk factors for developing mental illness are often greater in refugee, asylum-seeking, and irregular-migrant populations. Premigration risk factors include trauma such as torture, imprisonment, witnessing death of family members, direct combat, sexual violence, and human rights abuses and extreme economic hardship such as deprivation of basic needs (e.g., food, water, and shelter). The physical act of travel may involve bodily harm from environmental threats and perilous conditions such as unsafe boats or long journeys by foot, extortion, sexual violence, human trafficking, and separation from family.

Once resettled, migrant-related government policies such as those related to seeking asylum, limited access to services such as health care, ongoing family separation, social exclusion and discrimination, financial and housing insecurity, loss of social identity, and linguistic challenges negatively impact mental health (Nygren-Krug 2013; Priebe et al. 2016). Many countries have employed migration deterrence strategies that also exacerbate psychological symptoms, such as restricted access to legal services, housing, and health care; systematic dispersal of asylum seekers; forced detention, where many migrants are vulnerable to violations of their rights to food and health; extended processing times; and restricted economic opportunities. These factors compound premigratory and perimigratory trauma (Silove et al. 2017).

Mental Illness and Suicide Prevalence Among Migrant Populations

Rates of mental disorders have varied widely across the refugee populations studied, in part due to heterogeneous methodology and background characteristics with regard to countries of origin, exposure to trauma, host country characteristics, and other risk factors. A systematic review by Fazel et al. (2005) of 6,700 refugees resettled in Western countries found prevalence rates of generalized anxiety disorder (4%) and major depressive disorder (5%) comparable to prevalence rates in the general population of host countries. However, rates of PTSD were 9% compared to 1%–3% of the host population. PTSD rates have been reported as high as 17% among asylum seekers (Priebe et al. 2016). For children, family separation and parental loss, such as the forced family separation policy affecting U.S. borders, have shown to increase risk of death from suicide (Cleveland et al. 2012).

Asylum policies, including detention and delayed processing, have major impacts on psychopathology and suicide risk. Asylum seekers who have been in a host country for longer periods of time compared to recent arrivals are more likely to have symptoms of PTSD, depression, and anxiety. Longer periods of detention also worsen psychological symptoms (Priebe et al. 2016). An Australian study looking at self-harm behavior in detained asylum seekers found the rate of self-harm to be 22% during a 20-month period (Hedrick 2017). The reported overall prevalence of suicidal behavior among refugees ranged between 3.4% and 34%. Acute risk may be elevated during early displacement (less than 6 months) or with prolonged stays in refugee camps or detention centers.

The vulnerability of migrant populations can be viewed from two perspectives simultaneously—that of the individual or migrant group qualities and that of the structural causes within the host country. Poor mental health outcomes among refugees further reinforce that the solution not only lies in providing access and promoting use of mental health services but also in addressing social determinants such as education, housing, employment, and public policy, among others, as modes of prevention and treatment within the host country. This places immense pressure on communities receiving migration flows to help people realize their rights to health and well-being.

Case Example 2

Firuzeh is a 17-year-old Farsi-speaking adolescent who is referred to the crisis unit by one of her teachers, who overheard Firuzeh expressing suicidal thoughts to another student. She is a refugee from Afghanistan who moved to the United States with her family 2 months ago. She states that she misses her friends and finds it hard adjusting to school, mainly due to the language barrier. She endorses feelings of frustration but denies depression, anxiety, or symptoms of PTSD. She explains that her teacher most likely misunderstood her intentions and that, as a Muslim, she could never think of taking her own life.

From the point of view of a standard SRA, Firuzeh's overall suicide risk would be considered low. She does not belong to a demographic group with a high suicide rate, does not have a history of suicide attempts, and does not endorse current suicidal ideation, depression, or anxiety. Her religious beliefs and family connections are additional protective factors.

At the same time, a trauma-informed, cultural humility approach needs to be incorporated into Firuzeh's SRA, with sensitivity to the vulnerabilities she faced throughout the process of migration. Because this is her first interface with the mental health system, this would include permission-seeking and explanation of the purpose and implications of the evaluation she is undergoing. Given her prior experience of lack of agency over her forced migration, the safety, trust, and partnership building necessary in this process may be forfeited if this step is neglected, impacting the provider's ability to gather important information pertaining to an SRA. Use of cultural brokers, meetings with families, and consultation with religious and community organizations can be considered (Kirmayer et al. 2011) but should be balanced with the need for confidentiality. Confidentiality issues must be considered very carefully, especially in communities with smaller numbers of refugees of the same cultural group and the potential for fewer degrees of separation between the patient and members of the group who may become involved as brokers, consultants, or even translators.

> Firuzeh shares that her family was fortunate to be able to move directly from Afghanistan to the United States, avoiding the usual lengthy waiting period and serial migrations. Her mother describes Firuzeh, the oldest child, as being close to her younger five siblings and says that the family is feeling a sense of relief at having come to the United States. Firuzeh's father is unemployed but is looking for work. Meanwhile, the family receives Social Security income and housing assistance. Firuzeh is diagnosed with adjustment disorder and given a follow-up appointment at her local outpatient mental health clinic.
>
> Ten months later, Firuzeh is seen in the crisis unit again, this time after a suicide attempt by overdose. She has lost 15 pounds since her last evaluation. She reveals, very reluctantly, that she has been deeply depressed. She has continued to struggle in school and feels like a failure. She was never able to follow up with outpatient mental health services due to lack of transportation. Her parents remain unemployed, and the family is finding it difficult to make ends meet.

The Refugee Act of 1980 requires that host countries make public services, including mental health services, available to refugees (Kennedy 1981). However, this does not guarantee that the systems in place are accessible. Therefore, "treatment as usual" may be insufficient for vulnerable migrants, including refugees, who face many obstacles in accessing mental health care. Most refugees receive Medicaid insurance benefits and have to rely on already overburdened public mental health programs to access treatment. Unfortunately for this patient, her inability to access adequate care after a crisis led to worsening of her symptoms and a suicide attempt.

Although upstream factors related to pre- and perimigration may be impossible to address, more can be done to address postmigratory stressors to mitigate the risk for further trauma, mental illness, and death from suicide among refugees. Kirmayer et al. (2011) recommended systematic screening of patients' migration trajectory with regular follow-up on social, vocational, and family functioning over time. This allows clinicians to recognize developing problems and undertake appropriate preventive or treatment interventions before bad outcomes occur. These steps should be integrated into services provided for refugees rather than placing the burden of establishing care onto members of the vulnerable, disenfranchised, and disadvantaged groups.

Culturally Informed Interventions

Little research has examined interventions to prevent or reduce suicidal behavior in refugee and asylum-seeking populations, and whether strategies shown to be effective in the general population would be applicable to these groups is unknown. The main focus of recommended clinical practice has included fostering social inclusion through education, housing, and employment; coordination of care among multiple health systems; providing education on available entitlement programs; and creating methods to overcome language barriers. Alternatives to detention as used in France, Switzerland, and other countries include use of bail bonds, required reporting to immigration authorities, and other approaches that are less expensive and less likely to impinge human rights and adversely impact mental health (Priebe et al. 2016). In response to the spate of deaths from suicide among asylum seekers in Australia, Procter et al. (2018) advocated for trauma-informed collaborative safety planning, with the goal of helping migrant populations shift from the hopelessness associated with perceptions or reality of unbearable injustice that may lead to suicidal behavior to alternatives promoting life-affirming coping skills.

Conclusion

Culturally sensitive SRAs require a cultural humility approach that considers power imbalances in the patient–provider relationship. Implementing this approach requires that clinicians proactively engage in a lifelong process of self-reflection and learning. Providers need to develop structural competence by acquiring skills in recognizing upstream factors that contribute to suicide risk factors, rearticulating cultural formulations of suicidal thoughts and behaviors in structural terms, and identifying and advocating for appropriate interventions. This includes addressing upstream causes of risk factors, including social determinants of health, structural racism and discrimination, ACEs, and other systemic inequities. These approaches should also be used to address the increased risk of suicide death among various migrant populations with the added vulnerabilities to migration-related traumatic experiences.

Key Points

- Cultural humility is necessary for suicide risk assessment and management. This involves a lifelong process of self-evaluation and self-critique on the values, biases, and stereotypes providers bring to each clinical encounter and consideration of the inherent power imbalances in the patient–physician dynamic when evaluating suicidal ideation and risk.

- Providers need to develop structural competency to adequately address suicide risk. This includes recognizing the systemic upstream causes of mental illness and suicidal thoughts and behaviors; understanding how social determinants of health contribute to health inequities; and advocating for changes upstream to mitigate suicide risk that affect patients downstream.

- Adverse childhood experiences significantly impact mental health and risk of death from suicide in adulthood and are an important consideration in a suicide risk assessment.

- The intersectionality of cultural, gender, national, religious, and other identities is an important consideration when evaluating suicide risk factors.

- Refugees and asylum seekers are especially vulnerable to elevated risk of death from suicide due to disproportionate experiences of structural violence and trauma before, during, and after migration.

References

Anderson LM, Lowry LS, Wuensch KL: Racial differences in adolescents' answering questions about suicide. Death Stud 39(10):600–604, 2015 26083790

Bridge JA, Horowitz LM, Fontanella CA, et al: Age-related racial disparity in suicide rates among US youths from 2001 through 2015. JAMA Pediatr 172(7):697–699, 2018 29799931

Browne AJ, Varcoe C, Lavoie J, et al: Enhancing health care equity with indigenous populations: evidence-based strategies from an ethnographic study. BMC Health Serv Res 16(1):544, 2016 27716261

Cha CB, Tezanos KM, Peros OM, et al: Accounting for diversity in suicide research: sampling and sample reporting practices in the United States. Suicide Life Threat Behav 48(2):131–139, 2018 28276601

Chandler MJ, Lalonde CE: Cultural continuity as a moderator of suicide risk among Canada's First Nations, in Healing Traditions: The Mental Health of Aboriginal Peoples in Canada. Edited by Kirmayer LJ. Vancouver, British Columbia, UBC Press, 2008, pp 221–248

Cleveland J, Rousseau C, Kronick R: The Harmful Effects of Detention and Family Separation on Asylum Seekers' Mental Health in the Context of Bill C-31. Brief submitted to the House of Commons Standing Committee on Citizenship and Immigration concerning Bill C-31. Montreal, Quebec, Centre Integre Universitaire de Sante et de Services Socizux du Centre-Ouest-de-L'ile-de-Montreal, 2012

Craig SL, McInroy L: The relationship of cumulative stressors, chronic illness and abuse to the self-reported suicide risk of black and Hispanic sexual minority youth. J Community Psychol 41(7):783–798, 2013

Das-Munshi J, Thornicroft G: Failure to tackle suicide inequalities across Europe. Br J Psychiatry 212(6):331–332, 2018 29786494

Dube SR, Anda RF, Felitti VJ, et al: Childhood abuse, household dysfunction, and the risk of attempted suicide throughout the life span: findings from the Adverse Childhood Experiences Study. JAMA 286(24):3089–3096, 2001 11754674

Fazel M, Wheeler J, Danesh J: Prevalence of serious mental disorder in 7000 refugees resettled in Western countries: a systematic review. Lancet 365(9467):1309–1314, 2005 15823380

Gee GC, Ford CL: Structural racism and health inequities: old issues, new directions. Du Bois Rev 8(1):115–132, 2011 25632292

González HM, Tarraf W, Whitfield KE, et al: The epidemiology of major depression and ethnicity in the United States. J Psychiatr Res 44(15):1043–1051, 2010 20537350

Hansen H, Braslow J, Rohrbaugh RM: From cultural to structural competency—training psychiatric residents to act on social determinants of health and institutional racism. JAMA Psychiatry 75(2):117–118, 2018 29261827

Hedrick K: Getting out of (self-) harm's way: a study of factors associated with self-harm among asylum seekers in Australian immigration detention. J Forensic Leg Med 49:89–93, 2017 28601787

Kennedy EM: Refugee act of 1980. Int Migr Rev 15(1–2):141–156, 1981

Kirmayer LJ, Narasiah L, Munoz M, et al: Common mental health problems in immigrants and refugees: general approach in primary care. CMAJ 183(12):E959–E967, 2011 20603342

Lee SU, Oh IH, Jeon HJ, et al: Suicide rates across income levels: retrospective cohort data on 1 million participants collected between 2003 and 2013 in South Korea. J Epidemiol 27(6):258–264, 2017 28314637

Li LW, Gee GC, Dong X: Association of self-reported discrimination and suicide ideation in older Chinese Americans. Am J Geriatr Psychiatry 26(1):42–51, 2018 28917505

Machado DB, Rasella D, Dos Santos DN: Impact of income inequality and other social determinants on suicide rate in Brazil. PLoS One 10(4):e0124934, 2015 25928359

Merrick MT, Ports KA, Ford DC, et al: Unpacking the impact of adverse childhood experiences on adult mental health. Child Abuse Negl 69:10–19, 2017 28419887

Nygren-Krug H: International Migration, Health and Human Rights. Geneva, Switzerland, International Organization for Migration, 2013

Office of Disease Prevention and Health Promotion: Social determinants of health, in Healthy People 2020. Washington, DC, U.S. Department of Health and Human Services, 2018, pp 39.1–39.21. Available at: https://www.cdc.gov/nchs/data/hpdata2020/HP2020MCR-C39-SDOH.pdf. Accessed November 15, 2018.

Perry BL, Stevens-Watkins D, Oser CB: The moderating effects of skin color and ethnic identity affirmation on suicide risk among low-SES African American women. Race Soc Probl 5(1):1–14, 2013 23459264

Priebe S, Giacco D, El-Nagib R: Public Health Aspects of Mental Health Among Migrants and Refugees: A Review of the Evidence on Mental Health Care for Refugees, Asylum Seekers and Irregular Migrants in the WHO European Region. Copenhagen, Denmark, WHO Regional Office for Europe, 2016

Procter NG, Kenny MA, Eaton H, et al : Lethal hopelessness: understanding and responding to asylum seeker distress and mental deterioration. Int J Ment Health Nurs 27(1):448–454, 2018 28322492

Rockett IR, Wang S, Stack S, et al: Race/ethnicity and potential suicide misclassification: window on a minority suicide paradox? BMC Psychiatry 10:35, 2010 20482844

Silove D, Ventevogel P, Rees S: The contemporary refugee crisis: an overview of mental health challenges. World Psychiatry 16(2):130–139, 2017 28498581

Spicer RS, Miller TR: Suicide acts in 8 states: incidence and case fatality rates by demographics and method. Am J Public Health 90(12):1885–1891, 2000 11111261

Stone DM, Simon TR, Fowler KA, et al: Vital Signs: trends in state suicide rates—United States, 1999–2016 and circumstances contributing to suicide—27 states, 2015. MMWR Morb Mortal Wkly Rep 67(22):617–624, 2018 29879094

Suicide Prevention Resource Center: Suicide Among Racial/Ethnic Populations in the U.S.: American Indians/Alaska Natives. Waltham, MA, Education Development Center, 2013

Tervalon M, Murray-García J: Cultural humility versus cultural competence: a critical distinction in defining physician training outcomes in multicultural education. J Health Care Poor Underserved 9(2):117–125, 1998 10073197

United Nations General Assembly: Convention Relating to the Status of Refugees, United Nations, Treaty Series, 189:137-220, 1951, p.152

United Nations High Commissioner for Refugees: Figures at a Glance. Geneva, Switzerland, UNHCR, 2018. Available at: https://www.unhcr.org/en-us/figures-at-a-glance.html. Accessed November 15, 2018.

Walker R, Francis D, Brody G, et al: A longitudinal study of racial discrimination and risk for death ideation in African American youth. Suicide Life Threat Behav 47(1):86–102, 2017 27137139

World Health Organization: Closing the Gap in a Generation: Health Equity Through Action on the Social Determinants of Health. Geneva, Switzerland, Commission on the Social Determinants of Health, 2008

Yeager KA, Bauer-Wu S: Cultural humility: essential foundation for clinical researchers. Appl Nurs Res 26(4):251–256, 2013 23938129

PART II

Major Mental Disorders

CHAPTER 7

Depressive Disorders

Ryan Holliday, Ph.D.
Lindsey L. Monteith, Ph.D.
Sarra Nazem, Ph.D.
Hal S. Wortzel, M.D.

Depressive disorders are among the most common psychiatric diagnoses, with major depressive disorder (MDD) being the most prevalent mood disorder (Kessler et al. 2005a, 2005b). The 12-month prevalence of MDD in the United States is estimated to be approximately 7% (American Psychiatric Association 2013). The National Comorbidity Survey Replication found that approximately 16.6% of U.S. adults will experience MDD in their lifetime (Kessler et al. 2005a). Subsets of the general population also experience MDD with greater frequency. For example, women are twice as likely to experience MDD in their lifetime compared with men (American Psychiatric Association 2013).

Additional depressive disorders recognized by DSM-5 (American Psychiatric Association 2013) include disruptive mood dysregulation disorder, persistent depressive disorder (dysthymia), premenstrual dysphoric disorder, substance/medication-induced depressive disorder, depressive disorder due to another medical condition, other specified depressive disorder, and unspecified depressive disorder. Although all of these diagnoses share the essential feature of sustained sadness, emptiness, or irritability, MDD is unique in featuring diagnostic criteria that include suicidal ideation

This material is based upon work supported in part by the Department of Veterans Affairs; the Rocky Mountain Mental Illness Research, Education and Clinical Center (MIRECC) for Suicide Prevention; and the Office of Academic Affiliations, Advanced Fellowship Program in Mental Illness Research and Treatment, Department of Veterans Affairs. The views expressed are those of the authors and do not necessarily represent the views or policy of the Department of Veterans Affairs or the United States Government.

or recurrent thoughts of death. Hopelessness occurs more broadly across the depressive disorders and represents an important point of consideration when exploring the relationship between depressive disorders and risk of death from suicide.

Several studies reveal an association between depression and death from suicide, with MDD's relationship being among the strongest: MDD features in one-half to two-thirds of psychological autopsy cases (Hawton et al. 2013). Depressive disorders are also highly comorbid with several other psychiatric diagnoses (e.g., posttraumatic stress disorder [PTSD], anxiety disorders, substance use disorders) that carry their own independent associations with risk of death from suicide (Hawton et al. 2013).

This chapter offers conceptualizations of suicide risk among depressed patients based on predominant theories of suicide, with an emphasis on factors that may be identified and modified in clinical care. A therapeutic risk management framework is offered as an approach to assessing and managing suicide risk among patients with depressive disorders.

Transdiagnostic Conceptualization of Suicide Risk Among Patients With Depressive Disorders

Although MDD is a well-established, evidence-based risk factor for suicide, recognizing depressive symptoms or a depressive disorder alone is inadequate for stratifying and mitigating risk for death from suicide (Goldsmith et al. 2002). A patient's death from suicide is a complex and multidetermined occurrence that cannot be attributed to any single diagnosis or life event; a diagnosis of MDD, or any depressive disorder, is neither necessary nor sufficient in understanding any given death from suicide. Thus, to improve efforts at assessing, conceptualizing, and managing suicide risk, an approach that considers underlying drivers of suicide from a transdiagnostic lens is crucial.

One applicable theory is the *interpersonal-psychological theory of suicide* (IPTS; Joiner 2005; Van Orden et al. 2010). The IPTS posits that the desire to live is an inherent and evolutionary drive that is reduced in the presence of *thwarted belongingness* (TB), an unmet psychological need to belong, and *perceived burdensomeness* (PB), the perception that one's existence is burdensome to others. TB is engendered in the presence of loneliness, isolation, and perceptions of lack of social reciprocity. Given the propensity of patients with depressive disorders to enact interpersonal behaviors and attitudes that may increase rejection and social distance (Coyne et al. 1990), such as avoidance or excessive reassurance seeking, depressive dysphoria may further engender or exacerbate perceptions of TB. Additionally, self-hate is a central component of PB; thus, the low self-esteem and negative emotions commonplace in depressive disorders (American Psychiatric Association 2013) can further increase individuals' perceptions that they are a burden to those around them. The simultaneous presence of both PB and TB, particularly when expected to be persisting and unchanging, is theorized to result in the desire to die from suicide (Van Orden et al. 2010).

Beliefs that one does not belong or is a burden to others are likely to influence an individual's overarching "suicidal belief system," an aspect of the *fluid vulnerability theory* (Rudd 2006). Patients with MDD are likely to experience suicide-specific beliefs pertaining to themselves (e.g., "I am a bad person"), others (e.g., "No one likes me"), and the world (e.g., "The world is a cruel place"). Such thoughts are likely to be further reinforced as perceptions of PB and TB intensify. Additionally, the culmination of these beliefs with depressive symptomatology may precipitate perceptions of hopelessness. Indeed, research by Kleiman et al. (2014) found that hopelessness, PB, and TB each predict suicidal ideation, suggesting that an integrative framework that synthesizes perceptions of interpersonal functioning; views of self, world, and others; and hopelessness are integral to comprehensively elucidating suicide risk in patients with depressive disorders.

Nevertheless, perceptions of TB and PB, even when coupled with hopelessness and suicide-related beliefs, remain insufficient to result in patients engaging in suicidal behavior (Van Orden et al. 2010). Individuals must also develop the "acquired capability" to die from suicide. Within the IPTS framework, acquired capability develops and increases due to repeated exposure to painful and provocative events that diminish the fear of death and enhance physical pain tolerance (Van Orden et al. 2010), the conceptualized mechanisms that facilitate suicidal intent and behavior.

Building upon this framework, Klonsky and May (2014) also emphasized through their "ideation-to-action" framework the importance of concurrent *practice* aspects in increasing the likelihood of progression from ideation to behavior, suggesting that factors that ease the process from thinking about suicide to engaging in suicidal self-directed violence are more likely to result in suicidal behavior. Specifically, concrete factors (i.e., practical capacity) such as lethal means knowledge (e.g., proficiency in using a gun due to training, practice, and exposure) and access (e.g., having a loaded gun stored under one's bed) are considered to be associated with risk for suicidal behavior (Klonsky and May 2015). Therefore, within the "three-step theory," underlying factors driving risk for death from suicide must be weighed simultaneously with acquired capability, including prior exposure to fearful or painful stimuli as well as current access to lethal means, and particularly means with which the individual possesses facility (Klonsky and May 2015).

In addition to these factors, Rudd (2006) proposed that suicide-related beliefs driven by TB, PB, hopelessness, and psychosocial stressors are likely to fluctuate over time based on the patient's thoughts, feelings, behaviors, and physiology. This, in turn, is likely to result in periods of heightened suicide risk, based on the amalgamation of underlying, longstanding factors (e.g., chronic unemployment or ongoing interpersonal tumult) with more immediate, acute factors (psychosocial stressors such as being fired from one's job or divorce). Hence, baseline levels of risk of death from suicide are exacerbated by dynamic fluctuations in acute risk factors (Rudd 2006). Depressive symptomatology (e.g., decreased energy and ability to concentrate, insomnia) and automatic negative thoughts (e.g., "I can't do anything right") may further impact a patient's ability to function and cope with chronic and acute factors that drive risk of death from suicide.

Clinicians treating patients with depressive disorders (and other psychiatric disorders that increase the risk of death from suicide) should therefore bear in mind that this risk is dynamic. Underlying factors of PB, TB, and hopelessness, combined with acquired capability (Joiner 2005; Van Orden et al. 2010) and lethal means access and knowledge (Klonsky and May 2014), are important for informing the severity of a patient's immediate and long-term risk for suicide. These transdiagnostic approaches are helpful for improving conceptualization of suicidal desire and suicidal self-directed violence and also provide excellent approaches to inform evidence-based suicide risk assessment, management, and intervention for depressed individuals.

Therapeutic Risk Management: Risk Assessment and Intervention

Case Example

A 25-year-old veteran has been silently struggling with depression and PTSD symptoms since returning from his tour of duty. His fiancée has grown exasperated with his irritable and isolative behaviors and has been thinking of calling off the wedding. The veteran's distress at this development triggered some heavy alcohol consumption, during which he experienced suicidal ideation. Though the veteran has previously experienced thoughts of suicide, these thoughts were always very fleeting. The veteran found himself scared by these ideas for the first time.

The veteran presents to urgent care the following day in an effort to establish treatment for his depression and PTSD and reports recent suicidal ideation and a plan to shoot himself. The veteran has ready access to the stated means of death. The urgent-care clinician considers the recent suicidal ideation and its increased intensity, the presence of a plan with accessible means, and the absence of any established mental health treatment. The clinician deems the patient to be at high risk for death from suicide and quickly and unilaterally decides that psychiatric hospitalization is warranted, despite the patient's objection. Upon arriving on the inpatient unit, the patient is reticent to discuss circumstances leading up to his admission, pointing out that his initial efforts to obtain help for his distress "got me locked up."

Risk Stratification

Absent a familiar methodology for conducting suicide risk assessment and management, a clinician's anxiety about patient safety may influence, or potentially even substitute for, clinical judgment. This can result in unnecessary hospitalizations (Paris 2004) that may potentially damage rapport and trust with the patient, which in turn may compromise the ability to mitigate suicide risk in the long term. A therapeutic risk management approach, which stratifies and communicates suicide risk and facilitates interventions to mitigate risk and maximize protective factors, combines clinical judgment with structured risk assessment. Key components of the model involve augmenting clinical assessment with structured instruments, stratifying suicide risk in terms of both severity and temporality, and developing a safety plan (Wortzel et al. 2013). This approach results in a more objective assessment of risk and facilitates evidence-informed risk management, which may then be tracked over time to determine if implemented interventions have been effective in decreasing target symptoms, enhancing protective factors, and mitigating risk of death from suicide.

Stratifying Risk

Therapeutic risk management involves stratifying both acute and chronic suicide risk in terms of low, moderate, or high severity (Wortzel et al. 2014). Suicide risk is sufficiently nuanced such that a single term describing severity seldom suffices to capture the details regarding the nature of any individual's risk of death from suicide or how best to manage risk. A dual stratification of suicide risk in terms of severity and temporality better facilitates communication regarding risk over time and what is needed to manage and mitigate that risk. For example, interventions appropriate for acute risk of death from suicide—that is, risk of suicide in the immediate foreseeable future, spanning hours or days—are often unhelpful in terms of mitigating chronic risk—that is, risk over the long term, spanning weeks, months, and years. An involuntary hospitalization may afford the external support and safety that addresses acute risk but is less likely to afford the skill building and enhanced protective factors typically needed to optimize chronic risk, clinical accomplishments that usually require sustained treatment efforts on an outpatient basis.

Returning to the case example, the clinician's further inquiry prior to deciding to hospitalize the patient involuntarily might have revealed that the patient did not have intent or desire to die from suicide, was future oriented, wanted to establish mental health care and improve his emotional status and coping style, and was highly motivated to do so in an effort to repair the relationship with his fiancée. A dual designation of low acute and high chronic risk would then better capture the nature of his suicide risk and would enhance communication of that risk. For this patient, establishing outpatient management is the more appropriate treatment option, while simultaneously implementing appropriate treatment plans to augment coping skills, sustain sobriety, and develop a safety plan.

Augmenting Clinical Assessment With Structured Instruments

Risk assessment requires a robust clinical interview in which the clinician gathers data on psychiatric symptoms, functioning, and relevant suicide risk and protective factors (e.g., social support, coping skills, comorbidity, history of self-directed violence). However, relying solely on unstructured clinical interviews may result in missing important risk and protective factors (Wortzel et al. 2013) and thus potentially omitting crucial information that can inform the nature and level of suicide risk. Clinical interviews are best augmented with structured assessment tools that specifically assess key risk and protective factors (Homaifar et al. 2013). Although the following discussion reviews a number of appropriate structured assessment instruments, no particular instruments are being recommended. Selection should be guided by clinical needs and available resources because the time, training requirements, and costs across various instruments vary considerably.

Providers may benefit from using a structured clinical interview. Various options exist, including the Columbia Suicide Severity Rating Scale (Poster et al. 2008), the Self-Injurious Thoughts and Behaviors Interview (Nock et al. 2007), or the Lifetime-Suicide Attempt Self-Injury Count (Linehan and Comtois 1996). These measures can be used to assess recent and lifetime history of suicidal thoughts and behaviors and thus can be used to gather important suicide-related data (e.g., lethality of suicide attempts, suicidal intent). Many also assess nonsuicidal self-injury (NSSI). Although NSSI is easily missed during routine clinical interviews, it remains relevant to determining a patient's level of risk for both death from suicide and future NSSI, such as cutting or burning oneself without suicidal intent (see Chapter 24, "Self-Injurious Behavior").

In the case of depressive disorders, concurrent assessment of severity of depressive symptoms and suicidal ideation using a clinical interview and self-report measure (e.g., Patient Health Questionnaire–9 [Kroenke et al. 2001]; Beck Depression Inventory-II [Beck et al. 1996] for depressive symptoms; Beck Scale for Suicidal Ideation

[Beck and Steer 1991]; or C-SSRS for recent suicidal ideation severity) may increase detection of risk and inform treatment. Using both the interview and self-report instrument may facilitate detecting discrepancies between the two. For example, a patient may deny current suicidal ideation on interview but report it on the self-report instrument. For many individuals experiencing depression and suicidal ideation, acknowledging and disclosing these experiences may be difficult. The opportunity to offer a written response, as opposed to having to verbalize these experiences, affords another avenue for disclosure that may be more acceptable to individuals already in emotional distress.

Yet another advantage of this combined approach, particularly in systems of care wherein patients are likely to encounter different providers across various settings, is that it establishes baselines against which future improvements or exacerbations can be measured in quantifiable terms. A provider's clinical judgment of the severity of a patient's depression or intensity of suicidal ideation may be difficult to track and communicate in records across time or clinicians. Periodic use of structured tools to measure depression or suicidal thoughts and behaviors can create reference points for evaluators first meeting a patient.

This measurement-based care approach can be especially helpful in discerning between elevated suicide risk that constitutes an acute crisis and an elevated, but relatively stable, degree of chronic suicidal ideation. In other words, reviewing prior responses on structured assessments may facilitate recognizing baseline levels of acute suicide risk (e.g., stable levels of suicidal ideation severity) as opposed to an acute crisis (e.g., a meaningful increase in scores over the past few sessions) (Paris 2004). Although certain interventions do overlap, interventions targeting acute risk versus chronic risk generally vary significantly.

In addition to assessment of risk factors, protective factors that can be augmented to reduce risk of death from suicide must also be reviewed. Complementing their clinical interview, providers might consider administering the Reasons for Living Inventory (Linehan et al. 1983), a self-report measure that assesses for multiple factors that typically decrease patient's risk of suicide, including, for example, fear of suicide, moral objections, and family-related beliefs. Depressed patients often struggle to spontaneously identify positive aspects of their lives or reasons to keep living. A structured tool can facilitate identifying such positives in many instances.

Collateral Data

Clinicians should also consider the import of augmenting their interview and assessment data with appropriate collateral information obtained, for example, from a family member who knows the patient's history or the police officer who brought the patient into the emergency department. Patients may not be willing to disclose previous history or access to lethal means for multiple reasons. In addition, severe depression can at times result in symptoms such as psychosis or delusions that may preclude conducting an informative clinical interview or assessment or limit the validity of the information obtained in the interview. Absent psychosis, even acute depression and related cognitive distortions may sufficiently color the patient's worldview, such that they are unable to accurately portray various life circumstances.

Collateral data from third parties can be used to confirm the veracity of information and to identify inconsistencies between the patient's report of recent and past behavior and the reports of other firsthand observers. For example, a patient may deny prior suicide attempts, but a parent may be able to report that the patient attempted suicide twice during childhood. Even when permission to disclose has not been granted, certain emergency clinical situations allow for a good-faith breach of confidentiality and warrant obtaining collateral information. A risk-benefit assessment can help inform decisions about when breaching confidentiality is clinically appropriate (Petrik et al. 2015).

Suicide Risk Management for the Depressed Patient

Although depressive disorders are associated with increased risk of death from suicide, patients with various depressive disorders may experience any level of acute and chronic risk for suicide, depending on a myriad of factors. In addition, a patient's risk can also fluctuate over time, necessitating ongoing assessment of risk and potentially modifying the treatment plan accordingly. The tenet that risk assessment is a process, rather than an event, is broadly applicable, but especially so in the context of depressive disorders.

Depression and its treatment inherently involve circumstances that influence risk and that wax and wane. For example, even within the context of a single depressive episode, the avolition associated with a severe neurovegetative depressed state might be temporarily protective, with increased risk counterintuitively emerging in the setting of treatment and initial improvement. Similarly, some patients may experience paradoxical reactions to various treatment strategies, resulting in unanticipated spikes of acute risk. In short, the dynamic nature of depression and surrounding psychosocial circumstances make the level or acuity of suicide risk a moving target, such that risk assessment must be an ongoing process. Information about acute and chronic risk for suicide informs subsequent risk management (Table 7–1).

Providers should consider using several brief interventions to increase stability and maintain safety in the setting of heightened acute risk. High acute risk typically indicates a perceived inability to maintain safety absent external support, such that psychiatric hospitalization is usually warranted. Providers should collaboratively construct a safety plan with patients who are at elevated risk to assist them in identifying warning signs of increasing risk of death from suicide as well as appropriate coping strategies. In the setting of depression, the safety plan might incorporate symptoms and behaviors that the patient has historically experienced in the context of increasing depression (e.g., disrupted sleep, irritability, and isolative behavior).

Safety plans espouse a hierarchical approach to addressing suicide risk. These plans may further reinforce the patient's self-efficacy during acute distress by facilitating the patient's initial engagement of appropriate coping skills, followed by reaching out for social support and help (e.g., to a close family member or friend) and, as a last resort, accessing emergency resources (e.g., National Suicide Prevention Lifeline [800-273-8255 or https://suicidepreventionlifeline.org], 911, emergency department), should prior steps prove insufficient. If patients endorse preparatory behaviors or potential suicide plans (e.g., stockpiling excess medication or plans involving intentional overdose) or access to lethal means (e.g., firearm), providers should also consider lethal means restriction as an evidence-based strategy to reduce practical capacity for suicide.

TABLE 7–1. Stratification of suicide risk by temporality and severity

	Acute	Chronic
High	Suicidal ideation with intent to die and inability to maintain safety independent of external help or support. Likely presents with a suicide plan, access to lethal means, and potentially a history of ongoing preparatory behaviors or suicide attempt. May be exacerbated by psychiatric symptoms or an acute psychosocial stressor. Action: Psychiatric hospitalization (see Chapter 16)	Typically presents with prior suicide attempt(s), chronic health conditions, limited ability to cope, and few reasons for living. Typically is highly exacerbated by psychosocial stressors. Action: Routine mental health treatment that screens for suicide risk; suicide-specific intervention; coping skills–based intervention
Moderate	Suicidal ideation with potential intent. Able to maintain safety independent of external support or help. May present similar to high acute risk but endorses reasons for living; may have less history of preparatory behaviors or suicide attempt(s); and usually demonstrates an increased ability to abide by suicide-specific intervention(s) (e.g., safety plan, lethal means safety). Action: Consider psychiatric hospitalization or intensive outpatient management	Balance of protective factors, coping skills, and reasons for living with prior suicidal ideation or suicide attempt(s), chronic health conditions, and experience of psychosocial stressors. Action: Routing mental health treatment that screens for suicide risk; suicide-specific intervention
Low	No suicidal ideation or suicidal ideation with no intent, definite plan, or preparatory behavior. Capable of using resources, including coping strategies, suicide-specific interventions, and social support to maintain safety independently. Action: Management through current treatment regimen; referral to mental health treatment may be indicated if patient is not currently accessing mental health care	No history of suicidal ideation or history of suicidal ideation but demonstrated ability to manage stressors without resorting to self-directed violence. Coping skills, reasons for living, and protective factors appear to stably outweigh risk factors. Action: Management through current treatment regimen; referral to mental health treatment may be indicated if patient is not currently accessing mental health care

Interventional approaches to reduce chronic risk are available and important. For instance, should the patient endorse persistent difficulty navigating psychosocial stressors and distress, providers can consider structured interventions that facilitate problem solving, such as problem-solving therapy, as well as those that teach and reinforce use of coping skills and interpersonal effectiveness, such as dialectical behavior therapy (see Chapter 3, "Cognitive and Behavioral Therapy"). These interventional approaches may facilitate coping with distress related to suicide-related beliefs and hopelessness as well as potentially reduce difficulties with social interactions that may, in part, be driving TB.

Additionally, these interventions may help to prepare the patient for treatment specifically targeting underlying theory-driven factors associated with suicide risk. Several evidence-based psychotherapies for depression (e.g., cognitive-behavioral therapy, Acceptance and Commitment Therapy, interpersonal therapy) can assist the patient in identifying and attenuating suicide-related beliefs or unhealthy behaviors that perpetuate chronic suicide risk. For example, during cognitive-behavioral therapy, clinicians can work with patients to identify and reframe distorted beliefs pertaining to themselves (e.g., "I'm a failure") or others (e.g., "No one likes me") that may be maintaining depressive symptomatology as well as driving risk of death from suicide. During the course of these treatments, providers can also track and assess suicide risk, including monitoring patients' acute suicide risk, updating the patient's safety plan, and providing lethal means counseling. Similarly, endorsed protective factors during clinical assessment or over the course of treatment can be used to further reinforce reasons for living, especially during initial suicide-specific interventions (e.g., safety planning), when the patient is experiencing elevations in acute suicide risk, or to increase motivation and engagement throughout treatment.

Pharmacological Strategies for Depression and Suicide

Several effective pharmacological interventions for depression exist and are reviewed in more detail in Chapter 2 ("Psychopharmacology and Neuromodulation"). Relatively little evidence suggests that medication management in the setting of suicide risk should deviate substantially from practice guidelines applicable to depressive disorders more generally. For example, readers are directed to the American Psychiatric Association's *Practice Guideline for the Treatment of Patients With Major Depressive Disorder* (Gelenberg et al. 2010). Consistent with this guideline, factors that typically call for pharmacological interventions include a prior favorable response to antidepressant treatment, moderate to severe symptomatology, substantial disturbances in sleep or appetite, the presence of agitation, a need for ongoing maintenance therapy, and patient preference.

Given that clinical efficacy across classes of antidepressants is generally equivalent, selection is typically guided by various other considerations. This remains the case in the setting of suicide risk, although the safety of medications potentially becomes more important. Relative to other classes of antidepressants, selective serotonin reuptake inhibitors and serotonin norepinephrine reuptake inhibitors offer relatively favorable profiles in relation to safety, tolerability, side effects, and potential pharmacological interactions. This profile makes these agents typically good first-line choices for depressive disorders more generally as well as in the setting of increased suicide risk.

Risk-benefit analysis on a case-by-case basis may guide clinical decision making in the selection of appropriate medication. For example, a body of literature suggests that lithium offers some protection in relation to suicide risk, although the strength of that evidence is modest (Cipriani et al. 2013). At the same time, lithium is dangerous in overdose and potentially lethal. Hence, decision making around lithium use in the setting of suicide risk mandates attention to specifics relating to the individual patient. For example, in a patient with historically modest treatment adherence and a history of multiple impulsive suicide attempts involving overdose, the risks attendant to lithium would arguably outweigh the potential for modest protective effects. Alternatively, in a motivated patient with whom the clinician has a strong therapeutic relationship, and who has historically had excellent medication adherence and consistent willingness and ability to follow a safety plan, risk-benefit analysis arguably favors a trial of lithium. Providers should clearly document risk-benefit analysis and informed consent when collaboratively arriving at such clinical decisions with patients.

A growing body of literature also suggests a potential role for ketamine as a treatment for suicidal ideation in patients with depressive disorders (Wilkinson et al. 2018), although long-term data are generally lacking, as is information pertaining to various common comorbid conditions. Furthermore, the extent to which ketamine might favorably impact risk for suicide attempts or deaths from suicide remains unclear. Once again, providers considering this emerging intervention should carefully engage in and document a risk-benefit analysis specific to the individual as well as informed consent.

Conclusion

MDD and depressive disorders are some of the primary diagnoses associated with suicidal ideation, suicide attempts, and suicide deaths. Clinical assessment of depressive symptoms and suicidal thoughts and behaviors in these patients is important in order to reduce risk of suicide. A nuanced approach of balancing clinical interview with measures of depressive symptoms, suicidal ideation, and evidence-driven risk and protective factors can assist in developing a comprehensive understanding of the patient's acute and chronic suicide risk. By considering this information along with the patient's ability to maintain safety (e.g., coping skills, support system), providers can assess acute and chronic suicide risk and implement interventions to mitigate risk of death from suicide.

Key Points

- Major depressive disorder (MDD) and depressive disorders are some of the diagnoses associated most strongly with suicidal ideation, suicide attempts, and deaths from suicide.

- Assessment of suicide risk in patients with MDD and depressive disorders benefits from a therapeutic risk management approach that uses concurrent clinical interview, structured assessment, and collateral information to assess suicide risk.

- The will to live among depressed patients may be reduced in the presence of *thwarted belongingness*, which is an unmet psychological need to belong, and *perceived burdensomeness*, which is the perception that one's existence is burdensome to others.

- Suicide risk stratification capturing both temporality and severity allows for more effective assessment (and communication), which in turn better informs clinical decision making. This enables providers to balance suicide risk and protective factors with patients' ability to maintain safety outside of a therapeutic, inpatient setting.

- Several evidence-based psychotherapeutic and pharmacological treatments exist that can facilitate managing risk for suicide among patients with MDD and depressive disorders. Risk-benefit analysis on a case-by-case basis may help inform treatment selection.

References

American Psychiatric Association: Diagnostic and Statistical Manual of Mental Disorders, 5th Edition. Arlington, VA, American Psychiatric Association, 2013

Beck AT, Steer RA: Beck Scale for Suicide Ideation. San Antonio, TX, Psychological Corp, 1991

Beck AT, Steer RA, Brown GK: Beck Depression Inventory-II (BDI-II). San Antonio, TX, Psychological Corp, 1996

Cipriani A, Hawton K, Stockton S, et al: Lithium in the prevention of suicide in mood disorders: updated systematic review and meta-analysis. BMJ 346:f3646, 2013 23814104

Coyne JC, Burchill SAL, Stiles W: An interactional perspective on depression, in Handbook of Social and Clinical Psychology: The Health Perspective. Edited by Snyder CR, Forsyth SO. New York, Pergamon, 1990, pp 327–349

Gelenberg AJ, Freeman MP, Markowitz JC, et al: Practice Guideline for the Treatment of Patients With Major Depressive Disorder, 3rd Edition. Arlington, VA, American Psychiatric Association, 2010

Goldsmith SK, Pellmar TC, Kleinman AM, et al: Reducing Suicide: A National Imperative. Washington, DC, National Academies Press, 2002

Hawton K, Casañas I Comabella C, Haw C, et al: Risk factors for suicide in individuals with depression: a systematic review. J Affect Disord 147(1-3):17–28, 2013 23411024

Homaifar B, Matarazzo B, Wortzel HS: Therapeutic risk management of the suicidal patient: augmenting clinical suicide risk assessment with structured instruments. J Psychiatr Pract 19(5):406–409, 2013 24042246

Joiner TE: Why People Die by Suicide. Cambridge, MA, Harvard University Press, 2005

Kessler RC, Berglund P, Demler O, et al: Lifetime prevalence and age-of-onset distributions of DSM-IV disorders in the National Comorbidity Survey Replication. Arch Gen Psychiatry 62(6):593–602, 2005a 15939837

Kessler RC, Chiu WT, Demler O, et al: Prevalence, severity, and comorbidity of 12-month DSM-IV disorders in the National Comorbidity Survey Replication. Arch Gen Psychiatry 62(6):617–627, 2005b 15939839

Kleiman EM, Law KC, Anestis MD: Do theories of suicide play well together? Integrating components of the hopelessness and interpersonal psychological theories of suicide. Compr Psychiatry 55(3):431–438, 2014 24332385

Klonsky ED, May AM: Differentiating suicide attempters from suicide ideators: a critical frontier for suicidology research. Suicide Life Threat Behav 44(1):1–5, 2014 24313594

Klonsky ED, May AM: The Three-Step Theory (3ST): a new theory of suicide rooted in the "ideation-to-action" framework. Int J Cogn Ther 8(2):114–129, 2015

Kroenke K, Spitzer RL, Williams JBW: The PHQ-9: validity of a brief depression severity measure. J Gen Intern Med 16(9):606–613, 2001 11556941

Linehan MM, Comtois K: Lifetime Parasuicide History (unpublished). Seattle, WA, University of Washington, 1996

Linehan MM, Goodstein JL, Nielsen SL, et al: Reasons for staying alive when you are thinking of killing yourself: the reasons for living inventory. J Consult Clin Psychol 51(2):276–286, 1983 6841772

Nock MK, Holmberg EB, Photos VI, et al: Self-Injurious Thoughts and Behaviors Interview: development, reliability, and validity in an adolescent sample. Psychol Assess 19(3):309–317, 2007 17845122

Paris J: Is hospitalization useful for suicidal patients with borderline personality disorder? J Pers Disord 18(3):240–247, 2004 15237044

Petrik ML, Billera M, Kaplan Y, et al: Balancing patient care and confidentiality: considerations in obtaining collateral information. J Psychiatr Pract 21(3):220–224, 2015 25955265

Poster K, Brent D, Lucas C, et al: Columbia-Suicide Severity Rating Scale (C-SSRS). New York, Columbia University Medical Center, 2008

Rudd MD: Fluid vulnerability theory: a cognitive approach to understanding the process of acute and chronic suicide risk, in Cognition and Suicide: Theory, Research, and Therapy. Edited by Ellis TE. Washington, DC, American Psychological Association, 2006, pp 355–368

Van Orden KA, Witte TK, Cukrowicz KC, et al: The interpersonal theory of suicide. Psychol Rev 117(2):575–600, 2010 20438238

Wilkinson ST, Ballard ED, Bloch MH, et al: The effect of a single dose of intravenous ketamine on suicidal ideation: a systematic review and individual participant data meta-analysis. Am J Psychiatry 175(2):150–158, 2018 28969441

Wortzel HS, Matarazzo B, Homaifar B: A model for therapeutic risk management of the suicidal patient. J Psychiatr Pract 19(4):323–326, 2013 23852108

Wortzel HS, Homaifar B, Matarazzo B, et al: Therapeutic risk management of the suicidal patient: stratifying risk in terms of severity and temporality. J Psychiatr Pract 20(1):63–67, 2014 24419312

CHAPTER 8

Anxiety Disorders, Obsessive-Compulsive Disorder, and Posttraumatic Stress Disorder

Britta Klara Ostermeyer, M.D., M.B.A., FAPA

Rachel Funk-Lawler, Ph.D.

Jedidiah Perdue, M.D., M.P.H.

Suicide is an enormous public health problem (Sareen 2011). Suicidal behaviors, defined in this chapter as *suicidal ideation* (SI) and *suicide attempt* (SA), are highly prevalent in communities, with incidences of 11%–14% for the former and 2.8%–4.6% for the latter (Sareen et al. 2005).

Psychopathology is one of the most well-recognized suicide risk factors. Anxiety disorders are the most common class of psychiatric disorders, with a lifetime prevalence of 28.8% (Kessler et al. 2005). Converging empirical evidence supports that anxiety disorders are statistically significant risk factors for suicidal behaviors (Sareen 2011). Among inpatients who died from suicide, 79% were found to have experienced anxiety/agitation, and 92% of patients admitted from emergency departments after serious SAs had severe anxiety (Busch et al. 2003). Severe anxiety and agitation are often acute, immediate suicide risk factors, and higher anxiety and distress levels are associated with more intrusive SI (Schmidt et al. 2001).

The National Epidemiologic Survey on Alcohol and Related Conditions (NESARC) data showed that more than 70% of individuals with a lifetime history of SAs had an anxiety disorder and that anxiety disorders are independently associated with SAs

(Nepon et al. 2010). According to information from the U.S. Food and Drug Administration (FDA) patient databank, patients with minimal- to moderate-severity anxiety disorders and baseline minimal suicide risk were found to have a 10-fold increased suicide and SA risk compared to the general population (Khan et al. 2002). In comparison, patients with depressive and psychotic disorders have a suicide risk 60–70 times higher than the general population (Khan et al. 2002). Therefore, national organizations for the study and prevention of suicide, such as the American Association of Suicidality, the American Foundation for Suicide Prevention, and the National Prevention Lifeline, list anxiety as an important suicide risk factor (Bentley et al. 2016).

Notably, controversy exists regarding whether anxiety disorders independently increase suicide risk (Sareen 2011). Moreover, to date, information as to whether anxiety disorders increase suicidal behavior in older patients and whether treatment of such disorders reduces future suicidal behavior remains unclear (Sareen 2011).

In this chapter, we discuss the risk for suicidal behavior and suicide in patients with anxiety disorders, specifically with social anxiety disorder (SAD), panic disorder, and generalized anxiety disorder (GAD). We also include obsessive-compulsive disorder (OCD) and posttraumatic stress disorder (PTSD), which are no longer classified as anxiety disorders in DSM-5 (American Psychiatric Association 2013); research on anxiety disorders prior to DSM-5 included OCD and PTSD.

Anxiety Disorders and Suicidal Behavior

Strong and consistent evidence indicates that anxiety disorders, in particular panic disorder and PTSD, are independently associated with an increased risk of suicidal behaviors and death from suicide (Norton et al. 2008; Sareen 2011). In a prospective, population-based longitudinal study, baseline anxiety disorders were significantly associated with SI and SA even after adjusting for sociodemographic factors and all other psychiatric disorders. This suggests that untreated anxiety disorders might be missed opportunities for preventing suicidal behavior (Sareen et al. 2005).

In a large national study, disorders characterized by anxiety/agitation and poor impulse control emerged as the strongest risk factors among those with SI who moved on to develop suicide plans and make SAs (Nock et al. 2010). Nepon et al. (2010) published the first study with adequate adjustment for sociodemographic factors, mood and substance use disorders, schizophrenia spectrum disorders, and personality disorders, which showed that anxiety disorders, in particular panic disorder and PTSD (formerly classified as an anxiety disorder), are independently associated with SAs. No sex differences between each anxiety disorder and lifetime SAs were found. A recent meta-analysis of 42 studies further supports the finding that any anxiety disorder increased the incidence of suicide behaviors, SI, SA, and deaths from suicide (Kanwar et al. 2013). Raposo et al. (2014) published the first study to show strong and significant associations between individual past-year anxiety disorders and past-year SI, controlling for sociodemographic factors, depression, and substance use disorders in younger and older adults.

These findings are contrary to patients' fears of dying during panic attacks (Sareen 2011). Why would patients who are afraid of dying want to kill themselves? Although the exact mechanisms by which anxiety, suicidal behaviors, and death from suicide are associated is unclear, possible explanations for this paradoxical relationship are: 1) the "intolerable experience hypothesis," in which the person wants to escape from distress/suffering from anxiety and distress related to functional, social, and occupational losses or hopelessness about recovery (Schmidt et al. 2001); 2) the indirect impact from other comorbid psychiatric disorders, such as mood and substance use disorders, that may potentiate the relationship between anxiety disorders and suicidal behaviors (Norton et al. 2008; Sareen et al. 2005); or 3) the "depression-mediated hypothesis," which suggests that patients with anxiety disorders tend to also develop depression, which increases suicidal behavior risk (Schmidt et al. 2001). In addition, feelings of distrust in SAD and PTSD may lead to a lower sense of belonging, an important vulnerability factor in interpersonal models of suicide (Cougle et al. 2009).

Anxiety Disorders and Comorbid Nonanxiety Psychiatric Disorders

Comorbid psychiatric disorders are highly associated with anxiety disorders. One point of contention is whether this comorbidity of mood and substance use disorders, and not the anxiety disorder itself, increases suicidal behaviors (Nepon et al. 2010; Schmidt et al. 2001). Accordingly, after controlling for depression, the association between anxiety disorders and death from suicide was substantially reduced (Schmidt et al. 2001).

The presence of comorbid anxiety disorder in patients with other psychiatric disorders clearly amplifies suicidal behavior risk (Sareen 2011). Depressed patients with comorbid GAD had higher levels of SI when compared to patients with only depression (Zimmerman and Chelminski 2003). Persons with mood disorders in combination with anxiety disorders had the highest likelihood of SI and SAs compared with those with neither anxiety nor mood disorders in both cross-sectional and longitudinal evaluations (Sareen et al. 2005). Also, the presence of a combination of mood and anxiety disorder yielded a higher risk for SAs compared with mood disorder alone (Sareen et al. 2005).

Anxiety disorder and depression together conveyed an additive and interactive SI risk. Therefore, actual levels of depressiveness and anxiousness should be considered when assessing suicide risk, rather than simply making a distinction between having or not having an anxiety disorder or depressive disorder diagnosis (Norton et al. 2008). In addition, individuals with comorbid personality disorder with panic disorder and with PTSD demonstrated much stronger associations with SAs over either disorder alone (Nepon et al. 2010).

In outpatients with bipolar disorder, lifetime anxiety disorders were associated with a more than doubling of the odds of past SAs, while current anxiety comorbidity was associated with a more than doubling of the odds of current SI (Simon et al. 2007). The study concluded that comorbid anxiety disorders, specifically SAD, in outpatients with bipolar disorder are associated with current and lifetime suicidal behavior. Anxiety disorders may result in stress, affective instability, and impairment of social and role functioning that unleash an early onset of initial mood episodes, thereby increasing the likelihood of lifetime SAs (Simon et al. 2007).

These findings are consistent with previous research showing that the majority of people who die from suicide have had multiple comorbid psychiatric disorders (Sareen 2011) and that all patients need to be evaluated for comorbid anxiety as part of their suicide risk assessment and prevention (Simon et al. 2007).

Social Anxiety Disorder

SAD has a lifetime prevalence of 12.1% (Kessler et al. 2005). This disorder is relatively common, usually with an early onset, chronic course, and limited recovery (Keller 2006). Studies show significant association between SAD and SI through both cross-section surveys and lifetime accounts (Cougle et al. 2009; Norton et al. 2008; Raposo et al. 2014). Several studies suggest that the association between SAD and SI persisted even when accounting for comorbid conditions and demographic factors (Cougle et al. 2009; Sareen et al. 2005). Additionally, SAD has been shown to clearly predict subsequent SAs (Bentley et al. 2016; Cougle et al. 2009). Yet the risk of SAs appears to be less than that associated with SI, and the relationship between SAD and SAs became nonsignificant after accounting for comorbidities and covariates (Sareen et al. 2005).

Studies suggest that additional variables may explain the link between SAD and suicidal thoughts and behaviors (Nepon et al. 2010). Indeed, SAD generally has a high rate of comorbid conditions, chiefly depressive disorders, other anxiety disorders, and personality disorders (Keller 2006). The NESARC data demonstrated that comorbidity enhances the relationship between SAD and suicide (Nepon et al. 2010). Similarly, well-controlled studies of depressive disorders, PTSD, and bipolar disorder have each shown that persons with these disorders have an increase in suicidal behaviors with co-occurring SAD (McMillan et al. 2017; Norton et al. 2008; Simon et al. 2007). Moreover, comorbid SAD and alcohol use disorders have been associated with more frequent prior SI, suicide plans, and SAs (Oliveira et al. 2018).

Case Example 1

Jim was a 26-year-old computer technician who struggled at his job. He described himself as "forever shy." At work, he felt anxious, fearing his colleagues found him unlikeable. He spent most of his time at home alone. When socializing, Jim relied on drinking alcohol heavily and remained aloof toward others. He felt like "a burden" to his family and thought his brothers judged him for being less successful. He has recently begun to drink a six-pack every night to calm thoughts of inadequacy. Also, he felt as though his life "isn't worth much" and reported recurrent SI.

As suggested in Jim's case, SAD is a chronic, early onset condition that often exists comorbid with other conditions, such as alcohol use disorder. He acutely feared criticism across various social settings and relied on alcohol and avoidance to lessen his distress. His case demonstrates the negative impact of SAD on multiple areas of functioning leading to isolation, embarrassment, problematic behaviors, and, in many cases, ultimately SI. Social avoidance such as that demonstrated by Jim has been proposed as a contributor to the development of SI (Cougle et al. 2009). Behavioral inhibition, impaired social functioning, and negative self-appraisal typical of SAD reduce quality of life and limit social connections, leading to increased risk of suicide (Bentley et al. 2016; McMillan et al. 2017).

Panic Disorder

The lifetime prevalence of panic disorder is 4.7% (Kessler et al. 2005), and its association with suicidal behavior has received the greatest attention (Cougle et al. 2009). In the past, study results were not entirely consistent, likely due to methodological differences in adjusting for comorbid nonanxiety mental disorders (Sareen 2011). More recent studies support an independent association of panic disorder and suicidal behavior even when controlled for comorbid psychiatric disorders (Nepon et al. 2010; Norton et al. 2008; Schmidt et al. 2001).

Catastrophic cognitions and fear of dying during panic attacks were associated with a sevenfold increase in subsequent SAs in a large-scale prospective study, even after controlling for comorbid disorders and demographic factors (Yaseen et al. 2013). Fear of dying may be a unique marker of more severe panic attacks, with greater association to SAs. The fact that the average interval between SI and SA is merely 10 minutes in persons with panic disorder is consistent with panic state acuity and symptom acceleration (Yaseen et al. 2013).

A landmark study in the *New England Journal of Medicine* using data from the large-scale Epidemiologic Catchment Area study found that patients with a lifetime panic disorder diagnosis had a 47% rate of SI and a 20% rate of SAs (Weissman et al. 1989). This study also demonstrated that panic disorder is associated with an increased risk of suicidal behaviors even when controlling for comorbid psychiatric conditions. The prevalence of current SI in panic disorder patients without comorbid depression was 11.4%, which was three times higher than in those without panic disorder or depression, after controlling for demographic factors and substance use (Goodwin et al. 2001). An expansion of this primary-care study (Pilowsky et al. 2006) found that

1. 6.1% of primary care patients had SI.
2. Approximately one-fifth of patients with current panic disorder reported SI.
3. Panic disorder patients were about twice as likely to experience current SI as those without panic disorder, even after controlling for common co-occurring psychiatric disorders.
4. Panic disorder patients with comorbid depression were three times more likely to report SI than patients with panic disorder and no depression.
5. SI did not increase significantly in patients with both panic disorder and depression when compared to patients with depression only.

When panic disorder patients become depressed, their risk of SI may increase, and therefore, such patients warrant additional or repeated suicide risk reassessment (Pilowsky et al. 2006). Although this study evaluated current panic symptoms and current SI, which strengthened its association with panic disorder, the study did not evaluate for personality disorder. The authors opined that if they had assessed and controlled for personality disorder diagnoses, the panic disorder and SI association might have been attenuated.

Other studies also found a significant, independent association of panic disorder and SI (Cougle et al. 2009; Norton et al. 2008; Sareen et al. 2005) as well as a strong association of panic disorder with SAs (Sareen et al. 2005). Although Cougle et al. (2009)

TABLE 8–1. Additional suicidal ideation risk factors associated with panic disorder

Younger age

Early onset of illness (in one study)

Low socioeconomic status

Current alcohol use

More severe panic symptoms but not agoraphobic symptoms

Less social support

Source. Data from Huang et al. 2010. Adapted from Antar and Hollander 2012.

did not find an association of panic disorder with SAs, Nepon et al. (2010) did find a significant association of panic disorder with lifetime SAs in a study that controlled for comorbid psychiatric disorders, including all 10 personality disorders. In a small sample of 60 outpatients with panic disorder, 31.7% were found to have had SI in the preceding 2 weeks (Huang et al. 2010). Panic symptoms positively correlated to SI, but symptoms of agoraphobia did not. In addition, panic disorder patients had increased SI associated with other concurrent risk factors (Huang et al. 2010; Table 8–1).

Schmidt et al. (2001) studied whether anxiety or panic-specific factors may contribute to SI in patients with panic disorder and found several anxiety-related variables (Table 8–2).

Although the relationship between these variables and SI is unclear, suicide may represent an escape from these intolerable subjective experiences that amplify general patient distress. Higher anxiety levels are indeed associated with more intrusive SI (Schmidt et al. 2001). In addition, current comorbid mood symptoms were significantly related to current SI in 43% of panic patients with depression compared to only 10% of panic patients without depression (Schmidt et al. 2001).

Like other anxiety disorders, panic disorder is often accompanied by other psychiatric disorders that exacerbate suffering and significantly increase suicidal behavior risk (Antar and Hollander 2012). Comorbid disorders, such as mood and substance use disorders, carry their own suicidal behavior risk, and together with panic disorder they synergistically increase this risk (Antar and Hollander 2012). Comorbid panic disorder in bipolar patients also may confer an increased suicide risk (Kilbane et al. 2009), which indicates that all patients with panic disorder require screening and treatment for comorbid psychiatric disorders.

Case Example 2

Marie was a 21-year-old college student with progressively severe panic disorder symptoms since age 19. She came into the emergency center with her mother via ambulance after attempting suicide at home by taking "a couple of my mother's pills." She was distressed and crying and reported "about 10 severe" panic attacks weekly as well as significant behavior changes to the point that she could no longer leave her home without severe distress or without her mother. She feared "more panic attacks outside my home." During panic attacks, she experienced "going crazy, horrible fears of dying!"

After medical stabilization, Marie agreed to voluntary psychiatric hospital admission. Given her SA, significant distress, severe panic attacks, and panic-specific variable of fear of going crazy, she was transferred to a locked psychiatric inpatient unit. She was placed on 15-minute nursing safety checks, started on sertraline, and seen by mental health professionals for safety planning and progressive relaxation as well as support-

TABLE 8–2. **Anxiety-related variables associated with suicidal ideation in panic disorder**

Overall anxiety severity

Level of anticipatory anxiety

Avoidance of bodily sensations

Attentional vigilance toward bodily perturbations

Phrenophobia (fear of cognitive incapacitation)

Source. Data from Schmidt et al. 2001. Adapted from Antar and Hollander 2012.

ive and cognitive-behavioral therapy (CBT). She responded well to inpatient psychiatric treatment and was discharged home with outpatient mental health treatment follow-up with a psychiatrist to continue psychopharmacological management and a psychologist to continue CBT.

Generalized Anxiety Disorder

GAD has a lifetime prevalence of 5.7% (Kessler et al. 2005) and is frequently seen in primary care settings (Antar and Hollander 2012). It is associated with suicidal behavior and death from suicide (Cougle et al. 2009; Sareen et al. 2005), even when studies control for comorbid diseases (Sareen et al. 2005), and is also prominently associated with subsequent SI and SAs. Compared with depressed patients with no GAD, depressed patients with GAD had

1. Higher SI levels
2. Poorer social functioning
3. Greater frequency of other anxiety, eating, and somatoform disorders
4. Higher subscale scores on most self-report DSM-IV (American Psychiatric Association 1994) Axis I disorder measures
5. Greater pathological worry level
6. Higher risk of GAD in first-degree family members (Zimmerman and Chelminski 2003)

Case Example 3

Karen was a 25-year-old dental assistant who described herself as "anxious lifelong." She worried excessively on a daily basis and was unable to stop the worries. She was nervous "about everything in my life, all the time!" In addition, she was restless, easily fatigued, complained of muscle tension, and usually could not fall asleep without medication. As time went by, she became tormented by fear that "my anxiety will never improve," started to feel hopeless and depressed, and eventually developed SI.

GAD is well known to be associated with comorbid psychiatric disorders. This case illustrates the classic example of a patient who has struggled with GAD over years and then secondarily became depressed as well. She required treatment for anxiety, depression, and insomnia to alleviate her suffering and suicidal behavior risk. She started taking fluoxetine and received CBT. Additionally, she was educated on sleep hygiene and instructed to use pharmacy-grade melatonin as needed for insomnia.

TABLE 8–3.   **Suicide risk factors that increase risk in patients with obsessive-compulsive disorder**

High severity of depressive symptoms	Comorbidity: depression and schizophrenia
High severity of anxiety symptoms	Male sex
Aggressive obsessions	History of suicide attempt
Sexual obsessions	Adverse family relationships
Ordering compulsions	Single/Unpartnered marital status
Hoarding compulsions	Unemployment
Alexithymia	

Source.   Adapted from Angelakis et al. 2015; Antar and Hollander 2012; De La Vega et al. 2018.

Over several weeks, she gradually improved with less anxiety, less depression, and greater sleep quality.

Obsessive-Compulsive Disorder

OCD has a lifetime prevalence of 1.6% (Kessler et al. 2005). Early, cross-sectional OCD research suggested that the disease poses a low risk of death from suicide (Norton et al. 2008; Simon et al. 2007), which was confirmed by a large meta-analysis revealing that suicide risk was elevated for all anxiety disorders except OCD (Kanwar et al. 2013). Similarly, in a later review, Bentley et al. (2016) reported that a diagnosis of OCD was not associated with subsequent SAs and suicide deaths. Any initial associations between OCD and lifetime SI or SAs disappeared when accounting for relevant covariates and comorbidities (Sareen et al. 2005).

However, not all studies have found OCD to be a low suicide risk factor. Another systematic review reported that suicidal thoughts and behaviors in OCD were highly underestimated (Angelakis et al. 2015). Pooled effect sizes from this study revealed that OCD was significantly associated with SI and SA but not deaths from suicide. Furthermore, mental health comorbidity increased severity of suicide behaviors above that associated with OCD alone. High variance in outcomes of the individual studies may explain the significant discrepancy between findings across research review publications.

Additionally, this inconsistency in research findings could be attributed to advances in disease classification, because OCD is no longer included as an anxiety disorder in DSM-5. Some traits may be specific to impulse-control issues such as OCD; in fact, evidence for unique factors associated with suicide and OCD is available (Table 8–3). In particular, alexithymia has been associated with OCD severity, higher attitude of responsibility (perfectionism), and lower insight, which have all been associated with SI (Angelakis et al. 2015; De La Vega et al. 2018).

Case Example 4

Daron was a 41-year-old divorcé with two teenage daughters. He described himself as "perfectionistic with high standards" and struggled with sadness and unemployment after military retirement. He experienced daily intrusive thoughts about harm, such as sexual assault befalling himself or his family. He distracted himself by excessively cleaning his house. He insisted that his daughters follow the same daily routine "to prevent something bad from happening." Daron felt humiliated by his thoughts and behaviors and became increasingly depressed. He went to see his primary care physician because he began to think about taking his own life. He was started on a selective serotonin reuptake inhibitor and referred to a psychologist for psychotherapy.

Daron's experience demonstrates the intensity and destructiveness of OCD, including the impact on family. He has numerous risk factors for death from suicide, including comorbid depression, sexual obsessions, and ordering compulsions. Appropriate treatment for OCD, as in Daron's case, may include antidepressant use and exposure and relapse prevention, a subtype of CBT.

Posttraumatic Stress Disorder

PTSD has a lifetime prevalence of 6.8% (Kessler et al. 2005) and increases the risk of suicidal behavior and death from suicide. The National Comorbidity Survey–Replication (NCS-R), a cross-sectional study of 4,131 individuals assessed by structured diagnostic interview, demonstrated that 40.3% of persons with a lifetime PTSD history had experienced SI and that 18.8% had a prior SA, compared to rates of 14% and 4.5% in the general population, respectively (Cougle et al. 2009). Increased odds of SI (1.80) and SA (1.96) remained significant after adjustment for demographic variables and psychiatric comorbidity, supporting an independent association between PTSD and suicidal behavior (Cougle et al. 2009). This finding has been replicated in other epidemiological studies (Nepon et al. 2010; Raposo et al. 2014; Rojas et al. 2014; Sareen et al. 2005).

In addition, evidence for an independent association between PTSD and SI and SA extends beyond cross-sectional studies. In a meta-analysis of longitudinal studies that used an anxiety-specific variable to predict a suicide-related outcome, PTSD was associated with a 2.25-fold greater incidence of SI and 2.07-fold greater incidence of SA (Bentley et al. 2016).

Suicide deaths occur with greater frequency in patients with PTSD than the general population. Gradus et al. (2015) described a large Danish cohort involving 101,633 individuals with a stress or adjustment-related disorder and found a suicide rate of 0.61% among PTSD patients compared to 0.04% in the comparison cohort. After controlling for baseline psychiatric disorders and cumulative comorbidity, the association remained strongly significant (adjusted rate ratio 13). A recent study of veterans enrolled in the Agent Orange Registry demonstrated an increased risk of death from suicide among those with PTSD, with a hazard ratio (HR) of 7.1 after adjusting for covariates (Bullman et al. 2018). The highest suicide risk was observed among veterans with both depression and PTSD (HR 15.22).

Comorbid depression, personality disorder, and substance abuse diagnoses are associated with increased suicidal behavior risk in PTSD (Gradus et al. 2015; Nepon et al. 2010; Rojas et al. 2014). In the Danish cohort described earlier, those with depression and PTSD were 29 times more likely to die from suicide than those without either diagnosis (Gradus et al. 2015). Patients with PTSD and personality disorders demonstrated greater than three times the incidence of SA than those with PTSD alone in the NESARC trial (*n*=34,653; Nepon et al. 2010). In the NCS-R, lifetime alcohol dependence doubled the likelihood of endorsing past SI among individuals with a PTSD history and increased the likelihood of a prior SA sixfold (Rojas et al. 2014).

TABLE 8–4.	Suicide risk factors that increase risk in patients with posttraumatic stress disorder (PTSD)

Comorbidities
  Depression
  Personality disorders
  Substance abuse (especially alcohol)
PTSD symptom severity (especially negative alterations in cognition and mood)
Self-recrimination
  Guilt
  Remorse
  Self-blame
  Self-criticism
Childhood trauma
Benzodiazepine prescription

Source.   Bryan 2016; Gradus et al. 2015; Guina et al. 2017; Nepon et al. 2010; Rojas et al. 2014.

Recent studies have examined the impact of PTSD-related factors on the risk of suicidal behavior. In a study of 480 outpatients, SAs were significantly associated with increased overall PTSD symptom severity and each individual symptom cluster, with the strongest association to negative alterations in cognition and mood (Guina et al. 2017). Childhood trauma, especially childhood physical abuse, had the strongest association with SAs and was most strongly correlated with SAs (Guina et al. 2017). A correlation between benzodiazepine prescription and SAs was also demonstrated (Guina et al. 2017). Other factors potentially mediating the association between PTSD and suicidal behavior include guilt, remorse, self-blame, and self-criticism (Bryan 2016). Table 8–4 summarizes risk factors for suicidal behavior in PTSD.

Individuals with PTSD should be systematically assessed for suicide risk, with consideration of psychiatric hospitalization and initiation of evidence-based medication for those at high risk. Suicide-focused interventions, such as dialectical behavioral therapy or CBT for suicide prevention, should be the initial focus of psychotherapy, followed by trauma-specific treatment once risk is attenuated (Bryan 2016). Additionally, psychiatric and substance-related comorbidities should be addressed and risk-reduction strategies employed.

Case Example 5

Mark was a 62-year-old veteran who served two tours of duty as an infantryman. He witnessed the death of a friend and was himself wounded shortly thereafter. After an honorable discharge, he worked various jobs until opening up his own car repair shop. His wife noticed that he often seemed withdrawn, avoided violent television content, and often sat in the back of a room, scanning the environment. For several years, his doctor prescribed temazepam at bedtime for sleep.

After his children left home, Mark decided to retire and spend time engaged in hobbies. However, he found it even more difficult to distract himself from the intrusive thoughts and flashbacks associated with his trauma. He felt guilty to have survived while his friend died. He began to drink heavily and became increasingly depressed, feeling hopeless and tormented by the past. Weeks later, he decided to end his life, taking his boat to the middle of a lake with a pistol in hand. His plan was interrupted by an unexpected phone call from a friend. He voiced his despair, and his friend encouraged him to seek help. Mark went to the U.S. Department of Veterans Affairs' psychiatric emergency clinic and was diagnosed with PTSD, depression, and alcohol use disorder. Inpatient treatment was recommended initially, with subsequent outpatient follow-up.

By the time of discharge, Mark no longer expressed intent to harm himself and completed a safety plan collaboratively with his psychiatrist. It was agreed that his adult son would keep his firearms until he improved. After a course of CBT, 4 months of treatment with sertraline, and abstinence from alcohol, Mark demonstrated significant improvement in mood. His PTSD symptoms responded robustly to a subsequent course of cognitive processing therapy.

As this case exemplifies, untreated PTSD presents an independent risk factor for death from suicide. Mark's risk was amplified by comorbid alcohol abuse and depression as well as feelings of guilt, self-blame, and a high burden of PTSD symptoms. Upon entry into care, a crisis-response (safety) plan, an important element of CBT for suicide prevention, was developed, and the comorbidities of depression and alcohol were simultaneously addressed. In addition to the aim of successful suicide prevention, this therapy prepared him for the trauma-specific intervention of cognitive processing therapy, which successfully ameliorated his PTSD symptoms.

Conclusion

Strong research evidence indicates that anxiety disorders (especially panic disorder) and PTSD are independently associated with an increased risk of suicidal behaviors and death from suicide. Additionally, anxiety disorders significantly potentiate suicidal behavior risk when comorbid with other psychiatric disorders. All anxiety disorders, OCD, and PTSD require suicide risk assessments as well as screening and treatment for comorbid psychiatric disorders. Inpatient treatment may be required initially or intermittently to provide safety for patients while they start appropriate treatment with medications and psychotherapy. However, all patients with these disorders, especially those with comorbid disorders or symptoms that increase risk of death from suicide, should develop safety plans with their mental health professionals.

Key Points

- Anxiety disorders and posttraumatic stress disorder (PTSD) are independently associated with suicidal behaviors and death from suicide.

- Anxiety disorders and PTSD additively and interactively increase suicidal behavior risk when comorbid with other psychiatric disorders. All patients with anxiety disorders, obsessive-compulsive disorder (OCD), and PTSD require suicide risk assessments and screening for comorbid psychiatric disorders. All patients with nonanxiety psychiatric disorders require screening for comorbid anxiety disorders, PTSD, and OCD as well.

- Social anxiety disorder is associated with risk of suicide ideation (SI) and, to a lesser extent, suicide attempts (SAs). This risk is increased by comorbid psychiatric disorders and social isolation.

- Panic disorder is associated with increased suicidal behavior and risk of death from suicide. Patients with panic disorder must be evaluated for panic symptom severity and for comorbid psychiatric disorders because more severe panic symptoms and comorbid disorders increase the risk for suicidal behaviors.

- Generalized anxiety disorder (GAD) is associated with suicidal behavior. This disorder is often comorbid with depression or other psychiatric disorders, which significantly increases the risk of suicidal behavior. Patients must be treated for both GAD and comorbid disorders.

- It remains unclear whether OCD is associated with increased suicidal behavior and risk of death from suicide. However, specific risk factors, such as sexual obsessions, aggressive behavior, hoarding compulsions, and ordering compulsions, may increase suicide risk in these patients.

- PTSD increases the risk of SI, SAs, and suicide deaths. Psychiatric comorbidity, especially depression, personality disorders, and alcohol use disorder, greatly increases this risk. Inpatient hospitalization may be necessary for those at high risk, and suicide-specific psychotherapy should precede exposure-based interventions among these patients.

References

American Psychiatric Association: Diagnostic and Statistical Manual of Mental Disorders, 4th Edition. Washington, DC, American Psychiatric Association, 1994

American Psychiatric Association: Diagnostic and Statistical Manual of Mental Disorders, 5th Edition. Arlington, VA, American Psychiatric Association, 2013

Angelakis I, Gooding P, Tarrier N, et al: Suicidality in obsessive compulsive disorder (OCD): a systematic review and meta-analysis. Clin Psychol Rev 39:1–15, 2015 25875222

Antar LN, Hollander E: Anxiety disorders, in Textbook of Suicide Assessment and Management, 2nd Edition. Edited by Simon RI, Hales RE. Washington, DC, American Psychiatric Publishing, 2012, pp 539–552

Bentley KH, Franklin JC, Ribeiro JD, et al: Anxiety and its disorders as risk factors for suicidal thoughts and behaviors: a meta-analytic review. Clin Psychol Rev 43:30–46, 2016 26688478

Bryan CJ: Treating PTSD within the context of heightened suicide risk. Curr Psychiatry Rep 18(8):73, 2016 27314245

Bullman T, Schneiderman A, Gradus JL: Relative importance of posttraumatic stress disorder and depression in predicting risk of suicide among a cohort of Vietnam veterans. Suicide Life Threat Behav 2018 29926933 Epub ahead of print

Busch KA, Fawcett J, Jacobs DG: Clinical correlates of inpatient suicide. J Clin Psychiatry 64(1):14–19, 2003 12590618

Cougle JR, Keough ME, Riccardi CJ, et al: Anxiety disorders and suicidality in the National Comorbidity Survey Replication. J Psychiatr Res 43(9):825–829, 2009 19147159

De La Vega D, Giner L, Courtet P: Suicidality in subjects with anxiety or obsessive-compulsive and related disorders: recent advances. Curr Psychiatry Rep 20(4):26, 2018 29594718

Goodwin R, Olfson M, Feder A, et al: Panic and suicidal ideation in primary care. Depress Anxiety 14(4):244–246, 2001 11754133

Gradus JL, Antonsen S, Svensson E, et al: Trauma, comorbidity, and mortality following diagnoses of severe stress and adjustment disorders: a nationwide cohort study. Am J Epidemiol 182(5):451–458, 2015 26243737

Guina J, Nahhas RW, Mata N, et al: Which posttraumatic stress disorder symptoms, trauma types, and substances correlate with suicide attempts in trauma survivors? Prim Care Companion CNS Disord 19(5):17m02177, 2017

Huang MF, Yen CF, Lung FW: Moderators and mediators among panic, agoraphobia symptoms, and suicidal ideation in patients with panic disorder. Compr Psychiatry 51(3):243–249, 2010 20399333

Kanwar A, Malik S, Prokop LJ, et al: The association between anxiety disorders and suicidal behaviors: a systematic review and meta-analysis. Depress Anxiety 30(10):917–929, 2013 23408488

Keller MB: Social anxiety disorder clinical course and outcome: review of Harvard/Brown Anxiety Research Project (HARP) findings. J Clin Psychiatry 67(suppl 12):14–19, 2006 17092191

Kessler RC, Berglund P, Demler O, et al: Lifetime prevalence and age-of-onset distributions of DSM-IV disorders in the National Comorbidity Survey Replication. Arch Gen Psychiatry 62(6):593–602, 2005 15939837

Khan A, Leventhal RM, Khan S, et al: Suicide risk in patients with anxiety disorders: a meta-analysis of the FDA database. J Affect Disord 68(2–3):183–190, 2002 12063146

Kilbane EJ, Gokbayrak NS, Galynker I, et al: A review of panic and suicide in bipolar disorder: does comorbidity increase risk? J Affect Disord 115(1–2):1–10, 2009 19000640

McMillan KA, Asmundson GJG, Sareen J: Comorbid PTSD and social anxiety disorder: associations with quality of life and suicide attempts. J Nerv Ment Dis 205(9):732–737, 2017 28609312

Nepon J, Belik SL, Bolton J, et al: The relationship between anxiety disorders and suicide attempts: findings from the National Epidemiologic Survey on Alcohol and Related Conditions. Depress Anxiety 27(9):791–798, 2010 20217852

Nock MK, Hwang I, Sampson NA, et al: Mental disorders, comorbidity and suicidal behavior: results from the National Comorbidity Survey Replication. Mol Psychiatry 15(8):868–876, 2010 19337207

Norton PJ, Temple SR, Pettit JW: Suicidal ideation and anxiety disorders: elevated risk or artifact of comorbid depression? J Behav Ther Exp Psychiatry 39(4):515–525, 2008 18294614

Oliveira LM, Bermudez MB, Macedo MJA, et al: Comorbid social anxiety disorder in patients with alcohol use disorder: a systematic review. J Psychiatr Res 106:8–14, 2018 30236640

Pilowsky DJ, Olfson M, Gameroff MJ, et al: Panic disorder and suicidal ideation in primary care. Depress Anxiety 23(1):11–16, 2006 16245304

Raposo S, El-Gabalawy R, Erickson J, et al: Associations between anxiety disorders, suicide ideation, and age in nationally representative samples of Canadian and American adults. J Anxiety Disord 28(8):823–829, 2014 25306089

Rojas SM, Bujarski S, Babson KA, et al: Understanding PTSD comorbidity and suicidal behavior: associations among histories of alcohol dependence, major depressive disorder, and suicidal ideation and attempts. J Anxiety Disord 28(3):318–325, 2014 24681282

Sareen J: Anxiety disorders and risk for suicide: why such controversy? Depress Anxiety 28(11):941–945, 2011 22076969

Sareen J, Cox BJ, Afifi TO, et al: Anxiety disorders and risk for suicidal ideation and suicide attempts: a population-based longitudinal study of adults. Arch Gen Psychiatry 62(11):1249–1257, 2005 16275812

Schmidt NB, Woolaway-Bickel K, Bates M: Evaluating panic-specific factors in the relationship between suicide and panic disorder. Behav Res Ther 39(6):635–649, 2001 11400709

Simon NM, Zalta AK, Otto MW, et al: The association of comorbid anxiety disorders with suicide attempts and suicidal ideation in outpatients with bipolar disorder. J Psychiatr Res 41(3-4):255–264, 2007 17052730

Weissman MM, Klerman GL, Markowitz JS, et al: Suicidal ideation and suicide attempts in panic disorder and attacks. N Engl J Med 321(18):1209–1214, 1989 2797086

Yaseen ZS, Chartrand H, Mojtabai R, et al: Fear of dying in panic attacks predicts suicide attempt in comorbid depressive illness: prospective evidence from the National Epidemiological Survey on Alcohol and Related Conditions. Depress Anxiety 30(10):930–939, 2013 23281011

Zimmerman M, Chelminski I: Generalized anxiety disorder in patients with major depression: is DSM-IV's hierarchy correct? Am J Psychiatry 160(3):504–512, 2003 12611832

CHAPTER 9

Substance-Related Disorders

Rebecca A. Payne, M.D.

Substance use is a known risk factor for suicide attempts and death from suicide. In the United States, suicide is a leading cause of death among individuals with substance use disorders (SUDs; Substance Abuse and Mental Health Services Administration 2016). Between 43% and 65% of suicide attempts and completions are estimated to involve substance use (Steele et al. 2018). Internationally, SUDs are the second most common mental health disorder among suicide victims (Conner et al. 2014).

Precipitating or Predisposing Factor?

Commonly accepted and proposed models examining the association between suicide and substance use describe acute or subacute precipitating factors and chronic or static predisposing factors (Yuodelis-Flores and Ries 2015). Precipitating factors include events such as the loss of a job, fight with a spouse, or intoxication. Depression, family history of suicide, or a drug use disorder (DUD) are examples of predisposing factors. Within this model, substance use could be characterized as a precipitating factor, predisposing factor, or both.

A different model proposes that a risk factor or factors, such as substance use, lead to aggression, which is then directed toward oneself, another, or both oneself and another (Harford et al. 2018). Other models address the biological, psychological, and social effects of both acute intoxication with substances and an underlying SUD. For example, alcohol is a known depressant secondary to modulation of brain serotonergic and dopaminergic states. These effects cause or exacerbate a myriad of psychological and social difficulties including negative affect, hopelessness, cognitive impairment, interpersonal problems, worsening of impulsive traits, adverse life events, and poor social support (Hoertel et al. 2018).

Case Example 1

Patty, a 35-year-old, married, seventh-grade history teacher, presents for an initial evaluation at the insistence of her husband. Thirteen months ago, she reported persistent low mood, difficulty with sleep, anhedonia, weight gain, and lack of energy to her primary care physician. She declined an antidepressant at that time, attributing symptoms to dissatisfaction in her job. Two weeks ago, she was reprimanded by the school principal, who had received persistent complaints from her students' parents. That night, she went out with friends for drinks after work. She arrived home intoxicated, telling her husband that she had suicidal thoughts and was considering an overdose on his blood pressure medication. Currently, she drinks about once a week, usually on the weekend, consuming four or five glasses of wine per occasion.

Patty was initially diagnosed with depression at age 15 after a suicide attempt by ingesting over-the-counter cold medication. Afterward, she was referred for therapy to discuss a history of childhood sexual abuse and prescribed a selective serotonin reuptake inhibitor (SSRI), which had modest effects. She has a family history of depression on her mother's side.

Patty has several predisposing, or chronic, factors for suicide: a current untreated episode of a major depressive disorder, history of a suicide attempt, genetic predisposition to depression from her maternal family, and history of childhood sexual abuse. The precipitating, or acute, factors for the suicidal thoughts and plan include interpersonal problems with her employer and alcohol intoxication.

Research Challenges

The medical literature on substance use and suicide provides conflicting results and conclusions. Comorbid psychiatric conditions complicate the relationship between suicide and substance use, as do psychological traits, personality disorders, and psychosocial factors. Furthermore, risk factors vary among age groups, between the sexes, and in certain populations. In order to implement prevention, improve screening, and provide treatment, these factors must be delineated.

The heterogeneity of study populations, suicide events, and substance use terminology accounts for some of the disparate findings. Study populations vary widely, which limits the generalizability of results. For example, a large epidemiological study of the general population is a much different cohort than treatment-seeking individuals with an SUD, and the characterization of suicide events in each of these groups would differ. Additionally, although no longer true, women were typically excluded from studies on substance use in the past, resulting in a lack of data regarding sex-specific factors (Wilcox et al. 2004). Similarly, the specific type of suicide event that was examined varied considerably, from suicidal thoughts to suicide attempts or completions.

Lastly, terminology to describe substance use and SUDs runs the gamut from "use," "acute use," and "misuse," to abuse, dependence, and use disorder. For example, in 2013, DSM-5 defined the diagnosis of "substance use disorders," combining the former DSM-IV-TR diagnostic categories of abuse and dependence (American Psychiatric Association 2000, 2013; see Box 9–1). Intending to improve diagnostic accuracy and based on scientific studies, the criterion of "legal problems" was eliminated and the criterion of "craving or a strong desire or urge to use the substance" was added (Hasin et al. 2013). For purposes of this chapter, in order to accurately present and discuss this particular body of literature, the terminology used by the author of the original study to describe both the substance use and suicide event is used.

Box 9–1. Diagnostic Criteria for Alcohol Use Disorder

A. A problematic pattern of alcohol use leading to clinically significant impairment or distress, as manifested by at least two of the following, occurring within a 12-month period:

1. Alcohol is often taken in larger amounts or over a longer period than was intended.
2. There is a persistent desire or unsuccessful efforts to cut down or control alcohol use.
3. A great deal of time is spent in activities necessary to obtain alcohol, use alcohol, or recover from its effects.
4. Craving, or a strong desire or urge to use alcohol.
5. Recurrent alcohol use resulting in a failure to fulfill major role obligations at work, school, or home.
6. Continued alcohol use despite having persistent or recurrent social or interpersonal problems caused or exacerbated by the effects of alcohol.
7. Important social, occupational, or recreational activities are given up or reduced because of alcohol use.
8. Recurrent alcohol use in situations in which it is physically hazardous.
9. Alcohol use is continued despite knowledge of having a persistent or recurrent physical or psychological problem that is likely to have been caused or exacerbated by alcohol.
10. Tolerance, as defined by either of the following:
    a. A need for markedly increased amounts of alcohol to achieve intoxication or desired effect.
    b. A markedly diminished effect with continued use of the same amount of alcohol.
11. Withdrawal, as manifested by either of the following:
    a. The characteristic withdrawal syndrome for alcohol (refer to Criteria A and B of the criteria set for alcohol withdrawal, pp. 499–500).
    b. Alcohol (or a closely related substance, such as a benzodiazepine) is taken to relieve or avoid withdrawal symptoms.

Specify if:

In early remission: After full criteria for alcohol use disorder were previously met, none of the criteria for alcohol use disorder have been met for at least 3 months but for less than 12 months (with the exception that Criterion A4, "Craving, or a strong desire or urge to use alcohol," may be met).

In sustained remission: After full criteria for alcohol use disorder were previously met, none of the criteria for alcohol use disorder have been met at any time during a period of 12 months or longer (with the exception that Criterion A4, "Craving, or a strong desire or urge to use alcohol," may be met).

Specify if:

In a controlled environment: This additional specifier is used if the individual is in an environment where access to alcohol is restricted.

Code based on current severity: Note for ICD-10-CM codes: If an alcohol intoxication, alcohol withdrawal, or another alcohol-induced mental disorder is also present, do not use the codes below for alcohol use disorder. Instead, the comorbid alcohol use disorder is indicated in the 4th character of the alcohol-induced disorder code (see the coding note for alcohol intoxication, alcohol withdrawal, or a specific alcohol-induced mental disorder). For example, if there is comorbid alcohol intoxication and alcohol use disorder, only the alcohol intoxication code is given, with the 4th character indicating whether the comorbid alcohol use disorder is mild, moderate, or severe: F10.129 for mild alcohol use disorder with alcohol intoxication or F10.229 for a moderate or severe alcohol use disorder with alcohol intoxication.

Specify current severity:
   305.00 (F10.10) Mild: Presence of 2–3 symptoms.
   303.90 (F10.20) Moderate: Presence of 4–5 symptoms.
   303.90 (F10.20) Severe: Presence of 6 or more symptoms.

Source.   Reprinted from American Psychiatric Association: *Diagnostic and Statistical Manual of Mental Disorders*, 5th Edition. Arlington, VA, 2013, p. 222. Copyright © 2013 American Psychiatric Association. Used with permission.

Other challenges exist in research on suicide and SUD. The inherent ethical dilemma of enrolling individuals who have an elevated suicide risk into studies leads to a literature dominated by retrospective analysis of existing databases, analysis of large-scale epidemiological studies, psychological autopsies, and surveys of certain cohorts, such as treatment-seeking patients. A history of suicide attempts or current suicidal thoughts often excludes individuals from participation in nonsuicide research studies, although valuable information on suicide could be collected from secondary outcomes. Additionally, half of suicide deaths occur in individuals attempting suicide for the first time, which imposes natural limits outside the context of a certain type of evaluation, such as a psychological autopsy (Center for Substance Abuse Treatment 2009).

Another challenge involves the assessment of substance use. Alcohol use and alcohol use disorders (AUD) are often queried independently, whereas drug use and DUDs are commonly lumped together, making it difficult to gather information on specific substances (Harford et al. 2018; Icick et al. 2017). Furthermore, individuals with DUDs often use multiple drugs, resulting in limited knowledge of one particular drug or class. Therefore, the existing literature on suicide and SUDs largely focuses on alcohol use and AUDs.

Even characterizing and reporting a death as a suicide is a challenge, because substantial evidence such as a suicide note or history of a depressive disorder or other mood disorder is often required (Oquendo and Volkow 2018). When drug use or a DUD is involved in the death, the burden of proof needed to determine suicide is particularly high, and often the death is characterized as "undetermined" or "accidental" (Rockett et al. 2018).

Patient Assessment

Sex

The suicide rate for men in the general population is nearly four times higher than that for women, and men are also more likely to use substances (National Institute on Drug Abuse 2018; Substance Abuse and Mental Health Services Administration 2016). However, SUDs increase risk for both suicide attempts and suicide among men and women (American Psychiatric Association 2003). Most research points to a higher risk of suicide for women with AUD than men with AUD when compared to the general pop-

TABLE 9–1.   **Suicide risk factors in individuals with substance use disorder**

Demographics/History	Female sex
	Younger age
	Previous suicide attempt
Comorbid conditions	Traits:
	Impulsivity
	Aggression
	Psychiatric diagnoses:
	Major depressive disorder
	Bipolar disorder
	Posttraumatic stress disorder
	Additional substance use disorders
	Borderline or antisocial personality disorders
Social factors	Financial difficulty
	Unemployment
	Interpersonal conflicts (e.g., divorce or separation, conflict with family)
	Minimal social support
Symptom report	Describes feelings of hopelessness, being a burden, or a lack of belonging

ulation (Brady 2006; Table 9–1). One study estimated that the suicide rate for women with AUD was 20 times the expected rate versus 4 times that for men with AUD (American Psychiatric Association 2003; Wilcox et al. 2004). The increased risk of suicide among women with SUDs has been replicated in a meta-analysis of 24 international psychological autopsy studies. Female suicide decedents had an 8.34-fold risk of having an SUD compared to a 3.87-fold risk among male suicide decedents (Yoshimasu et al. 2008). However, some studies still have found that suicide decedents who used alcohol are more likely to be male (American Psychiatric Association 2003; Conner et al. 2003).

Age

Substance use is a risk factor for suicide at any age (Steele et al. 2018). Most studies suggest an association with younger age (late 30s to late 40s), whereas others suggest that suicide decedents with alcohol dependence are more likely to be older (American Psychiatric Association 2003; Brady 2006; Conner et al. 2003). In the general population, the geriatric population (defined as age 65 and older) has the highest risk for death from suicide, with white men 85 and older at the highest risk among all groups (Steele et al. 2018). The three most common psychiatric illnesses among geriatric suicide decedents are depression, anxiety, and substance use (Steele et al. 2018).

Race/Ethnicity

Alcohol is involved in a higher percentage of suicides among Native Americans compared with the general population, with psychiatric illness, cultural alienation, and lack of access to resources also probable contributors (Center for Substance Abuse Treatment 2009; Substance Abuse and Mental Health Services Administration 2016).

Deaths from suicide among African American males are highest in the 15- to 24-years-old age group (American Psychiatric Association 2003). Risk factors within this group include anxiety, access to a firearm, and substance abuse, with the availability of a firearm and concomitant cocaine abuse a particularly risky combination (Center for Substance Abuse Treatment 2009; Substance Abuse and Mental Health Services Administration 2016). Hispanic/Latinx population suicide rates mirror those of white persons, although Hispanic/Latinx adolescents and younger groups, particularly women, experience more suicidal behavior if acculturated to American culture (Center for Substance Abuse Treatment 2009).

Special Populations

Certain groups of substance-using individuals such as veterans, adolescents, incarcerated individuals, and those with HIV/AIDS should be assessed carefully and given particular consideration with regard to suicide risk. In large studies of veterans, a diagnosis of any SUD was associated with higher rates of suicide compared to the general population, with a specific diagnosis of opioid use disorder (OUD) increasing suicide risk six times that of the general population (Center for Substance Abuse Treatment 2009; Oquendo and Volkow 2018). For adolescents, risk factors for self-harm or suicidal behavior include drug use, polysubstance use, comorbid mood disorders, tobacco use, and alcohol misuse, particularly binge drinking (American Psychiatric Association 2003; Hawton et al. 2012; Shlosberg et al. 2014). Lesbian, gay, and bisexual adolescents display more suicidal behaviors and are at an increased risk for SUDs compared to their heterosexual peers, although the data regarding the association of SUDs and suicidal behaviors in this group are mixed (Shlosberg et al. 2014). Individuals who die from suicide in jail are more likely to be young, white, single men with a history of substance abuse (American Psychiatric Association 2003). Those with HIV/AIDS commonly have comorbid conditions, such as psychiatric disorders, SUDs, or social circumstances (e.g., stigma and lack of support) that play a role in suicidal behaviors (American Psychiatric Association 2003).

Previous Suicide Attempt(s)

In the general population, previous suicide attempts have been described as the most predictive risk factor for death from suicide (Yuodelis-Flores and Ries 2015). Likewise, in individuals with SUDs, previous suicide attempts are associated with an increased risk of death from suicide (Center for Substance Abuse Treatment 2009; Yuodelis-Flores and Ries 2015). For example, women with drug use and prior suicide attempts have an 87-fold increase in deaths from suicide when compared with the general population (Yuodelis-Flores and Ries 2015).

Social Circumstances

Various social circumstances, also described as life events, have been implicated as risk factors for death from suicide in individuals with SUDs. Life events with particular salience include financial difficulty, interpersonal problems, hopelessness, and poor social support (Conner et al. 2003, 2014; Kuramoto-Crawford and Wilcox 2016; Yuodelis-Flores and Ries 2015). Among individuals with alcohol dependence, current unemployment and divorced or separated status were associated with past suicide attempts (Brady

2006). Similarly, conflict with family within the past year was significantly associated with death from suicide in individuals with an AUD compared to those without an AUD (Kõlves et al. 2017). An interpersonal loss or conflict around the time of suicide has also been demonstrated in individuals with DUD (American Psychiatric Association 2003).

Comorbid Conditions

Comorbid mental illnesses and SUDs increase risk for death from suicide; the more psychiatric symptoms or psychiatric disorders present, the higher the risk of death from suicide (American Psychiatric Association 2003). Comorbid SUD and depression (whether substance-induced or otherwise) or bipolar disorder are associated with a higher risk of suicide attempts and death from suicide (Kuramoto-Crawford and Wilcox 2016). One study found that among suicide decedents with an AUD, 64.3% had a comorbid mood disorder (Kõlves et al. 2017). Estimates of the incidence of depression in suicide decedents with alcohol dependence range between 22% and 25% (Brady 2006).

Although studied less extensively, comorbid SUD and bipolar disorder increases suicide risk significantly, with an estimated doubling or tripling of the risk (Yuodelis-Flores and Ries 2015). As might be anticipated, the presence of both an AUD and a DUD in bipolar disorder presents a particularly increased risk of suicidal behaviors. One study found that 97% of individuals with these three diagnoses had a past history of a suicide attempt, compared with 93% and 89% of those with bipolar and either a DUD or AUD alone, respectively (Yuodelis-Flores and Ries 2015).

Less is known about other psychiatric disorders and comorbid SUD in regard to death from suicide. Posttraumatic stress disorder (PTSD), panic disorder, and generalized anxiety disorder have been associated with suicidal behaviors in individuals with SUDs, with PTSD a particularly potent risk factor (Center for Substance Abuse Treatment 2009; Kuramoto-Crawford and Wilcox 2016; Yuodelis-Flores and Ries 2015). SUD also increases suicide risk among persons with schizophrenia, conduct disorder, and eating disorders (American Psychiatric Association 2003; Kuramoto-Crawford and Wilcox 2016; Yuodelis-Flores and Ries 2015).

In general, the use of one substance increases the risk for death from suicide, and the use of multiple substances further increases that risk. Specifically, one study found that among individuals who use multiple substances, the suicide rate increases nearly 17-fold when compared with the general population (Yuodelis-Flores and Ries 2015). The specific substance used in suicide appears to play a less important role compared with the number of substances used (American Psychiatric Association 2003). Certain patterns of alcohol use further increase suicide risk, including early onset of drinking, longer duration of drinking, earlier onset of heavy drinking, and heavier drinking patterns over the duration of drinking (American Psychiatric Association 2003, 2018; Conner et al. 2014; Yuodelis-Flores and Ries 2015).

In the presence of an SUD, certain personality traits and disorders increase risk of suicidal behaviors. Impulsivity and aggression are common traits in individuals with suicidal behaviors and SUDs. Recent studies have demonstrated that higher levels of aggression and impulsivity in the context of substance use play a role in suicidal behavior. Among suicide decedents, those with an AUD had greater levels of aggression compared to those without an AUD (Kõlves et al. 2017). Similarly, depressed individuals with alcoholism reported greater levels of suicidal thoughts and behaviors and higher aggression and impulsivity over their lifetime compared with depressed individuals without alcoholism (Yuodelis-Flores and Ries 2015). Impulsivity and aggression are also common traits in individuals with antisocial and borderline personality disorder, which confer an increased risk of suicidal behavior even in the absence of substance use (American Psychiatric Association 2003). In borderline personality disorder, depression or substance use further increases the risk for suicidal behaviors (Yuodelis-Flores and Ries 2015). Interestingly, concomitant borderline and antisocial personality disorders have been described as "highly prevalent" in individuals with DUDs (Kuramoto-Crawford and Wilcox 2016).

Alcohol

Alcohol influences suicidal thoughts, suicide attempts, and deaths from suicide (Center for Substance Abuse Treatment 2009). Alcohol use has been estimated to be present in 30%–70% of those who attempt suicide and in 18%–66% of those who die from suicide (Sher et al. 2009). The proposed mechanism by which alcohol intoxication leads to death from suicide suggests that intoxication increases impulsivity, aggression, and psychological distress and inhibits cognition, thus creating an amalgam of circumstances in which suicidal thoughts are more likely to be acted upon and the cognitive ability to better cope with adversity is limited (Yuodelis-Flores and Ries 2015).

The degree to which alcohol is involved in death from suicide varies. In some cases, an individual may use alcohol to ameliorate fear or anxiety associated with the act of suicide but not necessarily meet criteria for a current or past diagnosis of an AUD. For example, in 2010, alcohol intoxication was involved in 22% of deaths from suicide (Substance Abuse and Mental Health Services Administration 2016). Kaplan et al. (2014) found intoxication (defined as a blood alcohol content of 0.08 g/dL or greater) increased risk of death from suicide by 6.18-fold for males and 10.04-fold for females. However, disordered use of alcohol, rather than intoxication or acute use alone, generally confers a higher risk of death from suicide. Individuals with an AUD have a 10-fold higher suicide risk compared with a control group, and the lifetime risk of death from suicide for individuals diagnosed with alcohol dependence ranges between 7% and 15% (Kõlves et al. 2017; Sher et al. 2009). In summary, alcohol use increases suicide risk regardless of whether an AUD is present (Yuodelis-Flores and Ries 2015).

Previous studies show that intoxicated individuals and those who drink heavily are more likely to use one of the more lethal means of suicide, such as firearms or hanging (Sher et al. 2009; Yuodelis-Flores and Ries 2015). However, a recent Australian psychological autopsy review of individuals older than age 35 found no significant differences among suicide decedents with and without an AUD in rates of firearm use (12.7% vs. 11.4%, respectively) or hanging (47.3% vs. 45.8%, respectively) (Kõlves et al. 2017).

Drugs

Among treatment-seeking individuals with any substance use diagnosis, 40% report a lifetime history of a suicide attempt (Yuodelis-Flores and Ries 2015). Those with

DUDs have 5.8-times greater odds of a past suicide attempt (Bohnert et al. 2010). According to data from the 2010 National Violent Death Reporting System, opiates were found in 20% of suicide decedents, marijuana in 10.2%, cocaine in 4.6%, and amphetamines in 3.4% (Substance Abuse and Mental Health Services Administration 2016). Although the presence of a substance at the time of suicide does not necessarily indicate a use disorder, drug use clearly plays a prominent role in death from suicide.

As mentioned earlier, the use of multiple drugs has been shown to be more predictive of death from suicide as opposed to the use of a specific drug or class of drugs (Substance Abuse and Mental Health Services Administration 2016). Individuals who attempt or die from suicide tend not to use their drug of choice in these acts (Bohnert et al. 2010). Most information available on the association of suicide attempts and completions and DUDs pertains to cocaine, nicotine, and opioids (both heroin and prescription pain medication) (Hughes 2008; Kuramoto-Crawford and Wilcox 2016). An association between current tobacco use and death from suicide has been fairly consistently demonstrated, whether studies have controlled for comorbid psychiatric and concomitant drug use or not (Hughes 2008). Studies examining cocaine use and death from suicide vary widely in regard to routes of cocaine administration, concomitant substance use, and comorbid medical conditions. Therefore, the generalizability of these results is limited (Degenhardt et al. 2011). Cocaine use, particularly when used with other substances such as alcohol and opioids, increases risk for both suicidal ideation and attempts (American Psychiatric Association 2003; Degenhardt et al. 2011).

Prior to the declaration of the opioid crisis as a public health emergency in 2017, meta-analyses of cohort studies and psychological autopsies found a strong association between suicide and OUD using standardized mortality ratios, which examine death rates of a specific cohort compared with those of the general population (American Psychiatric Association 2003; Wilcox et al. 2004). More recently, the 2014 National Survey on Drug Use and Health (NSDUH) found that risk of suicidal ideation increased between 40% and 60% in individuals with OUD, specifically prescription opioids (Oquendo and Volkow 2018). Compared to nonopioid users, regular opioid users are 75% more likely to formulate a plan for suicide and two times more likely to make a suicide attempt (Oquendo and Volkow 2018). As noted earlier, deaths ruled as "indeterminate" or "accidental," particularly those associated with opioid use, may actually represent suicide (Oquendo and Volkow 2018; Rockett et al. 2018).

In regard to other drugs, our understanding of their relationship with deaths from suicide is more limited. Sedative-hypnotic-anxiolytic dependence was found to have a similar standardized mortality ratio to use of multiple substances and, in one cohort of treatment-seeking outpatients, was associated with serious suicide attempts in both men and women (American Psychiatric Association 2003; Icick et al. 2017). Data collected from the NSDUH from 2008 to 2015 indicated that marijuana use disorders, AUD, OUD (specifically prescription pain medication), and nicotine dependence were associated with violence toward both self and others (Harford et al. 2018). According to an analysis of data from the National Epidemiologic Survey on Alcohol and Related Conditions, one-fifth of individuals with inhalant use disorders had attempted suicide and nearly 70% had past suicidal thoughts (Howard et al. 2010). Methamphetamine users age 24 and younger are at increased risk of mortality secondary to overdose and suicide (Marshall and Werb 2010).

Case Example 2

Thomas, a 42-year-old Army veteran with PTSD, depression, and some borderline traits, has been in outpatient treatment for the past 3 years. He is stabilized on sertraline and completed a successful course of cognitive processing therapy for PTSD several years ago. Thomas has a history of abusing prescription pain pills 10 years ago, beginning after he had surgery on his right leg for an injury sustained in an improvised explosive device blast. He made a serious suicide attempt via carbon monoxide poisoning before entering treatment for OUD. He was detoxified from opioids but declined maintenance medications for OUD.

His psychiatrist currently sees Thomas once every month and noticed that he has appeared withdrawn and less interactive the past two visits. He has separated from his wife of 12 years and misses seeing his children regularly. He has an appointment to be seen tomorrow for a routine visit. His mother, with whom he now lives, left a telephone message yesterday stating that she had found a bottle of pills in his dresser drawer and was worried that he might be using drugs again. She expressed concern about his increasing isolation and erratic behaviors for the past several months.

The following day, Thomas presents for his appointment. He is reluctant to engage with the interview but eventually admits to suicidal thoughts with a plan to use his firearm. He feels hopeless about his marriage and family and shares that he has not truly belonged anywhere since he left the military. He obtained a bottle of hydrocodone from a friend and has been taking up to 10 pills a day, sometimes 2 or 3 at a time to "forget about life."

Thomas has numerous risk factors including a prior suicide attempt, multiple psychiatric comorbidities, active substance use, interpersonal difficulty (marital separation), feelings of hopelessness and lack of belonging, being a veteran, and ready access to firearms. After considering Thomas's risk factors for death from suicide, the psychiatrist recommends hospitalization for safety, and Thomas agrees. He permits his psychiatrist to speak with his mother, and the psychiatrist recommends that she either remove or secure the firearm. A urine drug screen performed on admission to the hospital reveals hydrocodone, benzodiazepines, and cannabis. Medications for OUD are discussed while Thomas is hospitalized, and he opts for treatment with a buprenorphine/naloxone combination. Sertraline dosage is increased, and he is referred to substance abuse treatment as well as to psychotherapy to address his feelings of hopelessness, sense of lack of belonging, and marital separation.

Prevention and Treatment Recommendations

Preventative methods of addressing suicide may include limiting availability and accessibility to alcohol. Recent population-based studies have described a correlation between a decrease in alcohol intake and a decline in suicide rates (Substance Abuse and Mental Health Services Administration 2016). The minimum drinking age of 21 in the United States has been estimated to have reduced the number of suicides by 600 per year (Substance Abuse and Mental Health Services Administration 2016).

In regard to treatment, a thorough evaluation should include addressing medical and psychiatric health. Depending on the patient's history and presentation, a physical examination and testing for medical conditions associated with drug use, such as hepatitis C and HIV, may be warranted. Laboratory tests such as a thyroid panel, vitamin levels, and a urine drug screen should also be considered. The psychiatric assessment should include the components of a standard initial evaluation, such as psychiatric symptoms, past and current substance use, and suicide risk and protective factors. Pro-

TABLE 9–2.   **FDA-approved medications for substance use disorders**

Alcohol use disorder	Opioid use disorder	Tobacco use disorder
Acamprosate	Buprenorphine	Nicotine replacement therapies
Disulfiram	Methadone	Bupropion
Naltrexone	Naltrexone	Varenicline

Note.   FDA=U.S. Food and Drug Administration.

tective factors against death from suicide in an individual with SUD have been studied, although not as extensively as risk factors, and may include employment, a therapeutic relationship with a medical professional, being married, having children or having responsibility in the care of a child or children, religious beliefs, involvement with mutual self-help groups, sobriety, and possessing optimism as a trait (Center for Substance Abuse Treatment 2009). A comprehensive evaluation allows the provider to accurately diagnose and assess suicide risk and determine a treatment plan. A recommendation to at least temporarily limit or restrict access to weapons, particularly firearms, should be a part of the treatment plan as well.

Suicide risk may be increased in individuals with SUD at treatment initiation or during treatment (Center for Substance Abuse Treatment 2009; Hoertel et al. 2018). Issues that arise during treatment that may increase suicide risk include relapses or concerns regarding relapse, acute life stressors, and transitions in care (Center for Substance Abuse Treatment 2009). It is important to be aware that patients hospitalized psychiatrically for suicidal behaviors are discharged sooner if substances were involved compared with patients who had no substance involvement (Conner et al. 2014). Debate exists as to whether treatment for SUD impacts subsequent suicide and related behaviors (compared to not receiving treatment), although suicide attempts may be half as likely in the year after treatment for SUD compared to the year preceding the treatment (Conner et al. 2014). Nonetheless, close monitoring and frequent reassessment throughout the treatment duration are paramount to good clinical care.

Both contingency management and cognitive-behavioral therapy have consistently demonstrated efficacy in the treatment of SUD and are effective psychotherapies (Carroll and Kiluk 2017; Petry et al. 2017). Mindfulness-based therapies for the treatment of SUD are an area of expanding research, and studies to date have been positive (Li et al. 2017). In addition to psychotherapy, medications are available for the treatment of patients with SUDs (Table 9–2). Concerns regarding the depressogenic effects of naltrexone have been raised in the past. Clinical trials found no difference in rates of depression and anxiety between placebo and naltrexone (both oral and injectable formulations), although some reports indicated suicidal behaviors and deaths from suicide in postmarketing surveillance (American Psychiatric Association 2018). In trials with acamprosate, suicidal behavior and deaths from suicide were only minimally increased (0.13% of patients on acamprosate vs. 0.10% of patients on placebo), and this was not sufficient to make a determination about the association of acamprosate and suicide risk (American Psychiatric Association 2018).

U.S. Food and Drug Administration–approved medications for tobacco use disorder include nicotine replacement therapies, bupropion, and varenicline. After its approval in 2006 and subsequent release, reports accumulated that varenicline increased suicidal behaviors, leading to a black box warning in 2009 stating varenicline could cause "changes in…suicidal thoughts and behavior and attempted suicide" (Davies and Thomas 2017). Since that time, several studies have demonstrated that the risk of death from suicide or attempted suicide was similar between varenicline and placebo.

Conclusion

SUDs increase the risk for suicide attempts and deaths from suicide. Appreciating and assessing risk factors and protective factors for suicide in this population is necessary given the relatively high prevalence. Thoughtful consideration regarding the choice of psychotherapeutic and pharmacological treatments for both the SUD and comorbid psychiatric conditions is imperative. More research is needed to expand understanding of the complex relationship between SUDs and suicidal behaviors.

Key Points

- Substance use is a known risk factor for suicide attempts and deaths from suicide.

- Alcohol use increases risk of death from suicide regardless of whether an alcohol use disorder (AUD) exists.

- Multiple drug use is more associated with death from suicide than use of a specific drug or class of drugs.

- Unemployment, financial difficulty, interpersonal problems, hopelessness, and poor social support are risk factors associated with substance use disorder (SUD) and suicidal behaviors.

- Treatment should address suicidal thoughts and behaviors, psychiatric disorders, and SUDs concomitantly.

- Medications to treat AUD, opioid use disorder, and tobacco use disorder are generally safe with regard to suicidal thoughts and behaviors.

References

American Psychiatric Association: Diagnostic and Statistical Manual of Mental Disorders, 4th Edition, Text Revision. Washington, DC, American Psychiatric Association, 2000

American Psychiatric Association: Practice Guideline for the Assessment and Treatment of Patients With Suicidal Behaviors. Arlington, VA, American Psychiatric Association, 2003. Available at: https://psychiatryonline.org/pb/assets/raw/sitewide/practice_guidelines/guidelines/suicide.pdf. Accessed November 24, 2018.

American Psychiatric Association: Diagnostic and Statistical Manual of Mental Disorders, 5th Edition. Arlington, VA, American Psychiatric Association, 2013

American Psychiatric Association: Practice Guideline for the Pharmacological Treatment of Patients With Alcohol Use Disorder. Arlington, VA, American Psychiatric Association, 2018. Available at: https://psychiatryonline.org/doi/pdf/10.1176/appi.books.9781615371969. Accessed November 24, 2018.

Bohnert ASB, Roeder K, Ilgen MA: Unintentional overdose and suicide among substance users: a review of overlap and risk factors. Drug Alcohol Depend 110(3):183–192, 2010 20430536

Brady J: The association between alcohol misuse and suicidal behaviour. Alcohol Alcohol 41(5):473–478, 2006 16891335

Carroll KM, Kiluk BD: Cognitive behavioral interventions for alcohol and drug use disorders: through the stage model and back again. Psychol Addict Behav 31(8):847–861, 2017 28857574

Center for Substance Abuse Treatment: Addressing Suicidal Thoughts and Behaviors in Substance Abuse Treatment. Treatment Improvement Protocol (TIP) Series No 50, HHS Publ No (SMA) 154381. Rockville, MD, Substance Abuse and Mental Health Services Administration, 2009

Conner KR, Beautrais AL, Conwell Y: Risk factors for suicide and medically serious suicide attempts among alcoholics: analyses of Canterbury Suicide Project data. J Stud Alcohol 64(4):551–554, 2003 12921197

Conner KR, Bagge CL, Goldston DB, et al: Alcohol and suicidal behavior: what is known and what can be done. Am J Prev Med 47(3 suppl 2):S204–S208, 2014 25145740

Davies NM, Thomas KH: The Food and Drug Administration and varenicline: should risk communication be improved? Addiction 112(4):555–558, 2017 27558015

Degenhardt L, Singleton J, Calabria B, et al: Mortality among cocaine users: a systematic review of cohort studies. Drug Alcohol Depend 113(2-3):88–95, 2011 20828942

Harford TC, Yi HY, Chen CM, et al: Substance use disorders and self- and other-directed violence among adults: results from the National Survey on Drug Use and Health. J Affect Disord 225:365–373, 2018 28846958

Hasin DS, O'Brien CP, Auriacombe M, et al: DSM-5 criteria for substance use disorders: recommendations and rationale. Am J Psychiatry 170(8):834–851, 2013 23903334

Hawton K, Saunders KEA, O'Connor RC: Self-harm and suicide in adolescents. Lancet 379(9834):2373–2382, 2012 22726518

Hoertel N, Faiz H, Airagnes G, et al: A comprehensive model of predictors of suicide attempt in heavy drinkers: results from a national 3-year longitudinal study. Drug Alcohol Depend 186:44–52, 2018 29547760

Howard MO, Perron BE, Sacco P, et al: Suicide ideation and attempts among inhalant users: results from the National Epidemiologic Survey on Alcohol and Related Conditions. Suicide Life Threat Behav 40(3):276–286, 2010 20560749

Hughes JR: Smoking and suicide: a brief overview. Drug Alcohol Depend 98(3):169–178, 2008 18676099

Icick R, Karsinti E, Lépine JP, et al: Serious suicide attempts in outpatients with multiple substance use disorders. Drug Alcohol Depend 181:63–70, 2017 29035706

Kaplan MS, Huguet N, McFarland BH, et al: Use of alcohol before suicide in the United States. Ann Epidemiol 24(8):588–592.e1, 2, 2014 24953567

Kõlves K, Draper BM, Snowdon J, et al: Alcohol-use disorders and suicide: results from a psychological autopsy study in Australia. Alcohol 64:29–35, 2017 28965653

Kuramoto-Crawford SJ, Wilcox HC: Substance use disorders and intentional injury, in The Oxford Handbook of Substance Use and Substance Use Disorders, Vol 2. Edited by Sher KJ. New York, Oxford University Press, 2016, pp 322–346

Li W, Howard MO, Garland EL, et al: Mindfulness treatment for substance misuse: a systematic review and meta-analysis. J Subst Abuse Treat 75:62–96, 2017 28153483

Marshall BD, Werb D: Health outcomes associated with methamphetamine use among young people: a systematic review. Addiction 105(6):991–1002, 2010 20659059

National Institute on Drug Abuse: Substance Use in Women (website). Bethesda, MD, National Institute on Drug Abuse, 2018. Available at: https://www.drugabuse.gov/publications/research-reports/substance-use-in-women. Accessed October 1, 2018.

Oquendo MA, Volkow ND: Suicide: a silent contributor to opioid-overdose deaths. N Engl J Med 378(17):1567–1569, 2018 29694805

Petry NM, Alessi SM, Olmstead TA, et al: Contingency management treatment for substance use disorders: How far has it come, and where does it need to go? Psychol Addict Behav 31(8):897–906, 2017 28639812

Rockett IRH, Caine ED, Connery HS, et al: Discerning suicide in drug intoxication deaths: paucity and primacy of suicide notes and psychiatric history. PLoS One 13(1):e0190200, 2018 29320540

Sher L, Oquendo MA, Richardson-Vejlgaard R, et al: Effect of acute alcohol use on the lethality of suicide attempts in patients with mood disorders. J Psychiatr Res 43(10):901–905, 2009 19246050

Shlosberg D, Zalsman G, Shoval G: Emerging issues in the relationship between adolescent substance use and suicidal behavior. Isr J Psychiatry Relat Sci 51(4):262–267, 2014 25841222

Steele IH, Thrower N, Noroian P, et al: Understanding suicide across the lifespan: a United States perspective of suicide risk factors, assessment and management. J Forensic Sci 63(1):162–171, 2018 28639299

Substance Abuse and Mental Health Services Administration: Substance use and suicide: a nexus requiring a public health approach. In Brief, 2016. Available at: https://store.samhsa.gov/system/files/sma16-4935.pdf. Accessed November 23, 2018.

Wilcox HC, Conner KR, Caine ED: Association of alcohol and drug use disorders and completed suicide: an empirical review of cohort studies. Drug Alcohol Depend 76(suppl):S11–S19, 2004 15555812

Yoshimasu K, Kiyohara C, Miyashita K: Suicidal risk factors and completed suicide: meta-analyses based on psychological autopsy studies. Environ Health Prev Med 13(5):243–256, 2008 19568911

Yuodelis-Flores C, Ries RK: Addiction and suicide: a review. Am J Addict 24(2):98–104, 2015 25644860

CHAPTER 10

Bipolar Spectrum Disorders

Victoria Cosgrove, Ph.D.

Trisha Suppes, M.D., Ph.D.

Ayal Schaffer, M.D.

Alaina Baker, B.S.

Nicole Kramer, M.S.

Bipolar disorders (BDs), previously referred to as "manic depression," are common worldwide, often severely disabling, and potentially fatal psychiatric illnesses. BDs refer to several disorders of mood, energy, and thought characterized by cycles of major depressive and either manic or hypomanic episodes that may be separated by periods of euthymic mood. Depressive episodes are defined by low or irritable mood, anhedonia, reduced energy leading to diminished activity, and social withdrawal. Although manic and hypomanic episodes differ by duration and intensity, they are broadly defined by elevated or irritable mood coupled with increased energy or overactivity as well as pressured speech, inflated self-esteem, impulsivity, and decreased need for sleep.

Bipolar spectrum disorders include bipolar I disorder (BDI), bipolar II disorder (BDII), a more persistent and subthreshold cyclothymic disorder, and other specified and unspecified bipolar and related disorders. In the United States, the estimated lifetime prevalence is 0.6% and 0.8% for BDI and BDII, respectively. These disorders account for the highest percentage (82%) of serious disability and impairment among mood disorders (American Psychiatric Association 2013).

Clinical symptoms associated with increased risk from death from suicide in bipolar spectrum disorders include current depression or depressive episode, past severe depression, and hopelessness. Additional clinical factors such as illness subtype, first-degree family history of deaths from suicide, and polarity of first and most recent episode are also associated with suicide deaths and suicide attempts in BD (Schaffer et al. 2015a, 2015b). This chapter highlights BD-specific assessments, predictive risk factors, and treatments related to suicidal behaviors in patients with bipolar and related disorders.

Reconceptualization of a Bipolar Spectrum in DSM-5

Psychiatric science has moved toward a dimensional view of mood disorders. The publication of DSM-5 (American Psychiatric Association 2013) marked a shift in how BDs are conceptualized, toward a spectrum of disorders characterized by distinct episodes of depressive and manic symptoms with co-occurring symptoms from the opposite pole. Diagnostic criteria for "manic-like phenomena" due to substance use or other medical conditions are now separate from diagnostic criteria for the disorders.

DSM-5 also summarizes bipolar-like symptoms that do not fulfill BDI or BDII diagnostic criteria as other specified or unspecified bipolar and related disorders. In previous editions of DSM, only a period of abnormal and persistently elevated expansive or irritable mood was necessary to meet diagnostic Criterion A for a hypomanic or manic episode. In DSM-5, the aforementioned symptoms have to be present concurrently with increased goal-directed activity most of the day, nearly every day, for either 7 (manic episode) or 4 (hypomanic episode) consecutive days.

DSM-5 defines three primary types of BDs. BDI is the modern version of manic-depressive illness, and mania is its defining feature. BDII is marked by hypomanic episodes, which largely have the same diagnostic criteria as manic episodes but with less severity and duration and at least one depressive episode. Cyclothymia is marked by chronically mercurial mood patterns that fluctuate between subclinical hypomanic symptoms and depressive symptoms without ever fulfilling the criteria for an episode of mania, hypomania, or major depression. Additionally, DSM-5 defines other specified and unspecified bipolar and related disorders that describe varied clinical presentations in which characteristic symptoms cause clinically significant distress or functional impairment but do not meet the full diagnostic criteria for any of the disorders in this diagnostic class (American Psychiatric Association 2013).

To enhance accuracy of diagnosis and aid in earlier clinical detection, Criterion A for both hypomanic and manic episodes now includes an emphasis on changes in activity and energy as well as mood or irritability. The DSM-IV (American Psychiatric Association 1994) diagnosis of BDI mixed episode has been removed, and a new specifier, "with mixed features," was added. Additional criteria for both poles of mood disorders have been introduced as well as new specifiers, including "anxious distress." Additionally, a "mixed features" specifier, indicating the presence of at least three symptoms from opposite poles, allows consideration of the possibility of the presence of subsyndromal symptoms from opposite poles. This specifier can be used with diagnoses of hypomanic and depressive episodes in BDI and BDII as well as other specified and unspecified BDs (Betzler et al. 2017).

Suicide Risk in Patients With Bipolar Disorders

Although increased mortality rates in BD are often associated with comorbid substance use and medical conditions, BD accounts for the highest standardized mortality ratio (SMR) for deaths from suicide (Tondo et al. 2016). The estimated lifetime risk of suicide attempts in patients with BD ranges from 15% to 50% (Schaffer et al. 2015a).

Disease-Specific Risk Factors

Individuals with BD have a higher risk of suicide-related deaths than both the general population and those with other mental disorders. Suicide rates as SMRs in individuals with BDs (SMR=28) are higher than the rates for the general population and averages at a similar rate among patients with unipolar depression (SMR=20) and polysubstance use disorders (SMR=19) (Tondo et al. 2016).

Several factors may contribute to the elevated suicide risk associated with BD. First, despite mania and hypomania diagnostically delineating the disorder, considerable symptomatic time is spent in depressive episodes, in which suicidal ideation is a common symptom. Furthermore, the impulsivity associated with mania and hypomania may reduce inhibitions and heighten impulsive decision making. Importantly, mixed states are common in both manic/hypomanic and depressive episodes and also are often associated with impulsivity. Finally, a highly stressful disease course may contribute to the higher suicide risk associated with BD.

Sex Differences

Although lifetime risk of BD seems to be nearly equal in both men and women, suicide risk and symptom presentation often vary based on sex (Karanti et al. 2015). Women with BD are more likely to experience subdiagnostic depressed mood and dysphoria and more likely than men to be diagnosed with BDII (Karanti et al. 2015). Women are also more likely to have depressive symptoms, but depressive symptoms in women do not seem to increase lethality (Altshuler et al. 2010). Female sex is associated with a greater number of suicide attempts, and male sex is associated with greater attempt lethality and deaths from suicide (Schaffer et al. 2015a).

Lethality of Attempts

The lethality of suicide attempts (measured by the potential for fatality) involves both intent (how much the patient wishes to die) and means used (e.g., firearms, poisoning). More than 2% of patients with BD attempt suicide each year, and more than 20% of those die from suicide. The ratio of attempts to deaths from suicide in patients with BD is 8.1:1, while the same ratio in the general population is estimated to be 25:1. Deaths from suicide in BD are therefore more than three times as likely to occur (1 death to every 8 attempts) than in the general population (1 death to every 25 attempts) (Pompili et al. 2009).

Other Suicide Risk Factors

Age and Duration of Illness

In both unipolar and bipolar affective disorders, the SMRs for all deaths were highest in patients with first admission to treatment at younger ages (15–29 years of age) and the SMR for BD decreased with increasing age (Ösby et al. 2001). A meta-analysis showed age at illness onset was 2.99 years younger among those with a history of suicide attempts compared with those without a history of attempts (Schaffer et al. 2015b). In some studies, more than one-third of suicidal acts occurred within 1 year of illness onset and more than one-half occurred within the first 5 years of the illness, indicating the necessity of early diagnosis and intervention.

Clinical Subtypes and Presentation

BDII, which has more prominent depressive than hypomanic episodes, has been found to be associated with a higher risk of death from suicide (Angst et al. 2012). Mixed affective states, which occur when depressive and manic symptoms co-occur during an episode, are often complex presentations associated with higher risk of death from suicide, and those with BD are at highest risk of death from suicide during mixed episodes (Angst et al. 2012). BD episodes marked by increased anxious distress have also been associated with elevated suicide risk over more classic presentations (Goes 2015).

As BD progresses into more advanced stages, durations between depressive and manic/hypomanic episodes may become shorter, constituting a more serious and impairing disease course. Rapid cycling, specified when the patient has had at least four depressive, manic, or hypomanic episodes in the previous 12 months, is associated with increased risk of death from suicide. Rapid cycling is a more treatment-resistant variant of BDI and BDII and often reflects a worsening of the underlying disorder and potentially an end stage of the illness, because cycles may get closer together over time. In some cases, ultra-rapid cycling (cycles that last less than 24 hours) occurs, with switches typically occurring between morning and evening.

Demographic Risk Factors

A variety of demographic factors appear to be associated with increased risk of death from suicide in patients with BD (Table 10–1).

Both white ethnicity and unmarried relationship status seem to be associated with increased risk for death from suicide in BD. Other sociodemographic variables increase the likelihood of suicide attempts in patients with BD: more patients of female sex and a younger age are likely to attempt suicide, and those of older age and male sex are likely to make more lethal attempts (Schaffer et al. 2015a). Research on the influence of race and ethnicity in patients with BD who die from suicide is limited, but a 2006 study demonstrated that individuals identifying with a non-Hispanic white ethnicity who died from suicide had higher rates of BD (6.1%) compared with individuals identifying as non-Hispanic blacks (2.6%), Hispanic (2.3%), and others (1.6%) (Schaffer et al. 2015a). Individuals with BD who are single or divorced have a significantly higher rate of lifetime suicide attempts, and single parents have significantly higher rates of death from suicide than those who are married (Schaffer et al. 2015a).

Genetic Factors

Genetic factors appear to increase the risk of not only BD but also death from suicide in BD. If a family member has BD, biological relatives are at an increased risk of developing the disorder. Twin studies have estimated the heritability of BD to be in the realm of 80%, and depression and mania seem to have significant genetic overlap (McGuffin et al. 2010). Individuals with BD who have a family history of BD and suicidal thoughts and behaviors have different familial loading for suicide behaviors and attempts compared with patients with BD who have a family history of BD but no family history of suicide attempts or deaths (Turecki 2001). Furthermore, the interaction among BD polygenic risk scores in relation to deaths from suicide, suicidal behaviors, and traumatic stress leads to an increased risk for suicide attempts and ideation, especially if the relative is exposed to trauma, thus increasing genetic vulnerability (Wilcox et al. 2017).

TABLE 10–1. **Sociodemographic characteristics of patients with bipolar disorder who attempted suicide**

Variable	*N*	%
Sex		
Male	20	40
Female	30	60
Marital status		
Single	12	24
Married	24	48
Divorced	12	24
Widowed	1	2
Education		
University and college	19	38
Vocational school	9	18
No professional education	22	44
Work status		
Employed	27	54
Student	5	10
Unemployed	6	12
Disability pension	12	24
Bipolar type		
Bipolar I disorder	20	40
Bipolar II disorder	30	60

Note. Suicide attempters *N*=50.

Source. Adapted from Pallaskorpi et al. 2017.

Stress

Environmental stressors also appear to increase risk of death from suicide. Evidence continues to grow that incidences of childhood trauma and traumatic stress are frequent in the history of patients with BD and likely affect the clinical expression of the disorder and suicidal behaviors (Schaffer et al. 2015a, 2015b). The relationships between childhood trauma and BD suggest a multitude of interpretations, including neurodevelopmental consequences and intergenerational transmission of trauma. Increasing family dysfunction in multiple domains, including communication and problem solving, has also been associated with suicide attempts in BD (Berutti et al. 2016).

Acute Assessment of Suicide Risk in Bipolar Disorders

Unpredictability and variability of symptoms in BD make the assessment of suicide risk particularly challenging due to mood lability, intense emotional reactivity, impulsivity, inhibited behavioral control, and different levels of adherence to treatment.

Routine screenings of risk factors for death from suicide are essential steps to estimate and monitor suicide risk in BD. Although no standardized tools validated specifically for suicide risk assessment in BD are available, brief clinical interviewing can assess for risk factors specific to BDs.

Additionally, the Columbia Suicide Severity Rating Scale (C-SSRS) systematically assesses suicidal ideation in behavior and can detect suicidal behaviors that are subthreshold to actual suicide attempts (Interian et al. 2018). Although research is limited, studies have explored the utilization of the Concise Health Risk Tracking (CHRT) self-report to assess suicidal thoughts and behaviors in patients with BD. CHRT has been found to be highly correlated with other measures of suicidal thoughts and behaviors at baseline and a powerful predictor of suicide-related serious adverse events, thus indicating it could be a quick and robust self-report tool to assess suicidal risk (De La Garza et al. 2019).

Collecting information about protective factors in a collaborative manner for patients at risk of death from suicide is also important. Collaborative assessment and management of suicidal thoughts and behaviors has shown that the quality of the therapeutic relationship affects treatment retention and suicidal ideation. A stronger therapeutic alliance correlates with reduced suicidal ideation initially and at a 1-year follow-up (Bolton et al. 2015).

Case Example: Brief Assessment

A 24-year-old woman previously diagnosed with BDII presented to her primary care doctor for an annual wellness visit. She started the visit by asking to change her birth control pill; after several years of taking this medication, she felt that it was "making her crazy." She worried that she was on the verge of losing her job because she was reprimanded for "lashing out" verbally at a coworker, which had never happened before. She reported calling in sick to work frequently during the past month, after her partner of nearly a year broke up with her 2 months ago in a brief text message and then "ghosted" her, providing no explanation for the unforeseen and abrupt ending of the relationship.

Most days, she reported, she "cannot stop crying," has difficulty getting out of bed, and feels exhausted all the time. However, over the past week, she has felt the only way to cope with this hard time was to hit the mall for "retail therapy" that she cannot afford or to go out drinking with her friends. When asked about her alcohol use, she says that she is ordinarily not a big drinker, usually only having a glass or two of wine per month, but this week she has felt the need to "blow off steam" with friends at the bar, drinking four or five drinks during each outing. Upon questioning in a suicide risk assessment, the clinician elicited the information that the patient had been experiencing suicidal thoughts over the previous few days.

Mapping out symptoms and drawing timelines of episodes can be a useful way to structure a brief assessment of mood symptoms in patients in whom BD has been diagnosed or is suspected. Although suicidal ideation may be more diagnostically evident in entrenched depression, mania and hypomania symptoms also warrant risk assessment due to the impulsivity and energy that can prompt individuals to act on suicidal inclinations, particularly when patients are experiencing episodes of depression with mixed features as seen in this case example.

Patients with BD typically experience distinct mood states and alternate between depressive and manic/hypomanic episodes. In a mixed features episode, however,

TABLE 10–2.   **Recommendations for pharmacological management of acute mania**

First line	Monotherapy: lithium (Li), quetiapine, divalproex (DVP), asenapine, aripiprazole, paliperidone, risperidone, cariprazine
	Combination therapies with Li and DVP: quetiapine, aripiprazole, risperidone, asenapine
Second line	Combination therapies: olanzapine, carbamazepine, olanzapine + Li/DVP, Li + DVP, ziprasidone, haloperidol, electroconvulsive therapy
Third line	Carbamazepine/Oxcarbazepine + Li/DVP, chlorpromazine, clonazepam, clozapine, haloperidol + Li/DVP, tamoxifen, tamoxifen + Li/DVP
Not recommended	Allopurinol, eslicarbazepine, gabapentin, lamotrigine, omega-3 fatty acids, topiramate, valnoctamide, zonisamide

Source.   Adapted from Yatham et al. 2018.

depressive and manic/hypomanic symptoms co-occur. Mixed symptoms represent a more complex bipolar event and warrant routine suicide risk assessment. This presentation can be life threatening when symptoms of suicidal ideation, common during a depressive episode, are coupled with the impulsivity of hypomania/mania.

Treatments to Limit Suicide Risk in Patients With Bipolar Disorders

Psychopharmacological

Although research has continued to demonstrate the efficacy of a multitude of psychopharmacological treatments, clear, controlled prospective data for medication that specifically targets suicidal ideation and behaviors in BD and results in decreases in suicidal ideation and behaviors are not yet available. For a summary of medication recommendations for pharmacological management of acute mania, see Table 10–2.

Antidepressant Medications

Suicidal behaviors have been strongly associated with acute symptoms of depression, and antidepressants have been proven effective to varying degrees in treating depressive states in BD and in major depressive disorder with moderate severity and acute nonpsychotic symptoms (Undurraga and Baldessarini 2012). However, the value of antidepressant treatment in BD still remains a question, with inconsistent answers regarding efficacy and prophylactic effectiveness. Clinical experiences suggest effectiveness of antidepressants in short-term bipolar depression (Undurraga and Baldessarini 2012), but the efficacy of antidepressants for long-term nonacute depressive episodes and recurrences in BD remains uncertain.

Antidepressant medications are present in lethal levels in approximately 16% of people with BD who die from self-poisoning (Schaffer et al. 2017). Risk of dying from antidepressant medication overdose was once a major cause for concern in patients with BD and other psychiatric illnesses. The use of selective serotonin reuptake inhibitors (SSRIs) and other antidepressants instead of tricyclic antidepressants (TCAs) and monoamine oxidase inhibitors (MAOIs) has reduced risk of suicide from overdose (Undurraga and Baldessarini 2012). Relative to serotonin-norepinephrine reuptake inhibitors and SSRIs, TCAs and MAOIs are highly toxic and can be lethal in overdose (Valuck et al. 2016). Nevertheless, antidepressant effectiveness in directly lowering risk of death from suicide remains inconclusive in major depressive disorder and insufficient for bipolar depression (Undurraga and Baldessarini 2012).

In more vulnerable populations, antidepressant use can increase agitation, evoke adverse behavioral responses (e.g., insomnia and irritability), and even increase risk of impulsivity and suicidal behaviors (Undurraga and Baldessarini 2012). These possible adverse effects led the U.S. Food and Drug Administration (FDA) to include a black box warning requirement on the labels of all drugs used to treat depression. The addition of the black box warning impacted treatment adherence and led to inadequate dosing and duration of treatment for depressed patients (Undurraga and Baldessarini 2012). The fact that risk of suicide behavior is associated with more than simply a depressed mood could explain the relatively low benefit received from antidepressant treatments in individuals with suicidal thoughts and behaviors who have other, more prominent risk factors.

Lithium Salts

Lithium has demonstrated prophylactic efficacy in patients with BD for mood episodes and has the strongest evidence base for reduced suicide risks, attempts, and deaths than any other treatment of the disorder (Kleindienst and Greil 2003). Lithium likely reduces aggressive and impulsive behavior, including suicidal behavior, through enhancing functioning of central serotonin systems (Undurraga and Baldessarini 2012). The clinical use of lithium to reduce suicidal thoughts and behaviors may seem paradoxical, because lithium's therapeutic index margin of safety is limited and relatively small amounts can be extremely lethal in acute overdoses. Nevertheless, the choice of lithium as a means of self-poisoning suicide attempts is uncommon (Baldessarini et al. 2006). One meta-analysis examining the role of lithium in the prevention of suicide demonstrated that lithium is more effective than other treatments, including (but not limited to) fluoxetine, lamotrigine, olanzapine, and placebo, in reducing number of overall deaths from suicide and that lithium remains an effective long-term treatment for BD (Cipriani et al. 2013).

Anticonvulsant Agents

Antiepileptic or anticonvulsant drugs are frequently used in both the short-term and maintenance treatment of BD. One analysis indicated that anticonvulsant treatment was often initiated in response to suicide attempts in patients with BD but was not associated with increased risk of suicide attempts (Marcus et al. 2013). Several anticonvulsants have demonstrated efficacy for possible long-term mood-stabilizing effects that in turn deter emergence of suicidal symptoms in those with BD.

Antipsychotics

Recent treatment guidelines have included second-generation antipsychotics as a first-line treatment of BD both for depression and acute mania. Antipsychotic medications have short-term, acute antimanic effects in BD; their potential to impact suicide risk directly in the long term is still unknown. The FDA recently approved quetiapine as a first-line treatment of acute manic/mixed episodes in pediatric BD, and olanzapine and ziprasidone were approved as second-line treatments. Clozapine, a frequently prescribed antipsychotic, is not approved for use in the treatment of BD but is frequently prescribed "off-label" when other treatments have proven ineffective (Undurraga and Baldessarini 2012).

Combination Pharmacotherapy

In BD, pharmacological treatment typically involves two or more medications. The risk of developing side effects associated with any individual medication is increased by the addition of other medications. Second-generation antipsychotics have been associated with physical disorders including diabetes, obesity, thyroid disorders, cardiovascular disorders, musculoskeletal disorders, and renal diseases. Although higher dosages of medication, often prescribed for patients with suicidal ideation, have been associated with greater risk for the aforementioned conditions, many patients with more severe BD will be on two or more medications with positive life-changing effects.

Brain Stimulation Treatments

Electroconvulsive therapy is often used in treatment-resistant affective disorders and is often recommended for individuals who experience chronic suicidal ideation and behaviors. This intervention has been demonstrated to be effective in short-term treatment of severe mania and bipolar depression, but evidence has not yet demonstrated long-term protection against death from suicide in BD (Bolton et al. 2015).

Repetitive transcranial magnetic stimulation (TMS) is a noninvasive brain therapy with established efficacy for unipolar depression (George et al. 2010). TMS techniques continue to evolve and be refined. One study conducted in patients diagnosed with treatment-resistant BDs demonstrated that deep TMS is a potentially effective and tolerated adjunctive therapy (Tavares et al. 2017).

Psychosocial Interventions

Evidence-based psychosocial interventions specifically designed to target suicidal thoughts and behaviors in patients with BD currently are not available (Chesin and Stanley 2013). Notably, psychosocial interventions are not typically used to reduce suicidal thoughts and behaviors during a manic episode, which may require hospitalization due to the associated psychosis or impulsivity that defines mania. Rather, psychosocial treatments often target the depressive-episode symptoms present in both major depressive disorder and bipolar depression.

Dialectical behavior therapy (DBT) is an evidence-based treatment often used to stabilize life-threatening behaviors, increase distress tolerance, and manage suicidal thoughts (see Chapter 3, "Cognitive and Behavioral Therapy"). Specific suicide prevention and safety plans are necessary for suicidal patients in any treatment setting. One randomized controlled trial demonstrated that individuals with BD tend toward reduced depressive symptoms after 12 weeks of DBT psychoeducational groups (Van Dijk et al. 2013).

Conclusion

BD is highly prevalent, often severe, disabling, and potentially fatal. It is often characterized by cycles of major depressive and either manic or hypomanic episodes that may be separated by periods of euthymic mood. DSM-5 marked a shift in how BD is conceptualized, toward a spectrum of disorders characterized by distinct episodes of depressive and manic symptoms, with co-occurring symptoms from the opposite pole.

Key Points

- One half of patients with bipolar disorder (BD) are at risk for attempting suicide, and at least 15% will eventually die by suicide.

- Risk of death from suicide is highest in the early stages of BD.

- Mixed affective states, when depressive and manic symptoms co-occur, are often associated with higher risk of death from suicide.

- Patients with BD have high rates of substance use, anxiety disorders, impulsivity, lack of insight, and poor treatment adherence, all of which increase the risk of death from suicide.

- Most mood-altering medications and psychosocial therapies have little evidence of effectiveness in reducing long-term suicide risk in patients.

- Lithium has demonstrated efficacy in the treatment of BD and is supported by the strongest evidence base of reduced suicide risks, attempts, and deaths than any other treatment. It may have specific antisuicide effects in BD, but prospective data are still needed.

- Anticonvulsants are frequently used in short-term, acute, and maintenance treatment of BD. Modern antipsychotics have been included as a first-line treatment of BD for both depression and acute mania. Both anticonvulsants and modern antipsychotics are widely employed in treatment, but their potential to influence suicide risk requires further study.

References

Altshuler LL, Kupka RW, Hellemann G, et al: Gender and depressive symptoms in 711 patients with bipolar disorder evaluated prospectively in the Stanley Foundation bipolar treatment outcome network. Am J Psychiatry 167(6):708–715, 2010 20231325

American Psychiatric Association: Diagnostic and Statistical Manual of Mental Disorders, 4th Edition. Washington, DC, American Psychiatric Association, 1994

American Psychiatric Association: Diagnostic and Statistical Manual of Mental Disorders, 5th Edition. Arlington, VA, American Psychiatric Association, 2013

Angst J, Gamma A, Bowden CL, et al: Diagnostic criteria for bipolarity based on an international sample of 5,635 patients with DSM-IV major depressive episodes. Eur Arch Psychiatry Clin Neurosci 262(1):3–11, 2012 21818629

Baldessarini RJ, Tondo L, Davis P, et al: Decreased risk of suicides and attempts during long-term lithium treatment: a meta-analytic review. Bipolar Disord 8(5 Pt 2):625–639, 2006 17042835

Berutti M, Dias RS, Pereira VA, et al: Association between history of suicide attempts and family functioning in bipolar disorder. J Affect Disord 192:28–33, 2016 26706829

Betzler F, Stöver LA, Sterzer P, et al: Mixed states in bipolar disorder: changes in DSM-5 and current treatment recommendations. Int J Psychiatry Clin Pract 21(4):244–258, 2017 28417647

Bolton JM, Gunnell D, Turecki G: Suicide risk assessment and intervention in people with mental illness. BMJ 351:h4978, 2015 26552947

Chesin M, Stanley B: Risk assessment and psychosocial interventions for suicidal patients. Bipolar Disord 15(5):584–593, 2013 23782460

Cipriani A, Hawton K, Stockton S, et al: Lithium in the prevention of suicide in mood disorders: updated systematic review and meta-analysis. BMJ 346:f3646, 2013 23814104

De La Garza N, Rush AJ, Killian MO, et al: The Concise Health Risk Tracking Self-Report (CHRT-SR) assessment of suicidality in depressed outpatients: a psychometric evaluation. Depress Anxiety 36(4):313–320, 2019 30370613

George MS, Lisanby SH, Avery D, et al: Daily left prefrontal transcranial magnetic stimulation therapy for major depressive disorder: a sham-controlled randomized trial. Arch Gen Psychiatry 67(5):507–516, 2010 20439832

Goes FS: The importance of anxiety states in bipolar disorder. Curr Psychiatry Rep 17(2):3, 2015 25617037

Interian A, Chesin M, Kline A, et al: Use of the Columbia-Suicide Severity Rating Scale (C-SSRS) to classify suicidal behaviors. Arch Suicide Res 22(2):278–294, 2018 28598723

Karanti A, Bobeck C, Osterman M, et al: Gender differences in the treatment of patients with bipolar disorder: a study of 7354 patients. J Affect Disord 174:303–309, 2015 25532077

Kleindienst N, Greil W: Lithium in the long-term treatment of bipolar disorders. Eur Arch Psychiatry Clin Neurosci 253(3):120–125, 2003 12904975

Marcus SM, Lu B, Lim S, et al: Suicide attempts in patients with bipolar disorder tend to precede, not follow, initiation of antiepileptic drugs. J Clin Psychiatry 74(6):630–631, 2013 23842016

McGuffin P, Perroud N, Uher R, et al: The genetics of affective disorder and suicide. Eur Psychiatry 25(5):275–277, 2010 20462744

Ösby U, Brandt L, Correia N, et al: Excess mortality in bipolar and unipolar disorder in Sweden. Arch Gen Psychiatry 58(9):844–850, 2001 11545667

Pallaskorpi S, Suominen K, Ketokivi M, et al: Incidence and predictors of suicide attempts in bipolar I and II disorders: a 5-year follow-up study. Bipolar Disord 19(1):13–22, 2017 28176421

Pompili M, Rihmer Z, Innamorati M, et al: Assessment and treatment of suicide risk in bipolar disorders. Expert Rev Neurother 9(1):109–136, 2009 19102673

Schaffer A, Isometsä ET, Azorin JM, et al: A review of factors associated with greater likelihood of suicide attempts and suicide deaths in bipolar disorder: part II of a report of the International Society for Bipolar Disorders Task Force on Suicide in Bipolar Disorder. Aust N Z J Psychiatry 49(11):1006–1020, 2015a 26175498

Schaffer A, Isometsä ET, Tondo L, et al: International Society for Bipolar Disorders Task Force on Suicide: meta-analyses and meta-regression of correlates of suicide attempts and suicide deaths in bipolar disorder. Bipolar Disord 17(1):1–16, 2015b 25329791

Schaffer A, Weinstock LM, Sinyor M, et al: Self-poisoning suicide deaths in people with bipolar disorder: characterizing a subgroup and identifying treatment patterns. Int J Bipolar Disord 5(1):16, 2017 28332123

Tavares DF, Myczkowski ML, Alberto RL, et al: Treatment of bipolar depression with deep TMS: results from a double-blind, randomized, parallel group, sham-controlled clinical trial. Neuropsychopharmacology 42(13):2593–2601, 2017 28145409

Tondo L, Pompili M, Forte A, et al: Suicide attempts in bipolar disorders: comprehensive review of 101 reports. Acta Psychiatr Scand 133(3):174–186, 2016 26555604

Turecki G: Suicidal behavior: is there a genetic predisposition? Bipolar Disord 3(6):335–349, 2001 11843783

Undurraga J, Baldessarini RJ: Randomized, placebo-controlled trials of antidepressants for acute major depression: thirty-year meta-analytic review. Neuropsychopharmacology 37(4):851–864, 2012 22169941

Valuck RJ, Libby AM, Anderson HD, et al: Comparison of antidepressant classes and the risk and time course of suicide attempts in adults: propensity matched, retrospective cohort study. Br J Psychiatry 208(3):271–279, 2016 26635328

Van Dijk S, Jeffrey J, Katz MR: A randomized, controlled, pilot study of dialectical behavior therapy skills in a psychoeducational group for individuals with bipolar disorder. J Affect Disord 145(3):386–393, 2013 22858264

Wilcox HC, Fullerton JM, Glowinski AL, et al: Traumatic stress interacts with bipolar disorder genetic risk to increase risk for suicide attempts. J Am Acad Child Adolesc Psychiatry 56(12):1073–1080, 2017 29173741

Yatham LN, Kennedy SH, Parikh SV, et al: Canadian Network for Mood and Anxiety Treatments (CANMAT) and International Society for Bipolar Disorders (ISBD) 2018 guidelines for the management of patients with bipolar disorder. Bipolar Disord 20(2):97–170, 2018 29536616

CHAPTER 11

Schizophrenia and Other Psychotic Disorders

Kimberly Brandt, D.O.

Lindsey Schrimpf, M.D.

John Lauriello, M.D.

Suicide in patients with schizophrenia and other psychotic disorders can be a medical and societal challenge. Clinicians should be well versed in its detection and management. The literature has consistently demonstrated that the prevalence and frequency of suicide attempts in patients with schizophrenia are significantly higher than those of the general population. An estimated 4%–10% of this population will die from suicide and 25%–50% will make suicide attempts in their lifetime (Balhara and Verma 2012).

Our goal in this chapter is to demonstrate the assessment of suicide risk factors and treatment strategies in schizophrenia and other psychotic disorders by presenting two case studies that will guide the clinician through management of these complex disorders. After each case is a discussion of the important considerations to appropriately treat patients, adequately assess their suicide risk factors, and reduce these risk factors when possible. Following the case examples, we discuss the underlying psychopathology and recommended treatment options.

Epidemiology of Suicide in Schizophrenia and Psychotic Disorders

Much of the basic assessment and management of suicidal thoughts and behaviors in patients with schizophrenia is analogous to the management of these in other psychiatric conditions. Many risk factors increasing suicide risk in schizophrenia or other psychotic disorders mirror the risks found in the general population, such as previous

TABLE 11–1.   **Risk factors associated with suicide in schizophrenia**

Nonmodifiable	Modifiable
History of suicide attempt	Depressed mood/Depression
Male sex	Hopelessness
Younger age	Social isolation
Close to illness onset	Unemployment
Older age at illness onset	Limited external support
White race	Substance misuse or dependence
Family history of suicide	Deteriorating health with good premorbid functioning
Recent loss or rejection	
Childhood parental loss	Severe residual symptoms and impairment at hospital discharge
Chronic illness with numerous exacerbations	Realistic awareness of illness
	Fear of further deterioration
	Excessive treatment dependence or loss of faith in treatment
	Family stress

Source.   Balhara and Verma 2012; Popovic et al. 2014.

suicide attempts, comorbid depression, comorbid substance abuse, and male gender (Hawton et al. 2005; Limosin et al. 2007). However, certain risk factors are unique to schizophrenia and deserve special consideration while treating this patient population. These risk factors are listed in Table 11–1.

In psychotic disorders, suicide attempts are associated with substance abuse and severe depressive symptoms as well as physical violence against others (Suokas et al. 2010). Although the body of literature investigating suicidal thoughts and behaviors in psychotic disorders other than schizophrenia is less robust, it provides evidence that patients with brief psychotic disorder, delusional disorder, substance-induced psychotic disorders, and catatonia also have increased risk of suicidal ideation and behaviors (Castagnini and Bertelsen 2011; González-Rodríguez et al. 2014; Kleinhaus et al. 2012; Zarrabi et al. 2016).

Although the course of brief psychotic disorder is time limited and the prognosis is generally favorable, the risk of suicidal behavior in these individuals is high and should not be overlooked. Acute stress and substance use are significantly associated with suicidal behavior in patients who are diagnosed with acute transient psychotic disorder (ATPD), a diagnosis found in ICD-10 (López-Díaz et al. 2018). ATPD is similar to brief psychotic disorder, with some difference in onset, duration, and symptom criteria. Individuals with ATPD have been shown to have a 30.9% increased risk of death from suicide compared with the general population (Castagnini and Bertelsen 2011).

Historically, studies have not shown an increased risk of death from suicide in delusional disorder; however, a 2014 study found that 8%–21% of patients with delusional disorder exhibit suicidal behavior, with suicide attempts being more frequent in those with persecutory and somatic type delusions (Castagnini and Bertelsen 2011; González-Rodríguez et al. 2014). Substance-induced psychotic disorders have also been shown to have increased risk of suicidal thoughts and behaviors (Castagnini and Bertelsen 2011). Stimulant abuse, especially methamphetamine, can increase risk of violence, suicidal behavior, and fatal suicide attempts (Zarrabi et al. 2016).

Within the schizophrenia and psychosis spectrum, patients who have experienced catatonia have been shown in a cohort prospective study to have significantly elevated risk of future suicide attempts, with 44% attempting suicide in catatonic schizophrenia compared to 25% in other schizophrenia subtypes (pre DSM-5) (American Psychiatric Association 2013; Kleinhaus et al. 2012). Another prospective follow-up study demonstrated that adolescents who experienced catatonia had a 60-fold increased risk of premature death, including death from suicide, when compared with those of the same age and sex in the general population (Cornic et al. 2009).

Case Example 1: New-Onset Schizophrenia

J.B., a medically healthy, 19-year-old Caucasian male with no previous psychiatric history, was one of three children from an upper-middle-class family. His parents were both professionally accomplished and did not have mental health problems. At age 15, his mother developed breast cancer and died.

J.B. finished high school with honors and was admitted to a prestigious university to study engineering. Halfway through his freshman year, he started developing symptoms of depression. His mood was low, he was having difficulty focusing on his studies, he spent a significant amount of time sleeping, and he was not engaging socially. By the end of his freshman year his grade point average had dropped from 3.8 to 2.5. Over the summer, his family insisted he seek treatment for depression, and he was started on an antidepressant. He did somewhat better during the first semester of his sophomore year but then quickly deteriorated during second semester.

During his second semester, J.B.'s depression increased, and he started developing symptoms of paranoia. He believed his teachers were trying to make him fail his classes and his peers were intent on preventing him from succeeding. He was increasingly reclusive and stopped going to class. Peers in the dormitory observed him talking to himself. He had multiple instances of aggression with peers due to paranoia. J.B.'s sister came to visit and check on him and found his room covered with writings and drawings that were hard to understand but generally consisted of plans to expose a government conspiracy he had discovered.

J.B. reluctantly agreed to psychiatric admission after long conversations with his family. He was able to admit at one point that maybe his beliefs were not real and that he might need treatment. He improved quickly with antipsychotic medication while in the hospital and was discharged home to the care of his family.

J.B. returned to school in the fall and again deteriorated quickly. He completely stopped his medications and became very psychotic. He was admitted to the psychiatric hospital after threatening the life of one of his dormitory mates. This hospitalization did not go as smoothly as the first and required involuntary administration of medication. Although his psychosis resolved, he became very depressed.

J.B. was able to be discharged and was compliant with his medication but spoke occasionally about being "crazy" and expressed frustration with his medication and the side effects he experienced. However, he was able to return to college and complete the semester with passing grades. He had started to engage a little socially and seemed to be doing better. Over semester break, his family was encouraged that he was taking his medication and had been able to complete the semester. Then, one morning, he did not come out of his room. When family went to check on him, he had hanged himself in his closet.

This case involving first-episode schizophrenia and episodes of depression highlights a number of factors involved in increased suicide risk in the psychotic disorders patient population. As mentioned previously, patients with schizophrenia spectrum disorders are at higher risk of death from suicide. In addition to the risk associated with a psychotic disorder diagnosis, this patient's risk was heightened by the fact that he was experiencing a first episode of psychosis. First-episode psychosis patients demonstrate a three times higher risk of death from suicide compared with patients with chronic psychosis (Ventriglio et al. 2016).

Many studies have investigated the risk factors involved with the increased risk of suicide for first-episode psychosis. In a clinical study by Barrett et al. (2015), predictors of suicide in first-episode psychosis included longer durations of untreated psychosis, more depressive episodes prior to diagnosis, depression at 1-year follow-up, and more suicide attempts during the 6 months prior to 1-year follow-up. J.B. did not have a history of prior suicide attempts, but he did have a history of depression before his first episode of psychosis and during his treatment, which increased his risk.

Like so many patients with psychotic disorders, J.B. quickly became nonadherent with his medications after his first episode of psychosis resolved. He likely had a 4- to 5-month period of untreated symptoms (both depression and psychosis) that resulted in a much more severe psychosis that was then followed by a much more severe depression. He had also experienced a childhood trauma (the death of his mother), which can place the patient at increased risk for depression and development of psychosis (Barrett et al. 2015). In a systematic review by Hawton et al. (2005), additional risk factors for suicide in first-episode psychosis included drug misuse, agitation and motor restlessness, fear of mental disintegration, poor adherence to treatment, and recent loss (see also Nordentoft et al. 2015).

Insight into illness has long been a consideration with regard to suicide risk in psychotic disorder patients. Drake and Cotton (1986) described the "demoralization syndrome," where insight is related to increased suicide risk in patients with chronic schizophrenia. Patients who develop good insight into having a psychotic illness and who begin to realize the consequences of this illness can become demoralized, placing them at higher risk for death from suicide. Every psychiatrist has had patients worry about being "crazy." For patients with psychotic illness, the weight of the realization that they may struggle with symptoms of psychosis for the rest of their lives can make them feel dysphoric and demoralized. J.B. came from an upper socioeconomic background and was academically accomplished, but his psychosis severely impacted his academic and personal success. J.B.'s family may have been happy that he passed his classes and was engaging socially, but he may have felt despair over being unable to achieve his previous academic capabilities and social success.

More recent research has revealed a mixed relationship between insight and suicide risk, with some studies reporting that insight decreases suicide risk and others continuing to show that insight increases suicide risk. A 3-year follow-up study showed a dynamic time-related relationship between insight and suicide risk, with multiple explanations for this relationship being offered (Ayesa-Arriola et al. 2018). Barrett et al. (2015) found that insight at baseline (i.e., at beginning of treatment) increased the risk for suicidal thoughts and behaviors, but insight at 1-year follow-up decreased risk. J.B. expressed insight into his illness early in treatment, which increased his risk for death from suicide.

Despite his illness, J.B. continued attending college, reflecting that he had relatively high cognitive levels of functioning. Patients experiencing fewer cognitive deficits in first-episode schizophrenia have been found to be more depressed and have increased suicidal ideation, while in one study disruption in white matter integrity on neuroimaging was associated with greater cognitive deficits and comparatively less suicidal ideation (Long et al. 2018). Cognitive deficits can result in difficulty with executive functioning; therefore, individuals with severe cognitive impairment and disorganization of thinking may lack the ability to adequately plan and follow through with suicide.

Early interventions that involve the family can dramatically improve risk for death from suicide and overall patient outcomes. In a review by Mueser et al. (2013), family psychoeducation was found to have the best body of data supporting its effectiveness. Effective family psychoeducation was long term (9–24 months), was delivered by a mental health professional, focused on the whole family, educated the family about schizophrenia and treatment, taught strategies to reduce stress and improve communication and problem solving, and involved looking toward the future rather than delving into the past. J.B.'s family was supportive, but even they might have benefited from a family education.

In a patient like J.B., screening for suicide regularly and assessing for depression are essential. Patients who are intent on suicide often do not report their suicidal feelings without prompting. At least two validated screens for suicide assessment in the psychotic disorders population are available: the Columbia Suicide Severity Rating Scale (C-SSRS; Posner et al. 2011) and the International Suicide Prevention Trial (InterSePT) Scale for Suicidal Thinking (ISST; Lindenmayer et al. 2003).

Assessment of depression in schizophrenia or other psychotic disorders can be difficult because affective blunting and negative symptoms of psychosis can mask or hide the symptoms of depression. Depressive symptoms have a prevalence ranging from 25% to 81% among people with schizophrenia, and the presence of depression or depressive symptoms (particularly hopelessness, worthlessness, and pessimism) is associated with increased risk of suicidal thoughts and behaviors in this population (Balhara and Verma 2012). Typical depression screens such as the Beck Depression Inventory or the Hamilton Rating Scale for Depression have difficulty distinguishing between negative symptoms of schizophrenia and depression as well as difficulty distinguishing between depression and extrapyramidal symptoms from antipsychotic treatment (Kim et al. 2006). The Calgary Depression Scale for Schizophrenia was created to address these concerns and has been validated in multiple studies (Kim et al. 2006).

Case Example 2: Elevated Suicide Risk in a Patient With Chronic Schizophrenia and Comorbid Substance Abuse

T.W. is a 33-year-old single male who was diagnosed with schizophrenia at age 20. He has experienced fragmented psychiatric care, with brief periods of antipsychotic medication treatment on both an inpatient and outpatient basis. T.W. always struggled to find a psychiatrist whom he trusted and never formed an adequate therapeutic alliance with an outpatient treatment provider. He was often without ongoing psychiatric care. His illness was exacerbated by his inability to abstain from using methamphetamine, which started at age 23.

During periods when he took his prescribed medication and abstained from abusing methamphetamine, T.W. could hold a job and obtain housing. However, if he stopped his antipsychotic medication or began to use methamphetamine, he quickly deterio-rated and would lose his job and shelter. T.W.'s family, who had helped support him earlier in his adult life, had grown increasingly frustrated with his substance abuse and inability to hold down a job. Without a network of stable support, T.W. became home-less, frequently abusing methamphetamine.

T.W. brought himself to the emergency department reporting strong suicidal urges to jump off a bridge to his death. He reported derogatory auditory hallucinations con-stantly telling him to kill himself in violent ways. He reported he had been using meth-amphetamine heavily and had become increasingly depressed since his last use of methamphetamine 3 days ago. On examination, T.W. appeared disheveled, under-weight, withdrawn, and guarded. He exhibited psychomotor slowing and poverty of speech. His urine toxicology was positive for amphetamines. T.W. had a history of two prior suicide attempts: one via walking in traffic on a busy highway and one via an at-tempted hanging.

T.W. was involuntarily hospitalized for psychiatric evaluation and admitted to the inpatient psychiatric unit. The staff at the emergency department and the inpatient unit were very familiar with T.W. due to his frequent emergency visits and inpatient admis-sions due to his methamphetamine abuse, psychosis, depressed mood, and suicidal thoughts and behaviors. The staff tended to have strong negative feelings about T.W. because of his frequent admissions, continued drug abuse, and treatment noncompli-ance. Staff members accused him of "abusing the system" because he was homeless; they would assert that treating T.W. was futile because he continued to be readmitted for the same reason, and they often suggested a quick discharge.

T.W. expressed ambivalence about his hospital admission. In the past, T.W. had been open to receiving treatment with antipsychotic medication, but during this admission he was paranoid, defiant, oppositional, and refused to take the medication. He believed the psychiatrist was trying to control his mind with neuroleptics and that his family was forcing the psychiatrist to prescribe medication. At baseline, T.W. experienced au-ditory hallucinations and had frequent persecutory delusions but did not exhibit disor-ganization of thought or speech. He exhibited hostility toward others, especially those in a position of authority; however, he did not have a history of violence toward others. He continued to report suicidal ideation with a plan to jump off a bridge or jump in front of traffic.

The psychiatrist petitioned for a hearing to detain T.W. for additional time for invol-untary treatment. The petition was granted, and the psychiatrist decided to start T.W. on a second-generation long-acting injectable antipsychotic (SGA-LAI) to ensure treat-ment compliance. T.W. had taken the same atypical antipsychotic in its oral form during his last inpatient hospitalization, and this medication had adequately treated his psy-chotic symptoms without significant side effects. T.W. tolerated the injection well, and his symptoms diminished greatly after several days. On discharge, he was referred to an intensive community outpatient case management program that provided him with a psychiatrist, therapist, case manager, dual diagnosis treatment, and monthly visits with a nurse for administration of the SGA-LAI.

The case of T.W. illustrates important factors in assessing and treating suicidal thoughts and behaviors in a patient with a well-established diagnosis of schizophre-nia who also has comorbid substance abuse. For any patient, the expression of sui-cidal thoughts and behaviors can have multiple layers of meaning and intent. In the case of T.W., expression of suicidal thoughts and behaviors could be the means to temporarily obtain food and shelter, or it might be a primitive way for T.W. to express anger toward himself and others and his own uncertainty about his life.

Regardless of all the possible meanings behind his suicidal thoughts and behaviors, T.W. is clearly at high risk for death from suicide. He is male, single, abusing drugs, poorly compliant with psychotropic medication, and poorly compliant with outpatient treatment and has very limited social support. His frequent inpatient admissions, limited cooperation, and multiple psychosocial problems make treating him extremely frustrating. However, T.W.'s risk for death from suicide due to negative countertransference among the hospital staff should not be minimized. It can be helpful to use clinical rating scales in these situations, including the C-SSRS and the ISST.

T.W.'s intermittent use of illicit stimulants compounds his problems. Multiple studies have documented that comorbid substance abuse is a risk factor for death from suicide in schizophrenia (Balhara and Verma 2012; Suokas et al. 2010). The rate of substance abuse among people with schizophrenia remains very high: up to 50% use illicit drugs or alcohol and up to 70% use nicotine. Individuals who are acutely intoxicated are at high risk of death from suicide because of impaired judgment and increased impulsivity.

Psychostimulants such as cocaine or amphetamine increase suicide risk during acute intoxication and additionally during the acute withdrawal phase. Individuals who abuse psychostimulants often experience a severe withdrawal dysphoria and depressive syndrome after a period of regular psychostimulant intake, consisting of psychomotor slowing, increased sleep, and increased suicidal ideation (Kosten 2002). Given the high prevalence of comorbid substance abuse in this patient population and the increased risk of suicidal thoughts and behaviors with substance abuse, concurrent treatment for both psychotic disorders and substance use is essential.

Patients experiencing psychotic disorders, including schizophrenia, are also more likely to die from more violent means of suicide, such as jumping off a building, from a bridge, or in front of moving vehicles (Sinyor et al. 2015) as T.W. ideated. These patients more often have impulsive and aggressive traits, and their suicidal thoughts and behaviors may be provoked more by the symptoms of their mental illness than acute life stressors. In an observational study of coroner reports in Toronto in 2015, 55.8% of the patients with schizophrenia who died from suicide did so by jumping from a height or in front of vehicles (Sinyor et al. 2015). In addition, the group of patients with schizophrenia left fewer suicide notes, possibly indicating a diminished capacity to plan or write a note or increased impulsivity of the suicide. A study in Australia and New Zealand in 2010 showed 44% of survivors who attempted suicide by jumping from a distance of more than 3 meters were diagnosed with a psychotic illness (Nielssen et al. 2010). One in five of these survivors was experiencing an undiagnosed and untreated psychotic illness.

T.W. would have greatly benefited from early intervention and treatment of schizophrenia and the establishment of a trusting and collaborative relationship with a psychiatrist and the mental health system. T.W. expressed hostility toward his psychiatrist and mistrust of mental health workers and authority figures. Because T.W. does not connect with nor trust health care providers, unraveling a longstanding maladaptive pattern of behavior and helping him establish therapeutic connections present difficult challenges. More aggressive and earlier treatment of his paranoid delusions might have helped him establish healthier relationships in the medical system. A meta-analysis has shown that poor treatment compliance is associated with poor therapeutic alliance and insufficient discharge planning (Lacro et al. 2002). A multidisciplinary treatment approach that addresses social, behavioral, psychological, and psychoeducational needs of the patient early in the course of schizophrenia can improve treatment adherence (Dolder et al. 2003).

Underlying Psychopathology

A variety of possible pathologies may contribute to increased suicide risk in schizophrenia. The serotonin neurotransmitter system has been studied for possible implications in suicidal thoughts and behaviors in schizophrenia. Individuals with schizophrenia who die from suicide have a significantly lower concentration of 5-hydroxyindoleacetic acid, a serotonin metabolite, in their cerebrospinal fluid (Balhara and Verma 2012). Neuroimaging studies of patients with schizophrenia and patients who attempt suicide also show volumetric abnormalities in the limbic system (Balhara and Verma 2012). Hyperactivity among the hypothalamic-pituitary-adrenal axis resulting in glucocorticoid toxicity is hypothesized as a possible mechanism for neuroimaging abnormalities in patients with schizophrenia who have attempted suicide, and abnormal dexamethasone suppression tests have also been reported (Balhara and Verma 2012). Genetic polymorphisms also have been implicated as a possible association for suicidal thoughts and behaviors in patients with schizophrenia; however, subsequent research has not shown an association between polygenetic scores in suicide attempters compared with nonattempters with schizophrenia (Balhara and Verma 2012; Bani-Fatemi et al. 2019).

Treatment

Psychotherapeutic interventions for patients with schizophrenia who have suicidal behavior are not well studied. A recent study focusing on the role of social cognition and short-term prediction of suicidal ideation in schizophrenia found links between coexisting suicidal ideation and negative attribution biases, increased reactivity to negative stimuli, and augmented accuracy in recognition of negative affect versus positive affect. Depressive symptoms influenced social cognitive bias toward negative interpretation of interpersonal scenarios and negative stimuli. Further study may demonstrate that therapies aimed at interventions in social cognition may have a role in suicide prevention in patients with schizophrenia (Depp et al. 2018).

The role of antipsychotic medications and suicidal thoughts and behaviors in patients with schizophrenia has been more robustly studied compared to other interventions. Typical or first-generation antipsychotics such as haloperidol, at high dosages, may be responsible for blocking the function of the reward circuitry in the brain due to high levels of D_2 antagonism. This effect may cause patients to develop negative symptoms or cause negative symptoms to worsen in patients already experiencing them. There may be a therapeutic window of optimal D_2 receptor occupancy where the antipsychotic efficacy and dysphoric side effects are balanced (de Haan et al. 2000).

Antipsychotics are known to have significant side effects that may cause patients to discontinue them. Akathisia is one of the most common but underdiagnosed or misdiagnosed side effects associated with antipsychotics. Akathisia has been associated with poor medication adherence, exacerbation of psychiatric symptoms and agitation, aggression, violence, and suicidal ideation and behaviors (Lohr et al. 2015). A nested case control study in Sweden found lower suicide risk in patients with schizophrenia and a history of extrapyramidal symptoms and found no significant association between akathisia and suicide risk (Reutfors et al. 2016).

The atypical or second-generation antipsychotics have lower affinity for the D_2 receptor and more effects on the serotonin system and appear to better preserve the function of the neural reward circuitry. An abundance of research is available regarding the use of atypical antipsychotics in the treatment of depression. A meta-analysis showed efficacy of olanzapine, risperidone, quetiapine, and aripiprazole when each agent was used to augment an antidepressant medication (Nelson and Papakostas 2009). The American Psychiatric Association's *Practice Guideline for the Treatment of Schizoaffective Disorder and Schizophrenia With Mood Symptoms* (Lehman et al. 2004) recommends the use of atypical antipsychotics for the treatment of depression in schizophrenia.

Clozapine is well established to be associated with reduction in suicidal thoughts and behaviors for patients with schizophrenia. The InterSePT demonstrated clozapine to have superior efficacy compared to olanzapine in reduction of suicidal behavior in schizophrenia (Meltzer et al. 2003). Additionally, a case series study has documented that patients with schizophrenia died from suicide after abrupt discontinuation of clozapine treatment, and increased rates of suicide attempts have been reported with discontinuation of olanzapine and risperidone (Patchan et al. 2015; Pompili et al. 2016).

Emerging evidence indicates that other atypical antipsychotics, including olanzapine, quetiapine, ziprasidone, aripiprazole, and asenapine, may also possess antisuicidal properties, but they have not yet been adequately studied for this purpose (Lehman et al. 2004). Aripiprazole and brexpiprazole have unique receptor profiles when compared with the other atypical antipsychotics. They have partial agonist activity at the D_2 receptor, partial agonist activity at 5-HT_{1A}, and antagonist activity at 5-HT_{2A}. The activity at 5-HT receptors is likely responsible for the antidepressant property of these medications (Jordan et al. 2004). Currently, the atypical antipsychotics approved by the U.S. Food and Drug Administration for adjunctive treatment in major depressive disorder are aripiprazole, quetiapine, olanzapine-fluoxetine combination, and brexpiprazole.

LAIs can increase engagement with mental health services, improve compliance and treatment adherence, and may indirectly help improve insight and awareness of illness. LAIs may also decrease suicidal thoughts and behaviors by indirectly modifying risk factors for death from suicide in patients with schizophrenia. LAIs have been shown to reduce the risk of relapses in patients with schizophrenia, and regular contacts with health care professionals administering the injection may also aid in reducing suicide risk (Pompili et al. 2017). A study investigating the benefits of using SGA-LAIs in newly diagnosed patients with schizophrenia showed decreased severity and intensity of suicidal ideation, but reduction of suicidal thoughts and behaviors was not seen in the long-term patients with schizophrenia (Corigliano et al. 2018). LAIs may play a role in improving illness and outcomes, and early intervention appears to be important for every aspect of treatment in schizophrenia.

Conclusion

Patients with schizophrenia and other psychotic disorders are at increased risk of death from suicide. Many of the risk factors for death from suicide in patients with schizophrenia and other psychotic disorders are similar to those for patients with many other psychiatric diagnoses. However, some risk factors, both modifiable and nonmodifiable, are unique to this specific patient population. When treating this challenging population to reduce the risk of death from suicide, clinicians face many complexities and challenges. These require consideration of all aspects of multidisciplinary care to effectively treat patients with schizophrenia and psychotic disorders using the best evidence-based practices to help improve patient outcomes and decrease risk of suicidal thoughts and behaviors.

Key Points

- Patients with schizophrenia and other psychotic disorders have a high risk of suicidal thoughts and behaviors.

- The first few years after diagnosis represent a high-risk period of time for suicidal thoughts and behaviors.

- The presence of depression, substance abuse, higher cognitive ability, awareness of the loss of function inflicted by the illness, and difficulty accepting a decline in functioning and status are illness-specific risk factors for suicidal thoughts and behaviors.

- Detecting depression in schizophrenia is a clinical challenge due to the overlap in clinical presentation of negative symptoms. Validated suicide rating scales can aid in diagnosis.

- Early intervention can minimize duration and severity of psychosis and establish a nonadversarial alliance with the medical system to improve engagement and treatment compliance.

- Clozapine is the only medication treatment approved by the U.S. Food and Drug Administration to reduce suicidal ideation and behaviors in schizophrenia. Other antipsychotics may have a role, but additional research is needed.

- Treatment should use the lowest effective dosages of antipsychotics to minimize dopamine D_2 receptor blockade and reduce the risk of side effects. Psychiatrists should consider long-acting injectable antipsychotics, which may indirectly reduce multiple suicide risk factors.

- A multidisciplinary approach with frequent patient contact on an outpatient basis can decrease modifiable suicide risk factors.

References

American Psychiatric Association: Diagnostic and Statistical Manual of Mental Disorders, 5th Edition. Arlington, VA, American Psychiatric Association, 2013

Ayesa-Arriola R, Terán JMP, Moríñigo JDL, et al: The dynamic relationship between insight and suicidal behavior in first episode psychosis patients over 3-year follow-up. Eur Neuropsychopharmacol 28(10):1161–1172, 2018 30097249

Balhara YP, Verma R: Schizophrenia and suicide. East Asian Arch Psychiatry 22(3):126–133, 2012 23019287

Bani-Fatemi A, Tasmim S, Wang KZ, et al: No interaction between polygenic scores and childhood trauma in predicting suicide attempt in schizophrenia. Prog Neuropsychopharmacol Biol Psychiatry 89:169–173, 2019 30149093

Barrett EA, Mork E, Færden A, et al: The development of insight and its relationship with suicidality over one year follow-up in patients with first episode psychosis. Schizophr Res 162(1-3):97–102, 2015 25620119

Castagnini AC, Bertelsen A: Mortality and causes of death of acute and transient psychotic disorders. Soc Psychiatry Psychiatr Epidemiol 46(10):1013–1017, 2011 20697690

Corigliano V, Comparelli A, Mancinelli I, et al: Long-acting injectable second-generation antipsychotics improve negative symptoms and suicidal ideation in recent diagnosed schizophrenia patients: a 1-year follow-up pilot study. Schizophr Res Treatment 2018:4834135, 2018 30245878

Cornic F, Consoli A, Tanguy ML, et al: Association of adolescent catatonia with increased mortality and morbidity: evidence from a prospective follow-up study. Schizophr Res 113(2–3):233–240, 2009 19443182

de Haan L, Lavalaye J, Linszen D, et al: Subjective experience and striatal dopamine D(2) receptor occupancy in patients with schizophrenia stabilized by olanzapine or risperidone. Am J Psychiatry 157(6):1019–1020, 2000 10831489

Depp CA, Villa J, Schembari BC, et al: Social cognition and short-term prediction of suicidal ideation in schizophrenia. Psychiatry Res 270:13–19, 2018 30243127

Dolder CR, Lacro JP, Leckband S, et al: Interventions to improve antipsychotic medication adherence: review of recent literature. J Clin Psychopharmacol 23(4):389–399, 2003 12920416

Drake RE, Cotton PG: Depression, hopelessness and suicide in chronic schizophrenia. Br J Psychiatry 148:554–559, 1986 3779226

González-Rodríguez A, Molina-Andreu O, Navarro Odriozola V, et al: Suicidal ideation and suicidal behaviour in delusional disorder: a clinical overview. Psychiatry J 2014:834901, 2014 24829903

Hawton K, Sutton L, Haw C, et al: Schizophrenia and suicide: systematic review of risk factors. Br J Psychiatry 187:9–20, 2005 15994566

Jordan S, Koprivica V, Dunn R, et al: In vivo effects of aripiprazole on cortical and striatal dopaminergic and serotonergic function. Eur J Pharmacol 483(1):45–53, 2004 14709325

Kim SW, Kim SJ, Yoon BH, et al: Diagnostic validity of assessment scales for depression in patients with schizophrenia. Psychiatry Res 144(1):57–63, 2006 16904189

Kleinhaus K, Harlap S, Perrin MC, et al: Catatonic schizophrenia: a cohort prospective study. Schizophr Bull 38(2):331–337, 2012 20693343

Kosten TR: Pathophysiology and treatment of cocaine dependence, in Neuropsychopharmacology: The Fifth Generation of Progress. Edited by Davis K, Charney D, Coyle JT, et al. Baltimore, MD, Lippincott Williams and Wilkins, 2002, pp 1461–1473

Lacro JP, Dunn LB, Dolder CR, et al: Prevalence of and risk factors for medication nonadherence in patients with schizophrenia: a comprehensive review of recent literature. J Clin Psychiatry 63(10):892–909, 2002 12416599

Lehman AF, Lieberman JA, Dixon LB, et al: Practice guideline for the treatment of patients with schizophrenia, second edition. Am J Psychiatry 161(2 suppl):1–56, 2004 15000267

Limosin F, Loze JY, Philippe A, et al: Ten-year prospective follow-up study of the mortality by suicide in schizophrenic patients. Schizophr Res 94(1–3):23–28, 2007 17574389

Lindenmayer JP, Czobor P, Alphs L, et al: The InterSePT scale for suicidal thinking reliability and validity. Schizophr Res 63(1–2):161–170, 2003 12892870

Lohr JB, Eidt CA, Abdulrazzaq Alfaraj A, et al: The clinical challenges of akathisia. CNS Spectr 20(suppl 1):1–14, quiz 15–16, 2015 26683525

Long Y, Ouyang X, Liu Z, et al: Associations among suicidal ideation, white matter integrity and cognitive deficit in first-episode schizophrenia. Front Psychiatry 9:391, 2018 30210372

López-Díaz Á, Lorenzo-Herrero P, Lara I, et al: Acute stress and substance use as predictors of suicidal behaviour in acute and transient psychotic disorders. Psychiatry Res 269:414–418, 2018 30173049

Meltzer HY, Alphs L, Green AI, et al: Clozapine treatment for suicidality in schizophrenia: International Suicide Prevention Trial (InterSePT). Arch Gen Psychiatry 60(1):82–91, 2003 12511175

Mueser KT, Deavers F, Penn DL, et al: Psychosocial treatments for schizophrenia. Annu Rev Clin Psychol 9:465–497, 2013 23330939

Nelson JC, Papakostas GI: Atypical antipsychotic augmentation in major depressive disorder: a meta-analysis of placebo-controlled randomized trials. Am J Psychiatry 166(9):980–991, 2009 19687129

Nielssen O, Glozier N, Babidge N, et al: Suicide attempts by jumping and psychotic illness. Aust N Z J Psychiatry 44(6):568–573, 2010 20482416

Nordentoft M, Madsen T, Fedyszyn I: Suicidal behavior and mortality in first-episode psychosis. J Nerv Ment Dis 203(5):387–392, 2015 25919385

Patchan KM, Richardson C, Vyas G, et al: The risk of suicide after clozapine discontinuation: cause for concern. Ann Clin Psychiatry 27(4):253–256, 2015 26554366

Pompili M, Baldessarini RJ, Forte A, et al: Do atypical antipsychotics have antisuicidal effects? A hypothesis-generating overview. Int J Mol Sci 17(10):1700, 2016 27727180

Pompili M, Orsolini L, Lamis DA, et al: Suicide prevention in schizophrenia: do long-acting injectable antipsychotics (LAIs) have a role? CNS Neurol Disord Drug Targets 16(4):454–462, 2017 28240189

Popovic D, Benabarre A, Crespo JM, et al: Risk factors for suicide in schizophrenia: systematic review and clinical recommendations. Acta Psychiatr Scand 130(6):418–426, 2014 25230813

Posner K, Brown GK, Stanley B, et al: The Columbia-Suicide Severity Rating Scale: initial validity and internal consistency findings from three multisite studies with adolescents and adults. Am J Psychiatry 168(12):1266–1277, 2011 22193671

Reutfors J, Clapham E, Bahmanyar S, et al: Suicide risk and antipsychotic side effects in schizophrenia: nested case-control study. Hum Psychopharmacol 31(4):341–345, 2016 27108775

Sinyor M, Schaffer A, Remington G: Suicide in schizophrenia: an observational study of coroner records in Toronto. J Clin Psychiatry 76(1):e98–e103, 2015 25650686

Suokas JT, Perälä J, Suominen K, et al: Epidemiology of suicide attempts among persons with psychotic disorder in the general population. Schizophr Res 124(1–3):22–28, 2010 20934306

Ventriglio A, Gentile A, Bonfitto I, et al: Suicide in the early stage of schizophrenia. Front Psychiatry 7:116, 2016 27445872

Zarrabi H, Khalkhali M, Hamidi A, et al: Clinical features, course and treatment of methamphetamine-induced psychosis in psychiatric inpatients. BMC Psychiatry 16(44):44, 2016 26911516

CHAPTER 12

Personality Disorders

Juan José Carballo, M.D.

Paula Padierna, M.D.

Barbara Stanley, Ph.D.

Beth S. Brodsky, Ph.D.

Maria A. Oquendo, M.D.

Recent investigations have estimated a point prevalence of personality disorders in the general population of the United States ranging from 9% to almost 16% (Lenzenweger et al. 2007). These figures are consistent with the results of a recent meta-analysis that showed that the rate of personality disorders in community populations in Western countries is about 12.1% (Volkert et al. 2018). Psychological autopsy studies have helped recognize the importance of a personality disorder diagnosis as a risk factor for death from suicide. One meta-analysis (Isometsä 2001) has shown that as many as 57% of those who die from suicide had at least one personality disorder. Similarly, among psychiatric outpatients, half of those who died from suicide had a personality disorder (Brown et al. 2000).

The occurrence of suicide attempts and self-injurious behavior is an equally staggering clinical problem. Suicide attempts may occur in up to 90% of individuals with personality disorders (Zanarini et al. 2008). This estimate varies depending on the type of disorder (Cluster A, B, or C or individual disorders) and on the presence of comorbid disorders, especially mood and substance use disorders. Self-injurious behavior is an important risk factor for suicidal behavior: 55%–85% of patients with self-injurious behavior have made at least one suicide attempt (Stanley and Brodsky 2005).

Suicidal Behavior in Personality Disorders

Two different models may be used to understand suicidal acts and self-injurious behavior. For understanding suicidal acts in the context of Axis I and II psychiatric disorders, a stress-diathesis model explains how different risk factors interact, resulting in death from suicide or suicide attempts. According to this model, the *diathesis* refers to the propensity for manifesting suicidal behavior, is considered trait related, and appears to be independent of the main psychiatric diagnosis (Mann 2003). In contrast, *triggers* are precipitants or stressors that determine the timing and probability of suicidal acts. Thus, triggers may be considered state related.

Stanley and Brodsky (2005) proposed a parallel model for understanding the intrapsychic phenomena that lead to suicidal behavior and self-injury in borderline personality disorder (BPD). The self-regulation model posits that self-injury and suicidal behavior serve a dual function in BPD. They both inflict physical harm and regulate the self, particularly emotions, in order to restore a sense of equilibrium and well-being. In this model, unbearable emotions, particularly anxiety, and thoughts are experienced as out of control and never-ending, even though they may last only a few hours. Self-condemnation for feeling out of control frequently ensues.

In response to this state, individuals feel they must act to alter their affective state. A suicide attempt or self-injury is perceived as a reasonable solution. After the episode, individuals usually feel calmer and often regain a sense of emotional equilibrium. Thus, the suicide attempt or self-injury episode achieves its goal. This may explain why individuals with BPD feel better after self-injury episodes and suicide attempts and frequently repeat the behavior. It also explains why, in some cases, hospitalization after a self-destructive episode may not be clinically indicated.

Cluster A Personality Disorders

According to DSM-5 (American Psychiatric Association 2013), the main characteristics of a personality disorder are impairments in personality (self and interpersonal) functioning and the presence of pathological personality traits. DSM-5 groups different personality disorders into three clusters based on descriptive similarities within each cluster. For instance, Cluster A includes paranoid personality disorder, schizoid personality disorder, and schizotypal personality disorders. Personality disorders included in this cluster share some clinical features such as eccentricities of behavior, social withdrawal, and distorted thinking.

Schneider et al. (2006) showed a higher risk of death from suicide in subjects with paranoid or schizotypal personality disorder but not in subjects with schizoid personality disorder. Lentz et al. (2010) demonstrated that individuals with schizotypal personality disorder are more likely to attempt suicide compared to the general population.

Cluster C Personality Disorders

Cluster C includes the avoidant, dependent, and obsessive-compulsive personality disorders, all of which are characterized by high levels of anxiety. Dervic et al. (2007) compared depressed inpatients with and without "pure" Cluster C personality disorders (those with Cluster A or Cluster B personality disorders were excluded from the study) and found that those with comorbid Cluster C personality disorders had higher levels of suicidal ideation but not more previous suicide attempts compared with depressed inpatients without Cluster C disorders. On the other hand, Diaconu and Turecki (2009) reported greater suicidal ideation and frequency of attempts in subjects with obsessive-compulsive personality disorder compared with healthy control subjects.

Few studies have investigated the association between Cluster C personality disorders subtypes (obsessive-compulsive, avoidant, and dependent) and suicidal behavior. Results of the meta-analysis conducted by Latas and Milovanovic (2014) suggested that among individuals with social anxiety disorder and coexisting Cluster C personality disorders, those with avoidant personality disorder and dependent personality disorder have an increased risk of death from suicide.

Cluster B Personality Disorders

Cluster B includes BPD, narcissistic personality disorder (NPD), histrionic personality disorder, and antisocial personality disorder (ASPD). Deficits in impulse control and emotional dysregulation are common features among these personality disorders. Data regarding suicide and histrionic personality disorder are not available separately from data regarding suicide and Cluster B personality disorders. The following discussion addresses other Cluster B personality disorders.

Antisocial Personality Disorder

As many as 72% of patients with ASPD attempt suicide (Pompili et al. 2004), likely because of the presence of comorbid BPD. In this vein, a recent longitudinal study showed that the univariate relationship between ASPD and suicide attempts disappeared after controlling for other personality disorders (McCloskey and Ammerman 2018).

Narcissistic Personality Disorder

At present, no reliable estimates of suicidal behavior are available for the NPD population. Some authors postulate that suicidal behavior is an underestimated cause of mortality in individuals with NPD (Blasco-Fontecilla et al. 2009). However, contradictory findings have been reported. Blasco-Fontecilla et al. (2009) reported that subjects with NPD show specific features of suicidal behavior compared to the rest of Cluster B personality disorders. In their study, individuals diagnosed with NPD who attempted suicide were less impulsive, and their suicide attempts were characterized by higher lethality. In contrast, Coleman et al. (2017) concluded that among a sample of subjects with mood disorders, patients with NPD were 2.4 times less likely to make a suicide attempt compared with patients without NPD. In addition, NPD was not associated with attempts of greater lethality (Coleman et al. 2017).

Borderline Personality Disorder

BPD is the only personality disorder in which suicidal behavior and self-injurious behavior are part of the diagnostic criteria. Between 50% and 90% of subjects with BPD report at least one previous suicide attempt, and up to 10% of people with BPD die from suicide (McCloskey and Ammerman 2018). This rate is almost 50 times higher than that found in the general population (Bourvis et al. 2017). In addition, many individuals with BPD engage in frequent nonsuicidal self-injury (NSSI), make repeated threats of suicide, and experience chronic suicidal ideation and intermittent nonlethal suicide attempts. Therefore, most research on suicidal thoughts and behaviors in personality disorders has focused on this group.

Case Example

Ms. B is a 31-year-old woman with BPD who uses self-injurious behavior to manage overwhelming feelings of anger, anxiety, and guilt. She states that when she is angry, she immediately feels guilty because she does not have the right to be so angry. These feelings of guilt intensify her feelings of worthlessness and self-loathing. As these feelings intensify, Ms. B becomes convinced that she cannot tolerate the degree of self-hatred, and she scratches her skin to elicit physical pain. Sometimes the intense scratching draws blood. The sight of the blood gives her relief because, she reports, she now has "something to show" for how badly she feels. Ms. B feels "back in control" after the scratching. She is clear that this behavior has nothing to do with wanting to die; rather, she is just seeking relief from emotional pain.

However, Ms. B also describes a suicide attempt that she distinguishes from the self-injurious behavior. On the anniversary of her father's death, she became angry at her boyfriend because he appeared to have "no clue" that this anniversary was a very difficult day for her. Ms. B felt that not only was her boyfriend unable to understand her distress on this date but also that he would never "get it." She felt hopeless and was convinced that she would always feel the aching loss of her father. She could not imagine that anyone could help her recover from that loss, which seemed insurmountable. Overcome with grief, feelings of loss, emptiness, and anger, she decided to take an overdose to kill herself.

After taking a handful of pills, Ms. B felt relieved. The suicide attempt was an action that helped her feel like she did have some control and that she could "do something." Feeling more in control, Ms. B's wish to die subsided. She fell asleep until the next morning, when she felt much better.

Discussion

Following the self-regulation model, several aspects of self-destructive behavior should be evaluated. Rather than assuming that the intent of NSSI is purely manipulative and attention seeking, evaluation to detect other functions of the self-injury, such as emotion regulation, self-punishment, and self-validation, may be useful. Awareness of the multiple functions of self-harm behavior, as illustrated in the case of Ms. B in her wish to die and to escape unbearable feelings, can target treatment approaches focused on the development of skills to achieve these goals.

Moreover, patients may have distorted beliefs that lead to self-injury. For example, as mentioned by Ms. B in the vignette, patients may believe they cannot tolerate emotional pain or that the only way to handle their emotional state is through self-injury. Such beliefs can be modified through the cognitive-behavioral therapy (CBT) technique of cognitive restructuring (see Chapter 3, "Cognitive and Behavioral Therapy"). The therapeutic dyad can work together to understand how intense emotional arousal leads to distorted cognitions or interpretations of external events. Therapeutic interventions can increase awareness of how past traumatic events can distort perceptions of current reality.

Identifying reinforcing consequences of the behavior provides information about ways to modify these reinforcement patterns to promote more constructive behaviors. Distinguishing between intended and unintended consequences can aid both patient and clinician to clarify original intent compared with actual consequences of the self-injurious behavior. Patients can gain insight into how their behaviors affect people in their lives, providing an opportunity for improved interpersonal effectiveness.

Risk Assessment and the Decision to Hospitalize

When deciding whether to hospitalize a patient, the twin goals of decreasing suicide risk and increasing the patient's capacity to safely tolerate chronic suicidal ideation are paramount. Decisions regarding hospitalization can be complicated in cases in which a patient has a history of chronic suicidal ideation or NSSI behavior. On the one hand, if the family or the clinician experiences the self-harm as attention seeking, regardless of the patient's intention, reduced sensitivity to risk may ensue. Similarly, becoming inured to the day-to-day emotional pain experienced by individuals with BPD can lead to underrecognition of suicide risk. On the other hand, chronic suicidal ideation and NSSI also can lead to multiple hospitalizations that severely disrupt the individual's ability to function, in addition to not always being helpful in decreasing suicide risk (Stanley and Brodsky 2005). Thus, assessment of the subjective experience of deliberate self-harm can aid in the decision of whether hospitalization is needed to maintain patient safety.

As illustrated in the case of Ms. B, suicidal ideation and self-injurious behavior in BPD do not necessarily indicate a strong intent to die. Instead, they may represent the patient's attempt to relieve an intolerable emotional state. An outpatient treatment that addresses the need for relief and provides support for the individual to manage these states can safely reduce the need for frequent hospital admissions. However, if hospitalization or emergency department admission is needed, brief stays during times of extreme distress that might precede a suicide attempt are optimal (Liljedahl et al. 2017). Under these circumstances, hospitalization would decrease the risk of self-harm while helping the patient tolerate the emotions until they subside.

Treatment

Psychosocial Interventions

Two treatment models have been reported to lower rates of attempted suicide among BPD patients: psychodynamically oriented day treatment involving a mentalization-based model and dialectical behavior therapy (DBT). However, a recent systematic review has concluded that the effects of these interventions are small and that prospective studies are needed to determine long-term effects (Cristea et al. 2017).

Psychodynamic Therapy

A randomized controlled trial (RCT) compared the effectiveness of psychodynamically oriented partial hospitalization with that of standard care for patients with BPD (Bateman and Fonagy 2001). Patients who were partially hospitalized showed improvement in depressive symptoms, a decrease in suicidal and self-injurious acts, and reduced inpatient days compared with the the standard care group.

Chiesa et al. (2004) used a stepdown treatment approach to evaluate the effectiveness of treatment using a specialized psychodynamic program combined with a postdischarge psychodynamic psychotherapy group in patients with primarily Cluster B personality disorders. After 2 years, a significant reduction in suicidal behaviors was observed in this group compared with individuals who received 1 year of a specialized psychodynamic inpatient program only and with those who received standard care in the community. Additionally, a randomized controlled study concluded that mentalization-based treatment for patients with comorbid BPD and substance use disorder might be helpful in reducing suicide attempts (Philips et al. 2018).

Dialectical Behavior Therapy

In the early 1990s, DBT, a form of CBT, was developed as a treatment for chronic suicidal thoughts and behaviors and self-injuring behaviors (Linehan 1993). The most fundamental dialectic addressed by the treatment is that of acceptance and change. Treatment attempts to help these patients—who ordinarily have trouble accepting themselves and others—to develop acceptance-oriented skills and change-oriented skills.

DBT is resource intensive; it requires components of individual and group therapy, weekly meetings between the individual and group clinicians, and availability of the individual therapist at all times. Both individual and group components help patients develop skills to manage intense feelings, self-awareness, and interpersonal effectiveness, all of which decrease self-harm behaviors and death from suicide (Linehan et al. 2015).

Research regarding the efficacy of DBT in reducing suicidal behavior is ongoing. A two-site single-blind trial, the first rigorously controlled trial comparing two different lengths of DBT for individuals with BPD and chronic suicidal behavior, is examining the clinical efficacy and cost effectiveness of 6 versus 12 months of DBT (McMain et al. 2018). Given that BPD can be a severe disorder with high treatment costs, and the limited resources available for psychotherapy, findings have the potential to significantly impact clinical practice. The controlled study, begun in February 2015, will evaluate the frequency of suicidal or NSSI episodes as the primary outcome. The dissemination of final results at international meetings is expected by the fall of 2019. Publication of the findings is planned for 2020.

In recent years, interest in mindfulness-based group interventions as a central component to DBT has surged (Panos et al. 2014). However, to date, the relationship of mindfulness with BPD and suicidal behavior has not been studied.

Cognitive Therapy

Another type of psychotherapy that has been adapted to treat BPD is CBT. More than 20 published RCTs have supported CBT's efficacy across a number of behavioral problems. Most of these studies have examined BPD specifically, with reduction of suicidal behaviors as a primary outcome (Rizvi et al. 2013).

Safety Planning Intervention

Safety planning intervention is a brief clinical intervention that combines a variety of evidence-based strategies to reduce suicidal behavior by developing a prioritized list of coping skills and strategies. Stanley et al. (2018) conducted a study in which they combined safety planning intervention administered in the emergency department and telephone follow-up. They concluded that after 6 months, patients who received the intervention had 45% less suicidal behavior than those who received regular emergency care. However, this study was not specifically targeted to patients with BPD.

Other Psychosocial Interventions

The treatment gap for people with mental disorders exceeds 50% in all countries of the world (Patel et al. 2010). Exploring how access to effective treatments can be increased for people with mental disorders based on evidence of effective interventions and respect for human rights is an area of growing interest (Patel et al. 2010). Internet interventions are considered a viable option to help reduce the mental health treatment gap. In the future, a mobile platform for skills training has the potential to increase the access of persons with BPD and suicidal ideation/behavior to an important treatment component (Rizvi et al. 2016).

Early Intervention

The question of whether or not to diagnose personality pathology in adolescence remains unresolved. However, a 1-year prospective follow-up study showed a stronger long-term reduction in self-harm and a more rapid recovery in suicidal ideation in adolescents who received 19 weeks of DBT adapted for adolescents compared to enhanced usual care (Mehlum et al. 2016).

Common Factors in Treatment of Suicidal Thoughts and Behaviors

The Group for the Advancement of Psychiatry Psychotherapy Committee attempted to establish the six common factors in the effectiveness of psychotherapeutic approaches to suicidal ideation and behaviors, regardless of the orientation of the therapy (Sledge et al. 2014):

1. Negotiates a frame for treatment
2. Recognizes and has insight into the patient's responsibilities within the therapy
3. Provides the therapist a conceptual framework for understanding and intervening
4. Uses the therapeutic relationship to engage and address suicide actively and explicitly
5. Prioritizes suicide as a topic to be addressed whenever it emerges
6. Provides support for the therapist

Pharmacotherapy

The U.S. Food and Drug Administration (FDA) has not approved medications specifically for the treatment of BPD. The following discussion summarizes medication trials that have demonstrated effects on decreasing suicidal behavior or on behaviors known to be high-risk factors for death from suicide, such as aggression or impulsivity.

Selective Serotonin Reuptake Inhibitors

Several RCTs of selective serotonin reuptake inhibitors (SSRIs) for treating patients with BPD have been conducted (Bellino et al. 2011). Results of these investigations suggest that SSRIs may lessen symptoms of affective instability, anger, and impulsivity in subjects with BPD. However, one meta-analysis found little evidence of effectiveness for treatment with SSRIs in patients with BPD (Lieb et al. 2010).

Mood Stabilizers

To date, divalproex is one of the most-studied pharmacological therapies used to treat patients with BPD. Reductions in aggression and depression are reported among patients treated with divalproex sodium, but it is important to bear in mind that subjects with suicidal ideation are usually excluded from studies and that many investigations lack measures of suicidal thoughts and behaviors, which limits the generalization of the results to suicidal patients.

The combined therapy of valproic acid with omega-3 fatty acid has been evaluated in patients with BPD, with positive long-lasting results even after the interruption of other interventions such as anger management (Bozzatello et al. 2018). The use of lamotrigine has shown contradictory results with regard to clinical or cost effectiveness (Crawford et al. 2018). Finally, in regard to mood stabilizers, three RCTs have studied the effectiveness of topiramate in the treatment of subjects with BPD, with promising results in treating symptoms of anger, including impulsive aggression (Stoffers et al. 2010).

Antipsychotics

Although not approved by the FDA for treatment of BPD, the use of low-dose antipsychotics for the acute management of global symptom severity does have some support (American Psychiatric Association 2001). Moreover, antipsychotics significantly improve cognitive symptoms in patients with BPD (Bellino et al. 2011).

RCTs have suggested that olanzapine may reduce obsessive-compulsive symptoms, interpersonal sensitivity, depression, anger-hostility, anxiety, paranoia, psychoticism, and overall psychopathology in patients with BPD (Lieb et al. 2010). However, suicidal behavior per se was not used as an outcome variable in these studies. Similar reports exist from open studies of risperidone and quetiapine use, although controlled trials are not available to verify these findings (Lieb et al. 2010).

A double-blind, placebo-controlled study that evaluated the role of aripiprazole in the treatment of patients with BPD found this atypical antipsychotic significantly reduced certain core pathological symptoms of BPD, such as anger and impulsivity (Canadian Agency for Drugs and Technologies in Health 2018; Nickel et al. 2006). The prevalence of self-injury compared to the control group was also reduced.

Other Psychopharmacological Agents

Other medications at times are used in the treatment of patients with BPD. Opiate antagonists have been used in an attempt to diminish the analgesia and euphoria associated with self-injurious behavior, with the goal of reducing this behavior. Because partial agonists are related to stabilization of opioid signaling in patients with BPD, these drugs provide an alternative treatment avenue for future research (Bandelow et al. 2010). Double-blind, placebo-controlled studies also have shown positive effects of supplementation with omega-3 fatty acids in the treatment of BPD, including reducing self-harm and depression (Bozzatello et al. 2018).

Given the executive dysfunction, subtle deficits in memory and social cognition, dissociative symptoms, and refractory depressive symptoms experienced by patients with BPD, N-methyl-D-aspartate (NMDA) antagonists such as ketamine would seem likely to be of benefit due to their rapid antidepressant effects, which can occur in as little as 40 minutes. In the past decade, multiple studies and trials have studied this psychopharmacological intervention and shown that some patients experience a remission of suicidal ideation (De Berardis et al. 2018). NMDA antagonists' rapid onset of action suggests a potential for treatment in crisis and emergency situations for patients at high risk of death from suicide. However, the dissociative effects and the potential for abuse, among other negative effects associated with these agents, may limit their use. The use of ketamine in the treatment of patients with BPD is not yet recommended, pending completion of studies on its clinical use, safety, and appropriate dosage.

Several studies have highlighted the beneficial effects of oxytocin on the decrease of reactivity to social stress in patients with BPD, particularly in subjects with a history of childhood trauma and insecurity of attachment (Debbané 2018). However, no studies on the impact of this hormone on suicide are available. More research is needed before oxytocin's clinical implementation, given mixed research results (Debbané 2018).

Unfortunately, only a few controlled studies of available psychopharmacological agents have reported benefits in reducing the risk of suicidal behavior associated with BPD. Clinicians should base treatment interventions on expert consensus practice guidelines. The National Institute for Health and Care Excellence's (2009) clinical guideline for BPD recommended: "Drug treatment should not be used specifically for borderline personality disorder or for the individual symptoms or behaviour associated with the disorder (for example, repeated self-harm, marked emotional instability, risk-taking behaviour and transient psychotic symptoms)." Similarly, The American Psychiatric Association's (2001) *Practice Guideline for the Treatment of Patients With Borderline Personality Disorder* states that the primary treatment for BPD is psychotherapy, complemented by symptom-targeted pharmacotherapy.

Conclusion

Patients with personality disorders, especially BPD, have an increased risk of death from suicide. In the treatment of BPD, self-harm behaviors must be addressed as the highest priorities. Therapists should evaluate risk for these behaviors as well as help the patient find ways to maintain safety. Psychiatrists can reduce the underrecognition of suicide risk in patients with BPD by identifying the various functions of deliberate self-harm, assuming the patient's self-harming behaviors are not intended solely to manipulate others, and maintaining awareness of the day-to-day emotional pain experienced by individuals with BPD. The primary treatment for BPD is psychotherapy, complemented by symptom-targeted pharmacotherapy. Empirically tested treatments for self-harm in BPD suggest that psychodynamically oriented day treatment involving a mentalization-based model and DBT may lower rates of attempted suicide among BPD patients, but more studies are needed.

Key Points

- Recent investigations have shown the importance of personality disorder as a risk factor for death from suicide.

- Between 50% and 90% of subjects with borderline personality disorder (BPD) report at least one previous suicide attempt, and up to 10% of people with BPD die from suicide. In addition, many individuals with BPD engage in frequent nonsuicidal self-injury (NSSI), experience chronic suicidal ideation, and have a history of incidents of nonlethal suicidal self-directed violence.

- Suicidal ideation and self-injurious behavior in BPD do not necessarily indicate a strong intent to die. Instead, they may be the patient's attempt to relieve an intolerable emotional state.

- Identifying the various functions of deliberate self-harm can reduce the underrecognition of suicide risk.

- Management includes establishing and maintaining a therapeutic framework and alliance as well as providing crisis intervention and monitoring patient safety.

- Psychodynamically oriented day treatment involving a mentalization-based model and dialectical behavior therapy have been reported to lower rates of attempted suicide among BPD patients, although prospective studies are needed to determine long-term effects.

References

American Psychiatric Association: Practice guideline for the treatment of patients with borderline personality disorder. Am J Psychiatry 158(10 suppl):1–52, 2001 11665545

American Psychiatric Association: Diagnostic and Statistical Manual of Mental Disorders, 5th Edition. Arlington, VA, American Psychiatric Association, 2013

Bandelow B, Schmahl C, Falkai P, et al: Borderline personality disorder: a dysregulation of the endogenous opioid system? Psychol Rev 117(2):623–636, 2010 20438240

Bateman A, Fonagy P: Treatment of borderline personality disorder with psychoanalytically oriented partial hospitalization: an 18-month follow-up. Am J Psychiatry 158(1):36–42, 2001 11136631

Bellino S, Rinaldi C, Bozzatello P, et al: Pharmacotherapy of borderline personality disorder: a systematic review for publication purpose. Curr Med Chem 18(22):3322–3329, 2011 21728970

Blasco-Fontecilla H, Baca-Garcia E, Dervic K, et al: Specific features of suicidal behavior in patients with narcissistic personality disorder. J Clin Psychiatry 70(11):1583–1587, 2009 19607766

Bourvis N, Aouidad A, Cabelguen C, et al: How do stress exposure and stress regulation relate to borderline personality disorder? Front Psychol 8:2054, 2017 29250007

Bozzatello P, Rocca P, Bellino S: Combination of omega-3 fatty acids and valproic acid in treatment of borderline personality disorder: a follow-up study. Clin Drug Investig 38(4):367–372, 2018 29302857

Brown GK, Beck AT, Steer RA, et al: Risk factors for suicide in psychiatric outpatients: a 20-year prospective study. J Consult Clin Psychol 68(3):371–377, 2000 10883553

Canadian Agency for Drugs and Technologies in Health: Treatment of Personality Disorders in Adults With or Without Comorbid Mental Health Conditions: Clinical Effectiveness and Guidelines (CADTH Rapid Response Report: Summary of Abstracts). Ottawa, Canada, CADTH, 2018

Chiesa M, Fonagy P, Holmes J, et al: Residential versus community treatment of personality disorders: a comparative study of three treatment programs. Am J Psychiatry 161(8):1463–1470, 2004 15285974

Coleman D, Lawrence R, Parekh A, et al: Narcissistic personality disorder and suicidal behavior in mood disorders. J Psychiatr Res 85:24–28, 2017 27816770

Crawford MJ, Sanatinia R, Barrett B, et al: The clinical effectiveness and cost-effectiveness of lamotrigine in borderline personality disorder: a randomized placebo-controlled trial. Am J Psychiatry 175(8):756–764, 2018 29621901

Cristea IA, Gentili C, Cotet CD, et al: Efficacy of psychotherapies for borderline personality disorder: a systematic review and meta-analysis. JAMA Psychiatry 74(4):319–328, 2017 28249086

De Berardis D, Fornaro M, Valchera A, et al: Eradicating suicide at its roots: preclinical bases and clinical evidence of the efficacy of ketamine in the treatment of suicidal behaviors. Int J Mol Sci 19(10):2888, 2018 30249029

Debbané M: Treating borderline personality disorder with oxytocin: an enthusiastic note of caution. Commentary to Servan et al. The effect of oxytocin in borderline personality disorder. Encephale 44(1):83–84, 2018 29402386

Dervic K, Grunebaum MF, Burke AK, et al: Cluster C personality disorders in major depressive episodes: the relationship between hostility and suicidal behavior. Arch Suicide Res 11(1):83–90, 2007 17178644

Diaconu G, Turecki G: Obsessive-compulsive personality disorder and suicidal behavior: evidence for a positive association in a sample of depressed patients. J Clin Psychiatry 70(11):1551–1556, 2009 19607764

Isometsä ET: Psychological autopsy studies—a review. Eur Psychiatry 16(7):379–385, 2001 11728849

Latas M, Milovanovic S: Personality disorders and anxiety disorders: what is the relationship? Curr Opin Psychiatry 27(1):57–61, 2014 24270478

Lentz V, Robinson J, Bolton JM: Childhood adversity, mental disorder comorbidity, and suicidal behavior in schizotypal personality disorder. J Nerv Ment Dis 198(11):795–801, 2010 21048469

Lenzenweger MF, Lane MC, Loranger AW, et al: DSM-IV personality disorders in the National Comorbidity Survey Replication. Biol Psychiatry 62(6):553–564, 2007 17217923

Lieb K, Völlm B, Rücker G, et al: Pharmacotherapy for borderline personality disorder: Cochrane systematic review of randomised trials. Br J Psychiatry 196(1):4–12, 2010 20044651

Liljedahl SI, Helleman M, Daukantaité D, et al: A standardized crisis management model for self-harming and suicidal individuals with three or more diagnostic criteria of borderline personality disorder: the Brief Admission Skåne randomized controlled trial protocol (BASRCT). BMC Psychiatry 17(1):220, 2017 28619050

Linehan MM: Cognitive-Behavioral Treatment of Borderline Personality Disorder. New York, Guilford, 1993

Linehan MM, Korslund KE, Harned MS, et al: Dialectical behavior therapy for high suicide risk in individuals with borderline personality disorder: a randomized clinical trial and component analysis. JAMA Psychiatry 72(5):475–482, 2015 25806661

Mann JJ: Neurobiology of suicidal behaviour. Nat Rev Neurosci 4(10):819–828, 2003 14523381

McCloskey MS, Ammerman BA: Suicidal behavior and aggression-related disorders. Curr Opin Psychol 22:54–58, 2018 28829989

McMain SF, Chapman AL, Kuo JR, et al: The effectiveness of 6 versus 12 months of dialectical behaviour therapy for borderline personality disorder: the feasibility of a shorter treatment and evaluating responses (FASTER) trial protocol. BMC Psychiatry 18(1):230, 2018 30016935

Mehlum L, Ramberg M, Tørmoen AJ, et al: Dialectical behavior therapy compared with enhanced usual care for adolescents with repeated suicidal and self-harming behavior: outcomes over a one-year follow-up. J Am Acad Child Adolesc Psychiatry 55(4):295–300, 2016 27015720

National Institute for Health and Care Excellence: Borderline Personality Disorder: Recognition and Management (Clinical Guideline CG78). London, National Institute for Health and Care Excellence, 2009. Available at https://www.nice.org.uk/guidance/cg78. Accessed February 13, 2019.

Nickel MK, Muehlbacher M, Nickel C, et al: Aripiprazole in the treatment of patients with borderline personality disorder: a double-blind, placebo-controlled study. Am J Psychiatry 163(5):833–838, 2006 16648324

Panos PT, Jackson JW, Hasan O, et al: Meta-analysis and systematic review assessing the efficacy of dialectical behavior therapy (DBT). Res Soc Work Pract 24(2):213–223, 2014 30853773

Patel V, Maj M, Flisher AJ, et al: Reducing the treatment gap for mental disorders: a WPA survey. World Psychiatry 9(3):169–176, 2010 20975864

Philips B, Wennberg P, Konradsson P, et al: Mentalization-based treatment for concurrent borderline personality disorder and substance use disorder: a randomized controlled feasibility study. Eur Addict Res 24(1):1–8, 2018 29402870

Pompili M, Ruberto A, Girardi P, et al: Suicidality in DSM IV cluster B personality disorders: an overview. Ann Ist Super Sanita 40(4):475–483, 2004 15815115

Rizvi SL, Steffel LM, Carson-Wong A: An overview of dialectical behavior therapy for professional psychologists. Prof Psychol Res Pr 44(2):73–80, 2013

Rizvi SL, Hughes CD, Thomas MC: The DBT Coach mobile application as an adjunct to treatment for suicidal and self-injuring individuals with borderline personality disorder: a preliminary evaluation and challenges to client utilization. Psychol Serv 13(4):380–388, 2016 27797571

Schneider B, Wetterling T, Sargk D, et al: Axis I disorders and personality disorders as risk factors for suicide. Eur Arch Psychiatry Clin Neurosci 256(1):17–27, 2006 16133739

Sledge W, Plakun EM, Bauer S, et al: Psychotherapy for suicidal patients with borderline personality disorder: an expert consensus review of common factors across five therapies. Borderline Personal Disord Emot Dysregul 1(1):16, 2014 26401300

Stanley B, Brodsky B: Suicidal and self-injurious behavior in borderline personality disorder: a self-regulation model, in Understanding and Treating Borderline Personality Disorder: A Guide for Professionals and Families. Edited by Gunderson J, Hoffman PD. Washington, DC, American Psychiatric Publishing, 2005, pp 43–63

Stanley B, Brown GK, Brenner LA, et al: Comparison of the safety planning intervention with follow-up vs usual care of suicidal patients treated in the emergency department. JAMA Psychiatry 75(9):894–900, 2018 29998307

Stoffers J, Völlm BA, Rücker G, et al: Pharmacological interventions for borderline personality disorder. Cochrane Database Syst Rev (6):CD005653, 2010 20556762

Volkert J, Gablonski TC, Rabung S: Prevalence of personality disorders in the general adult population in Western countries: systematic review and meta-analysis. Br J Psychiatry 213(6):709–715, 2018 30261937

Zanarini MC, Frankenburg FR, Reich DB, et al: The 10-year course of physically self-destructive acts reported by borderline patients and Axis II comparison subjects. Acta Psychiatr Scand 117(3):177–184, 2008 18241308

CHAPTER 13

Sleep and Suicide

Antonio Fernando, M.D., ABPN

Kieran Kennedy, M.B.Ch.B., B.Sc.

Recently, disorders of sleep have been identified as another possible risk factor for death from suicide (Singareddy and Balon 2001). Sleep is one of the most important of all human biological processes. In addition to spending about one-third of our lives asleep, the quality of our sleep influences the quality of our waking lives and our psychological health. Increasing evidence indicates that sleep and sleep disorders also influence suicidal thinking and behavior. This chapter presents evidence of the growing understanding of the link between disordered sleep and suicide; considers possible mechanisms for why disordered sleep is linked to suicide; and discusses practical ways of assessing and managing sleep disorders, particularly in regard to mitigating suicide risk.

Sleep and Suicide Link

Normal sleep is a multifaceted biological process resulting from a delicate balance of sensory, neurological, physiological, and psychological factors. Research continues to elucidate the complex mechanisms behind sleep. However, current evidence demonstrates that we derive mental and physical benefits from consistent and healthy sleep (Moszczynski and Murray 2012). Disordered sleep, conversely, is significantly linked to a range of physical and mental health disorders (Bernert and Joiner 2007).

DSM-5 (American Psychiatric Association 2013) contains a category of diagnoses, "sleep-wake disorders," that defines identified sleep abnormalities. Sleep-wake disorders exist in a multitude of forms that have both physical and mental causes (Moszczynski and Murray 2012). Separating the physical and mental causes and results of disordered sleep can be challenging. Abnormalities in sleep arise from medical and psychiatric conditions, and disordered sleep, in turn, affects both medical and psychological outcomes.

Although studies vary in terms of the extent of the association between disordered, attenuated, and poor sleep and risk for death from suicide—as well as in study design, population, and specific outcome measures reported (Pigeon et al. 2013; Singareddy and Balon 2001)—disordered sleep appears to be a significant factor in increased risk for death from suicide (Bernert and Joiner 2007). The influence of disordered sleep on suicide may be independent from that of psychiatric disorders (Bernert and Joiner 2007). Disordered sleep states now linked to suicide include insomnia, nightmares, hypersomnolence, sleep apnea, restless legs syndrome, rapid eye movement (REM) sleep behavior disorder, circadian rhythm misalignment, subjectively reported poor sleep, and abnormal sleep polysomnography (Bernert and Joiner 2007; Pigeon et al. 2013; Singareddy and Balon 2001). Although a number of these have demonstrated some association with increased risk of death from suicide, insomnia and nightmares have demonstrated the strongest independent links with risk of death from suicide (Singareddy and Balon 2001).

Only two meta-analyses have reviewed the literature on the connection between disordered sleep and suicide (Malik et al. 2014; Pigeon et al. 2013). Together, these analyses reviewed 58 original studies, with a combined total of more than 250,000 individual subjects, of disordered sleep states and risk of suicide-related outcomes. Both indicated a significant independent effect of disordered sleep and increased risk of suicide-related outcomes across several risk-related measurements, including suicidal ideation, attempted suicide, and deaths from suicide. These results were consistent even when controlling for possible confounding factors, including comorbid major depressive disorder.

Insomnia

Insomnia disorder is one of the most robustly studied and quantified links between disordered sleep and risk of death from suicide (Singareddy and Balon 2001). Review of the current literature reveals a significant risk of suicide conferred by the presence of insomnia-related symptomatology (Woznica et al. 2015). This likely reflects, at least in part, the prevalence of insomnia, with surveys revealing 1-year prevalence rates of up to 45% in the general population (Sadock et al. 2014). A significant positive relationship between the presence of insomnia and risk of both attempted suicide and death from suicide has been demonstrated after controlling for confounding variables (Bjørngaard et al. 2011; Pigeon et al. 2013; Zuromski et al. 2017).

DSM-5 defines *insomnia disorder* as a disorder of sleep initiation or maintenance whereby an individual fails to achieve an adequate quality or quantity of restorative sleep (American Psychiatric Association 2013). The DSM-5 diagnostic criteria include abnormal quality or quantity of sleep despite ample opportunity, significant distress or impairment in function, disturbance occurring on at least 3 nights per week, and presence for at least 3 months. The problem cannot be explained by other physical disorder, mental disorder (including other sleep-wake disorder), or substance use.

In fact, research has demonstrated an increased risk of suicide-related outcomes in the presence of symptoms of insomnia across unadjusted and adjusted samples. These studies range in longitudinal design from 1 week to 20 years (Chu et al. 2017; Malik et al. 2014). Several robust studies showed significance of effect even when adjusting for important areas of potential bias, including major depressive disorder, anxiety disorders, and alcohol use (Bjørngaard et al. 2011; Nadorff et al. 2013; Zuromski et al. 2017). One prospective study using data collected from 75,000 Norwegian adults between 1984 and 1986 and then following their causes of death over the ensuing 20-year period found that the presence of insomnia was a positive risk factor for death from suicide (Bjørngaard et al. 2011). Despite some limitations, a dose relationship was noted between sleep problem frequency and risk of dying from suicide, with those displaying insomnia to some degree "nearly every night" showing a risk of dying from suicide that was 4.9 times greater than in those who did not report insomnia (Bjørngaard et al. 2011).

Similarly, a study attempting to quantify whether increases in severity of insomnia correlated with increases in risk for suicidal thoughts and behaviors found that insomnia significantly increased risk of suicidal ideation in an incremental and unidirectional relationship (Zuromski et al. 2017). Another study examining insomnia, comorbid psychiatric disorders, and suicidal ideation in 6,700 active Canadian Armed Forces members found a significant link between insomnia and suicidal ideation in those without or with only one comorbid condition, but not in individuals with two or more psychiatric diagnoses (Richardson et al. 2017). Interestingly, individuals with insomnia may be more likely to attempt to take their own lives using more high-lethality means compared with those presenting with suicidal thoughts and behaviors without insomnia (Pompili et al. 2013).

Nightmares

The presence of nightmares is emerging as a unique and potentially powerful suicide risk factor. Studies have investigated this link without clear adjustment for possible mediators, such as posttraumatic stress disorder or major depressive disorder. However, studies in which an attempt has been made to control for these possible confounding factors continue to show an independent association between the presence of nightmares and increased suicidal ideation and behaviors (Bernert and Joiner 2007).

Those who have more frequent dreams with negative affective content are at an increased risk of not only suicidal ideation but also both attempted suicide and dying from suicide (Bernert and Joiner 2007; Singareddy and Balon 2001). Several studies have found a significant positive correlation between the presence of nightmares and an increased risk for suicidal thoughts and behaviors (Bernert and Joiner 2007). A meta-analysis including 14 studies in which nightmares were investigated as a potential suicide risk factor has reinforced this finding (Pigeon et al. 2013). Research is also demonstrating emerging support for frequency of nightmares, their timing within the sleep cycle, and the affective intensity of dream content as possible contributory factors that further increase the risk of suicidal thoughts and behaviors (Bernert and Joiner 2007).

Other Sleep Disorders

Research investigating other disordered sleep states and conditions that influence sleep is marked by scarcity of replicated findings as well as heterogeneity of methods and results. At present, disordered sleep states with potentially significant links to increased risk of death from suicide include disorders of hypersomnolence, REM and non-REM sleep disorders, disorders of nocturnal hypoventilation, and nocturnal panic attacks (Malik et al. 2014; Pigeon et al. 2013).

Medically based disturbances in sleep also appear to confer higher risk of an individual contemplating or attempting suicide or dying from suicide, independent of the presence of a psychiatric disorder, although further investigation is required. Current evidence demonstrates a significant link between suicide risk and a range of medical conditions with sleep pathologies (Ahmedani et al. 2017). Chronic pain and fibromyalgia may be linked specifically to disordered sleep (Ahmedani et al. 2017; Calandre et al. 2011; Racine et al. 2014). Such findings demonstrate the increasing awareness and evidence of the importance of sleep disturbances to increased risk of suicide, whether associated with psychiatric disorders or primary medical problems.

Alongside a range of diagnosable sleep disorders, objective and subjective abnormal sleep states also have been investigated and linked to risk of death from suicide. Objective measurements of sleep abnormality have displayed more defined links to states of disordered sleep and risk of death from suicide (Singareddy and Balon 2001). Measurement of electroencephalographic states during sleep, with abnormal sleep wave morphology including less slow wave activity, reduced latency to initiation of REM sleep, and an increased duration and activity of REM overall, have been linked to increased risk of suicidal thoughts and behaviors (Singareddy and Balon 2001). A heterogeneous group of subjective sleep disturbance measurements has also demonstrated that disturbed or abnormal sleep states have significant links to an increasing risk of death from suicide (Malik et al. 2014; Pigeon et al. 2013). Although the potential for bias and confounding variables is present in these studies, an adjusted and independent increased risk is indicated in the setting of subjective reports of sleep difficulty and perception of poorly restorative sleep (Pigeon et al. 2013; Singareddy and Balon 2001).

Mechanisms Mediating Disordered Sleep and Suicide Risk

Several potential mechanisms to explain the unique connection between sleep and suicide risk have been proposed. At present, however, underlying mechanisms remain firmly within the realm of hypothesis.

The majority of models seeking to explain an independent association between disordered sleep and suicide involve abnormalities in serotonin (5-HT) neurophysiology (Bernert and Joiner 2007; Singareddy and Balon 2001). In addition to its role in mood and anxiety states, serotonin pathways in the brain have a vital role in normal and adaptive sleep physiology, with abnormalities in serotonin neurotransmission being noted in those with a range of sleep disorders (Singareddy and Balon 2001). Similarly, suicidal ideation and behaviors as an independent variable itself has been linked to a reduction in cerebrospinal fluid levels of 5-HT and 5-hydroxyindoleacetic acid (HIAA; a breakdown metabolite of neural 5-HT) in individuals who have suicidal ideation, have attempted suicide, or have died from suicide (Singareddy and Balon 2001). Abnormal serotonergic balance may be a common denominator for disordered sleep and increased risk of death from suicide, alongside particular states of psychopathology.

A range of neurochemical and physiological markers have also been found to be common to increased suicide risk, mental disorders, and disordered sleep states (Bernert and Joiner 2007; Singareddy and Balon 2001). Although causality currently cannot be explained, increased hypothalamic-pituitary-adrenal axis activity and increased circulating proinflammatory cytokines have been found in both states of disordered sleep and increased suicidal thoughts and behaviors (Bernert and Joiner 2007).

Lastly, psychological explanations that link disordered sleep and increased risk of death from suicide are worthy of attention. The experience of insomnia, sleep disruption, and poor-quality, nonrestorative sleep can be highly distressing and bring a range of psychological, social, and physical consequences (Bernert and Joiner 2007). Psychological distress linked to disturbed sleep, and most prominently insomnia, has included increased negative rumination (e.g., "I really need at least 8 hours to get through tomorrow" or "I can't do this anymore"), anxiety, distress, frustration, and impaired coping (Bernert and Joiner 2007; Holdaway et al. 2018; Littlewood et al. 2017; Singareddy and Balon 2001). Ruminations regarding anxious, catastrophic cognitions or hopeless themes during and after the experience of disrupted sleep may underlie an individual's increased risk of experiencing distress, hopelessness, and isolation, all of which may be risk factors for suicidal thoughts and behaviors (Holdaway et al. 2018; Littlewood et al. 2017).

Assessment and Management of Insomnia and Nightmares

As discussed, various pathological sleep states are linked to suicidal thoughts and behaviors. However, insomnia and nightmares have demonstrated the strongest link to suicide risk.

Insomnia Assessment

Insomnia is one of the most common sleep complaints in the general population, with about one-third reporting its presence at any one time (American Psychiatric Association 2013). Although definitions may differ, insomnia usually refers to poor-quality sleep, broken sleep, delay in sleep onset, and early awakening. These symptoms rise to the level of a diagnosable disorder when they are frequent (at least 3 nights a week), chronic (lasting at least 3 months), and result in distress or impaired functioning.

Insomnia can occur in the absence of other disorders. However, the majority of individuals reporting insomnia have underlying psychiatric, medical, and other sleep disorders. Clinically, people with insomnia report symptoms such as broken sleep, delay in falling asleep, or early morning awakening. These can occur singly or in combination. Patients with insomnia often report fatigue and poor cognitive functioning. Nevertheless, most do not report excessive sleepiness or daytime somnolence; rather, many patients report feeling "wired" or overly activated despite having poor sleep. This subjective symptom might be related to the cognitive arousal that often accompanies insomnia.

Assessment of insomnia requires a systematic approach that includes taking a clinical history, obtaining sleep diary data, and using validated patient questionnaires. Sleep study or polysomnography is not often indicated for the diagnosis of insomnia because results offer little additional information beyond that reported by the patient. Nevertheless, such studies should be considered and used if symptoms suggestive of other sleep disorders, including restless legs or sleep apnea, are present. For example, if a patient reports significant sleepiness during the day in addition to insomnia, other possible pathologies including sleep apnea must be investigated and ruled out. Screening with an instrument such as the Epworth Sleepiness Scale (Johns 1991) can assist in estimating the severity of daytime sleepiness; any score above 10 on this scale is suggestive of significant pathology requiring investigation with an overnight sleep study.

Clinical interview of a patient with insomnia includes questions about sleep and bedtime routines, sleep hygiene, external factors related to insomnia (e.g., ambient noise or light), and screening for psychiatric, medical, and sleep disorders that may underlie the sleep disturbance. Sleep diaries can assist in documenting longitudinal sleep patterns with more accuracy than patients' recall of their sleep and bed routines; patients with insomnia tend to overestimate their problematic sleep and underestimate "good nights." Significant data, including average total sleep time and average total time in bed, both crucial in the behavioral management of insomnia, can be better obtained through use of a sleep diary than by relying entirely on patient memory and verbal reports. Table 13–1 outlines questions that assist in the diagnosis and management of insomnia complaints.

As Table 13–1 demonstrates, the complete assessment of a patient with insomnia requires gathering a lot of information. Validated patient questionnaires such as the Auckland Sleep Questionnaire (Arroll et al. 2011; Goodfellow Unit 2019) screen for insomnia symptoms, common sleep disorders, comorbid anxiety and mood pathologies, and substance use. These can assist clinicians in collecting needed data.

Insomnia Management

Insomnia disorder can be managed with psychological, behavioral, and pharmacological approaches. Clinicians should work with patients to address obvious factors contributing to insomnia, including stress, suboptimal physical surroundings, use of substances, and medical or psychiatric conditions. However, many patients with insomnia continue to experience poor-quality sleep long term. In these cases, use of psychological and behavioral interventions should be prioritized before using sedative or sleep-related medications (Cunnington and Qian 2017).

Effective behavioral approaches include sleep restriction therapy and stimulus control therapy (Lack and Lovato 2017). Many insomnia patients spend a much longer time in bed than they spend actually sleeping. Sleep restriction therapy advises patients to restrict the amount of time they spend in bed to approximate the actual amount of time they normally sleep. For example, a patient who sleeps for only 7 hours but spends 9 hours in bed is advised to limit the time spent lying down to 7 hours. A patient's sleep time can be obtained from a sleep diary kept by the patient for at least 1 week. Stimulus control therapy involves advising patients to go to bed only when sleepy, for example, when they are nodding off or unable to keep eyes open, and to get out of bed if they do not feel sleepy within 15 minutes.

Both behavioral approaches work by limiting the time spent in bed, thereby increasing sleep pressure, which then reduces wakefulness at night (Lack and Lovato 2017).

TABLE 13–1.   **Assessment of insomnia**

Assess bed-related routines	Activities before bedtime (2 hours before going to bed)
	Bedtime
	Sleep onset latency
	Middle of the night awakening (frequency and duration)
	Estimated total time spent in bed
	Estimated total sleep time (usually different from time spent in bed)
	Sleep time or napping outside of usual bedtime
	Time spent in bed outside of evening bedtime
	Use of gadgets/devices 2 hours before sleep or while in bed
Assess for external sleep disruptors	Noise and light in bedroom
	Pets, other humans causing sleep disruption
	Alcohol, cigarettes, stimulants, amphetamines, caffeine, energy drinks
Screen for other sleep disorders	Obstructive sleep apnea, restless legs syndrome, parasomnias
Screen for mood, anxiety disorders	
Screen for medical disorders	For example, gastroesophageal reflux disease, chronic obstructive pulmonary disease, chronic pain, fibromyalgia
Have patient keep a sleep diary for 2 weeks	
Use Auckland Sleep Questionnaire	Available at https://www.goodfellowunit.org/sites/default/files/insomnia/Main_Sleep_Questionnaire_final_version_2014.pdf
Screen for daytime sleepiness using Epworth Sleepiness Scale	

In both, patients also are advised that napping outside the prescribed or recommended bedtime should be strictly avoided. Typically, after 2–3 weeks of sleep restriction or stimulus control therapy, sleep becomes more consolidated and sleep onset shortens (Lack and Lovato 2017). Although behavioral interventions are considered a first-line treatment in most cases of chronic insomnia, this treatment is not recommended for patients with bipolar disorder because a manic or hypomanic episode may be precipitated by mood elevation from the partial sleep deprivation.

Many patients with insomnia develop cognitive distortions around their sleeping. They believe that sleep should be continuous and uninterrupted. Individuals with insomnia also commonly display "catastrophic" thinking. For example, they equate a disrupted night's sleep to being severely impaired the next day, followed by thoughts that they will lose their job and will never be successful in life. These distortions and negative thinking need to be addressed through therapy and psychoeducation.

Ideally, patients with chronic insomnia can obtain psychological and behavioral treatments from medical and psychological sleep specialists. However, psychiatrists treating patients with insomnia and suicidal thoughts and behaviors are advised to become familiar with behavioral and psychological treatment techniques, because insomnia is a common symptom in multiple psychiatric disorders and an independent risk factor for death from suicide, and access to sleep specialists and psychologists may be limited. In the absence of a medical specialist or sleep-trained psychologist, web-based platforms (e.g., Sleepio, www.sleepio.com) provide an alternative option that incorporate well-designed, evidence-based cognitive and behavioral programs for chronic insomnia.

Use of sleep-promoting medications in chronic insomnia is controversial because of the limited availability of long-term data (more than 6 weeks) regarding their safety and efficacy. Apart from eszopiclone (U.S. Food and Drug Administration 2014), almost all studies addressing the use of these medications evaluate their short-term rather than long-term use, hence the typical recommendation that medications be used for a short period of time. However, many chronic insomnia patients require ongoing off-label use of sleep medications in addition to psychological and behavioral interventions (Schutte-Rodin et al. 2008).

Identifying the best psychopharmacological agent for a patient with chronic insomnia requires a systematic trial and observation approach. No medication has been identified as a single drug treatment of choice, and many medication families contain agents that can be used to reduce symptoms of insomnia. Benzodiazepines (e.g., temazepam, lorazepam, oxazepam) are commonly used first-line hypnotics. They change neurotransmitter activity at γ-aminobutyric acid (GABA) receptors to promote sleep and muscle relaxation as well as decrease anxiety. However, long-term use of benzodiazepines raises significant concerns regarding patients' risk of developing tolerance and dependence.

The benzodiazepine receptor agonists family, which includes zolpidem and zopiclone, are also common first-line agents of choice. These medications are pharmacologically more specific to the GABA receptor involved in sleep when compared with traditional benzodiazepines. Zolpidem and zopiclone tend to have a quick onset of action and appear to pose less risk for dependence compared to benzodiazepines (Cunnington and Qian 2017). However, benzodiazepine receptor agonists do not have the antianxiety effects of benzodiazepines helpful in decreasing anxiety-related insomnias.

Other types of psychoactive agents such as certain antidepressants (mirtazapine, trazodone, amitriptyline) and antipsychotics (quetiapine, olanzapine) that cause sedation as a secondary effect are also commonly used as sleep medications. Clinicians may prefer use of these agents over benzodiazepines and benzodiazepine receptor agonists because they pose less risk of tolerance and dependence. However, clinicians should consider the metabolic issues and daytime side effects associated with these medications as well as the limited data on their efficacy in sleep treatment.

Some sedating medications, available without prescription, also have been used to treat symptoms of insomnia. Sedating antihistamines such as doxylamine and diphenhydramine are available without prescription. However, like antidepressants, they may cause daytime sedation, and evidence for their long-term efficacy is limited. Melatonin is a widely used over-the-counter medication that, in its natural form, is released 2 hours before sleep onset. At doses ranging from 0.5 mg to 6 mg, it can be helpful short term with circadian-related insomnia (e.g., jet lag) and insomnia in the elderly, but it has limited evidence in chronic insomnia (Bartlett 2017; Cunnington and Qian 2017; Olde Rikkert and Rigaud 2001).

Assessment of Nightmares

Nightmares, a common form of parasomnia, are generally defined as dreams with disturbing, vivid, or frightening content that awaken an individual from sleep (Nadorff et al. 2014). Nightmares constitute a separate diagnosable disorder and are also an often significant component of other psychiatric disorders and sleep disturbances. Nightmares mostly occur within the REM stage of the sleep cycle and thus are more likely to occur during the latter hours of sleep (Nadorff et al. 2014). Although related in content and disturbance to sleep terrors, nightmares differ from sleep terrors in that they usually occur within the second half of the sleep cycle, are associated with a sudden waking and remembrance of dream content, and are not associated with abnormal movements or vocalizations (Sadock et al. 2014).

Nightmares are more prevalent among children than among adults, with as many as 10%–50% of 3- to 6-year-olds experiencing nightmares regularly (Sadock et al. 2014). Within the general adult population, nightmares are relatively rare, with a prevalence rate for nightmare disorder ranging between 2% and 6% (Nadorff et al. 2014). Notably, clinical cohorts, including those with posttraumatic stress disorder (PTSD), mood disorders, and schizophrenia, are reported to have higher rates of nightmares than the general population (Nadorff et al. 2014). Clinicians should be aware that many widely prescribed medications such as antidepressants (e.g., SSRIs), β-blocker antihypertensives (e.g., propranolol), dopaminergic agonists (e.g., methylphenidate), and a number of antimicrobial agents (e.g., ciprofloxacin) can also cause nightmares as a common side effect (Zak and Karippot 2018).

Nightmare disorder is included in DSM-5 as a form of REM sleep–related parasomnia in which the individual has repeated and well-remembered nightmares. These usually occur during the second half of the sleep cycle and are followed by a rapid return to orientation and alertness upon awakening. In addition, nightmare disorder includes a significant impairment in expected functioning and significant distress due to disturbed sleep, and diagnosis requires that the disturbances are not directly caused or better explained by a physiological disturbance, substance use, or a coexisting mental disorder (American Psychiatric Association 2013). Specifiers are used to denote whether nightmares occur at the onset of sleep; alongside other disorders; as acute (less than 1 month), subacute (less than 6 months), or persistent (more than 6 months); and as mild (less than once weekly), moderate (at least once weekly), or severe (nightly).

Assessing nightmares thus requires a thoughtful exploration of dream content, frequency, severity, and disturbance of an individual's sleep and wake periods. As outlined earlier in the assessment of insomnia, exploration of an individual's routine sleep-wake patterns and sleep hygiene is required. Clinicians also need to assess the impact that the dream content and sleep disturbance might be having in terms of distress and functional impairment (American Psychiatric Association 2013; Zak and Karippot 2018).

The assessment of nightmares also requires screening of potential associated conditions, including possible mood disorder, trauma, acute stress reaction, PTSD, psychosis, and substance abuse. Similarly, a review of the patient's medical and psychiatric medications, and any recent changes therein, may offer insight into possible contributors. Gaining collateral information from family and bed partners can be invaluable in discerning nightmares from other parasomnias or sleep disturbances.

Objective means of sleep assessment or investigation, such as polysomnography, are rarely useful unless features or history suggest other sleep disturbances or disorders such as REM sleep behavior disorder or obstructive sleep apnea. Rarely, nocturnal seizures, which involve frightening and distressing sensory experiences, can present as nightmares. Seizures should be excluded if a patient has any history of seizure disorder or stereotyped seizure-related movements during sleep (Zak and Karippot 2018).

Nightmare Management

Increasing evidence linking the presence of nightmares to risk of suicidal ideation and behaviors indicates that management of frequent and severe nightmares is important. Depending on the outcome of the assessment, various therapeutic approaches to manage nightmares are available.

Identification and treatment of associated and underlying conditions is key to treatment. Comorbid psychiatric disorders that present with nightmares, including acute stress reaction, PTSD, depression, and schizophrenia, must be optimally treated. Should medication be a possible cause of nightmares, a careful exploration of other pharmacological options and a risk-benefit analysis related to possible reduction in dosage or cessation of likely agents must be explored with the patient (Zak and Karippot 2018). Addressing and consolidating sleep disturbance through improved sleep hygiene, optimized bed schedule, and lifestyle factors should also always be included (Zak and Karippot 2018).

Psychological management of nightmares includes approaches that range from more analytic means of content exploration to cognitive and behavioral interventions. Imagery rehearsal therapy (IRT) is a form of trauma-focused cognitive-behavioral therapy specifically used to target nightmares occurring in the context of trauma-related conditions (Nadorff et al. 2014; Zak and Karippot 2018). IRT focuses on allowing patients to gradually work toward imagining and reexperiencing nightmare-related content, writing content down in detail, and then making more favorable and less distressing imagined changes and alterations to dream content (Zak and Karippot 2018). IRT requires a trained therapist and regular rehearsals by the patient. Although developed from working primarily with those experiencing significant nightmares in the context of PTSD, treatment with IRT results in positive outcomes for both trauma-related and non-trauma-related nightmares (Zak and Karippot 2018).

Further psychological interventions with emerging evidence of therapeutic benefit in treating nightmares also include exposure, relaxation, and rescribing therapy; systematic desensitization and exposure therapy; and (particularly in the setting of nightmares related to disorders of trauma) eye movement desensitization and reprocessing therapy (Nadorff et al. 2014). Lucid dreaming has emerged as a novel means of potentially improving nightmares; however, empirical evidence is lacking in regard to significant clinical effects (Nadorff et al. 2014).

Pharmacological means of nightmare management most notably includes the use of the α_1-adrenergic receptor antagonist prazosin, which is currently deemed to be the only pharmacological treatment with reasonable empirical evidence for nightmare treatment (Nadorff et al. 2014). With consideration of prazosin's effects on blood pressure, dosing is usually commenced at 1 mg nightly before bed and gradually titrated over weeks to a usual dosage range between 6 and 10 mg nightly (Zak and Karippot

2018). Data from a number of trials, randomized controlled trials, and meta-analyses have generally been favorable with regard to prazosin's positive effect on reducing nightmare occurrence and severity (Nadorff et al. 2014). However, more recent studies have called the effectiveness of prazosin for posttraumatic nightmares into question (Waltman et al. 2018). Evidence for other pharmacological interventions has largely centered on populations with PTSD but is less robust. Some evidence suggests the possible benefit of various other agents, including clonidine, trazodone, gabapentin, topiramate, terazosin, olanzapine, and risperidone, for improvement of nightmares in these populations (Nadorff et al. 2014; Zak and Karippot 2018).

Conclusion

Research has increasingly established sleep disorders as a significant independent risk factor for suicidal thoughts and behaviors. Although further research and insight are required, a growing understanding of the importance of identifying and treating disturbed sleep in the setting of suicidal thoughts and behaviors is clear. Disorders of sleep and sleep-related symptoms are often readily modifiable and may mitigate risk of death from suicide. Of the various sleep disturbances found to potentially increase an individual's risk for suicidal thoughts and behavior, insomnia and nightmares have the strongest association to suicide risk.

Exploration of underlying mechanisms to explain this link are ongoing and at present remain largely hypothetical. Key neurobiological links between sleep, mental disorder, and suicidal thoughts and behaviors likely mediate this connection. Nevertheless, important psychological and behavioral impacts of disturbed sleep also likely influence an individual's risk profile. A thorough sleep assessment, particularly when comorbid mental and physical disorders are present or suspected, is vital.

Key Points

- Growing evidence shows a significant and independent association between disordered sleep and increased risk of suicidal thoughts and behaviors.

- Mechanisms to explain an independent link between disordered sleep and suicidal thoughts and behaviors at present include abnormal serotonergic transmission and psychological consequences to sleep disturbance.

- Basic assessment for the presence of disordered sleep, particularly insomnia and nightmares, should be included in any evaluation of psychiatric risk, with efforts made to intervene and improve sleep wherever possible.

- Insomnia, a common psychiatric condition, can be treated effectively using basic behavioral and psychological means that psychiatrists can implement.

- In the treatment of primary insomnia, prioritize use of psychological and behavioral interventions before using sedative or sleep-related medications.

- Identification and treatment of associated and underlying conditions is key to treatment of nightmares.

References

Ahmedani BK, Peterson EL, Hu Y, et al: Major physical health conditions and risk of suicide. Am J Prev Med 53(3):308–315, 2017 28619532

American Psychiatric Association: Diagnostic and Statistical Manual of Mental Disorders, 5th Edition. Arlington, VA, American Psychiatric Association, 2013

Arroll B, Fernando A 3rd, Falloon K, et al: Development, validation (diagnostic accuracy) and audit of the Auckland Sleep Questionnaire: a new tool for diagnosing causes of sleep disorders in primary care. J Prim Health Care 3(2):107–113, 2011 21625658

Bartlett D: Delayed sleep phase disorder, in Sleep Medicine. Edited by Mansfield DR. Melbourne, IP Communications, 2017, pp 321–332

Bernert RA, Joiner TE: Sleep disturbances and suicide risk: a review of the literature. Neuropsychiatr Dis Treat 3(6):735–743, 2007 19300608

Bjørngaard JH, Bjerkeset O, Romundstad P, et al: Sleeping problems and suicide in 75,000 Norwegian adults: a 20 year follow-up of the HUNT I study. Sleep (Basel) 34(9):1155–1159, 2011 21886352

Calandre EP, Vilchez JS, Molina-Barea R, et al: Suicide attempts and risk of suicide in patients with fibromyalgia: a survey in Spanish patients. Rheumatology (Oxford) 50(10):1889–1893, 2011 21750003

Chu C, Hom MA, Rogers ML, et al: Insomnia and suicide-related behaviors: a multi-study investigation of thwarted belongingness as a distinct explanatory factor. J Affect Disord 208:153–162, 2017 27770645

Cunnington D, Qian M: Pharmacotherapy for insomnia, in Sleep Medicine. Edited by Mansfield DR. Melbourne, IP Communications, 2017, pp 311–317

Goodfellow Unit: Auckland Sleep Questionnaire. Auckland, New Zealand, University of Auckland, 2019. Available at: https://www.goodfellowunit.org/sites/default/files/insomnia/Main_Sleep_Questionnaire_final_version_2014.pdf. Accessed January 30, 2019.

Holdaway AS, Luebbe AM, Becker SP: Rumination in relation to suicide risk, ideation, and attempts: exacerbation by poor sleep quality? J Affect Disord 236:6–13, 2018 29704657

Johns MW: A new method for measuring daytime sleepiness: the Epworth sleepiness scale. Sleep 14(6):540–545, 1991 1798888

Lack L, Lovato N: Cognitive and behavioural therapy for insomnia, in Sleep Medicine. Edited by Mansfield DR. Melbourne, IP Communications, 2017, pp 303–310

Littlewood D, Kyle SD, Pratt D, et al: Examining the role of psychological factors in the relationship between sleep problems and suicide. Clin Psychol Rev 54:1–16, 2017 28371648

Malik S, Kanwar A, Sim LA, et al: The association between sleep disturbances and suicidal behaviors in patients with psychiatric diagnoses: a systematic review and meta-analysis. Syst Rev 3(18):18, 2014 24568642

Moszczynski A, Murray BJ: Neurobiological aspects of sleep physiology. Neurol Clin 30(4):963–985, 2012 23099125

Nadorff MR, Nazem S, Fiske A: Insomnia symptoms, nightmares, and suicide risk: duration of sleep disturbance matters. Suicide Life Threat Behav 43(2):139–149, 2013 23278677

Nadorff MR, Lambdin KK, Germain A: Pharmacological and non-pharmacological treatments for nightmare disorder. Int Rev Psychiatry 26(2):225–236, 2014 24892897

Olde Rikkert MGM, Rigaud ASP: Melatonin in elderly patients with insomnia. A systematic review. Z Gerontol Geriatr 34(6):491–497, 2001 11828891

Pigeon WR, Pinquart M, Conner K: Meta-analysis of sleep disturbance and suicidal thoughts and behaviors. J Clin Psychiatry 73(9):e1160–e1167, 2013 23059158

Pompili M, Innamorati M, Forte A, et al: Insomnia as a predictor of high-lethality suicide attempts. Int J Clin Pract 67(12):1311–1316, 2013 24246209

Racine M, Choinière M, Nielson WR: Predictors of suicidal ideation in chronic pain patients: an exploratory study. Clin J Pain 30(5):371–378, 2014 23887336

Richardson JD, Thompson A, King L, et al: Insomnia, psychiatric disorders and suicidal ideation in a National Representative Sample of active Canadian Forces members. BMC Psychiatry 17(1):211, 2017 28583100

Sadock BJ, Sadock VA, Ruiz P: Kaplan and Sadock's Synopsis of Psychiatry: Behavioural Science/Clinical Psychiatry, 11th Edition. Alphen aan den Rijn, The Netherlands, Wolters Kluwer, 2014

Schutte-Rodin S, Broch L, Buysse D, et al: Clinical guideline for the evaluation and management of chronic insomnia in adults. J Clin Sleep Med 4(5):487–504, 2008 18853708

Singareddy RK, Balon R: Sleep and suicide in psychiatric patients. Ann Clin Psychiatry 13(2):93–101, 2001 11534931

U.S. Food and Drug Administration: Lunesta Medication Guide (Reference ID: 3506700). Silver Spring, MD, U.S. Food and Drug Administration, 2014. Available at: https://www.accessdata.fda.gov/drugsatfda_docs/label/2014/021476s030lbl.pdf. Accessed March 27, 2019.

Waltman SH, Shearer D, Moore BA: Management of post-traumatic nightmares: a review of pharmacologic and nonpharmacologic treatments since 2013. Curr Psychiatry Rep 20(12):108, 2018 30306339

Woznica AA, Carney CE, Kuo JR, et al: The insomnia and suicide link: toward an enhanced understanding of this relationship. Sleep Med Rev 22:37–46, 2015 25454672

Zak R, Karippot A: Nightmares and nightmare disorder in adults. Up to Date, March 16, 2018. Available at: https://www.uptodate.com/contents/nightmares-and-nightmare-disorder-in-adults. Accessed January 30, 2019.

Zuromski KL, Cero I, Witte TK: Insomnia symptoms drive changes in suicide ideation: a latent difference score model of community adults over a brief interval. J Abnorm Psychol 126(6):739–749, 2017 28557509

PART III

Treatment Settings

CHAPTER 14

Emergency Services

Dexter Louie, M.D.
Divy Ravindranath, M.D., M.S., FACLP

Evaluation of patients with suicidal ideation or behavior in emergency departments (EDs) presents unique challenges. The Emergency Medical Treatment and Active Labor Act requires that any patient presenting to an ED receive an evaluation for and stabilization of life-threatening conditions, including mental health conditions (Quinn et al. 2002). Moreover, an ED is at the juncture between outpatient and inpatient care and also at the intersection between different disciplines: psychiatry, general medicine, and emergency services. This nexus requires speedy yet thorough evaluations of patients and close collaboration with other providers.

The ED psychiatrist's primary responsibility toward a suicidal patient is to perform a suicide risk assessment and determine the most appropriate intervention(s) to ensure the patient's safety. In the context of suicide, an "emergency" is defined as an acute increase in risk of harm to self, thus increasing the odds that harm to self is imminent. This evaluation is not trivial: one retrospective study found that 40% of individuals who died from suicide had presented to the ED at least once during the year prior to their death (Da Cruz et al. 2011).

Multiple interventions are available for patients with suicidal ideation or behavior, including hospitalization. However, not all crises or emergencies are best treated in a hospital setting: *chronic suicide risk* may be better managed in other ways. Therefore, assessment in the ED is characterized by *acute crisis management*. This process is dynamic, unpredictable, unique to each patient, and fundamentally different from the demographic and statistical risk factors that predominate in actuarial and epidemiological analyses.

Case Example

Ms. J is a 25-year-old woman with a history of major depressive disorder and a suicide attempt 4 years ago who presented to the ED with her sister. According to her sister, the patient has been increasingly dysphoric and quiet over the past month despite regular follow-up with her therapist and psychiatrist. Recently, she and her boyfriend broke up, and she has been under increasing stress at work. Earlier today, Ms. J confided to her sister that she felt worthless and had impulses to cut in order to punish herself for "never having accomplished anything." On arrival to the ED, the patient reports suicidal ideation to the triage nurse. After a search to ensure she has no weapons, Ms. J is directed to a secure ED bay within sight of the nursing station to wait for medical and mental health evaluations.

On interview, Ms. J is cooperative but guarded and withdrawn. She confirms worsening mood, a pervasive sense of worthlessness, and thoughts about death. When asked about a plan to attempt suicide, she does not respond. In her prior attempt, she took an overdose of alcohol and drugs in the context of feeling lonely and rejected. She denies owning a firearm or having strong religious beliefs. The interview demonstrates that she still finds the thoughts of death to be disturbing but also hypnotic.

Upon contacting her outpatient psychiatrist, the ED psychiatrist learns that the patient has not endorsed a concrete suicidal plan but has become more depressed recently. She has had multiple medication trials without robust effect. She agrees to keep working with her outpatient psychiatrist and reassures the ED psychiatrist that she will not engage in suicidal behaviors if discharged home. However, Ms. J is unable to offer any strategy as to how she might manage future moments of crisis.

After conducting a complete risk assessment, the ED psychiatrist is concerned about Ms. J's safety. Although she is not at imminent risk of suicide, she is fragile, has worsening depression despite appropriate treatment, has recent stressors, has a history of suicidal behavior, and cannot construct a suicide safety plan. Therefore, the ED psychiatrist recommends that Ms. J might benefit from psychiatric hospitalization, to which Ms. J agrees.

Triaging of Suicidal Patients in the Emergency Department

Initial triage is defined as the rapid assessment of a patient's most immediate needs and integration into the ED workflow for the purpose of addressing both mental and physical health concerns. Patients with active suicidal ideation (SI) should be considered high priority due to the risk that they may abscond or harm themselves while in the ED. Patients with psychiatric symptoms but without report of either SI or warning signs of suicidal behavior or intent may be considered lower priority. In light of the rising rate of suicide in the United States (Centers for Disease Control and Prevention 2019) and its place as the tenth leading cause of death in the country (Centers for Disease Control and Prevention 2018), one of The Joint Commission (2019)'s National Patient Safety Goals is using a validated screening instrument for suicide risk in all patients who present with behavioral health concerns and subsequently managing that risk.

Most EDs in the United States use the Emergency Severity Index (McHugh et al. 2012) to assign triage tiers to patients who present to the ED; however, other systems exist. One example, the Australasian triage system (Australasian College for Emergency Medicine 2002), contains descriptors of mental illness within its scoring rubric.

Valuable information can be gained as soon as the patient arrives. For example, does the patient arrive alone, accompanied by a friend or family member, or with the police? The first is more likely to maximize symptoms; the second is more likely to minimize.

Whether the patient has arrived voluntarily is also important, because this not only informs the context of the interview but also may impact disposition. If available, obtain information from collateral informants. This information may be almost as important as the patient interview, because patient self-reports vary widely in reliability.

Triage can occur in a number of locations, each with advantages and disadvantages. The waiting room is the most accessible location, but the least private and contained. A "safe" room allows for maximum privacy and containment in case the patient has problematic behavioral issues but demands a dedicated space. An ED medical bay or triage room represents a middle ground between these two alternatives. When possible, consider minimizing long waiting times because they are a negative for both staff and patients (Derlet and Richards 2000).

Risk Management in the Emergency Department

Once identified to be at risk, patients who present with SI should not be left unsupervised, either in the waiting area before they have been triaged or after triage if they have been deemed to present a danger to themselves. Therefore, sitters or a standby security presence play a vital role in maintaining safety in the ED. Ideally, sitters and security personnel are unobtrusive and nonthreatening. Sometimes, a trusted family member can supervise a suicidal patient in lieu of a sitter; however, this must be determined on a case-by-case basis according to clinical judgment.

Medical evaluations are a critical part of the ED assessment process for patients who present with suicidal ideation or behavior. Agitation, depression, or psychosis are often mistaken as psychiatric in origin when in fact the causative factor is an underlying nonpsychiatric problem, for example, dementia or delirium. Furthermore, active, comorbid medical issues may also require acute intervention or assessment. These may range from problems unrelated to psychiatric issues, for example, unmanaged diabetes, to those intimately connected to mental health, such as surface wounds due to self-cutting, high blood pressure due to medication nonadherence secondary to crippling depression, or active alcohol use that may develop into alcohol withdrawal if the patient is admitted to a psychiatric facility. EDs are required to perform a general medical screening evaluation of all admitted patients. These assessments should include

- Evaluation for medical conditions present because of suicidal thoughts and behaviors
- Evaluation for chronic medical conditions poorly controlled secondary to the patient's mental condition
- Evaluation for chronic medical conditions that may impact the patient's psychiatric care
- Evaluation for comorbid medical conditions that may develop into medical calamities if not addressed

Checklists are available in the literature to aid the ED physician in conducting a brief but thorough medical assessment, which may ultimately be needed for "clearance" if the patient should be admitted to a psychiatric unit (Shah et al. 2012; Sood and Mcstay 2009).

The need for nonpsychiatric hospitalization usually supersedes the need for psychiatric hospitalization. Patients who have simultaneous acute psychiatric and nonpsychiatric issues should be maintained in the ED on close observation with suicide precautions, which includes removal of items that may be used for self-harm, such as scissors or metal cutlery (The Joint Commission 2016). Many hospitals have psychiatric or other mental health consultation available for monitoring, treatment, and disposition of patients admitted to medical/surgical wards with concomitant SI.

Substance Use Disorders and Suicidal Ideation

Patients who present to EDs with acute SI and active intoxication pose a significant challenge for ED personnel. Intoxication can alter one's risk for intentional self-injury: for example, in alcohol intoxication, emotional lability and behavioral disinhibition may prompt rash behaviors. Withdrawal may also influence risk for death from suicide, as exemplified by the profound depression experienced during cocaine withdrawal. Thus, both intoxication and withdrawal represent states in which risk of death from suicide is altered.

At the same time, identifying and modifying patients' risk factors for death from suicide may prove difficult if substance intoxication or withdrawal interferes with their capacity to engage in the interview. Thus, keeping the patient safe until the intoxication or withdrawal state can improve to a standard of clinical sobriety may be a precondition to a comprehensive patient evaluation.

Some knowledge of patients' typical behavior when intoxicated or in withdrawal may help provide context for their behavior and guide interventions to maintain safety. If substance use constitutes the patient's main risk factor, then maintaining the patient in a safe space until the patient is no longer acutely intoxicated or in active withdrawal may be the best means of reducing the risk of death from suicide. In some cases, inpatient psychiatric or medical hospitalization may be necessary to prevent medical complications of substance use or to address a prolonged withdrawal.

When a patient with a history of substance use disorder presents in a nonintoxicated and nonwithdrawal state but still demonstrates acute SI, suspect a primary psychiatric disorder. These "dual diagnosis" patients require treatment for both their substance use disorders and their primary mental illness. Conceptualize the two problems separately and devise independent treatment plans for both. For patients who are precontemplative about their readiness to cut back or discontinue substance use, consider a motivational interviewing approach (Miller and Rollnick 2002).

Suicide Risk Assessment in the Emergency Department

Psychiatric interviews in the ED face obstacles that may leave psychiatrists with the need to act based on incomplete information. Both the patient and the provider are often meeting each other for the first time and have no therapeutic relationship upon which to draw. Patients often present after business hours, making timely contact with their treating mental health providers, if any, difficult.

In addition, patients often arrive in an emotionally or behaviorally activated state that may worsen in the ED. The environment of the ED is not private and is often noisy and chaotic. Patients may be resentful or angry if compelled to have a mental health evaluation in the ED, for example, if SI was detected while evaluating an unrelated chief complaint. Furthermore, police often bring patients involuntarily to the ED as a result of their behavioral disturbances.

If the patient is behaviorally activated, safety of both the patient and the practitioner is the most important consideration. ED staff should attempt verbal deescalation by use of validating statements in a calm tone of voice (Holloman and Zeller 2012). Clinicians can also redirect patients by addressing their immediate needs, starting with, for example, food, water, and physical comfort. Clinicians should avoid hot beverages, which can be used as weapons.

If these interventions fail to decrease the patient's agitation, emergent medications may become necessary. Clinicians should first offer medications by mouth, although if the patient refuses or rapid effect is needed, clinicians may need to use intramuscular injections (Table 14–1) or physical restraints. Restraints are indicated by immediate risk of (Coburn and Mycyk 2009):

- Harm to patient
- Harm to other patients
- Harm to caregivers/staff
- Serious disruption or damage to the environment

Individual institutions have their own policies and procedures regarding restraints. The utmost care should be taken to avoid injury to the patient and staff and to ensure that patients are not left in restraints indefinitely.

The goal of the psychiatric interview is to clarify risk factors contributing to a patient's acute suicide risk state. Critical data to gather in a suicidal patient include the following acute risk factors: active SI, active plan or intent to die, rehearsal behaviors, and access to means (including firearms). Important chronic risk factors include a personal and family history of suicide attempt.

However, although understanding a patient's global risk of dying from suicide is important, their acute risk state is the focus of clinical attention. Pisani et al. (2016) proposed a formulation process for suicide risk that separately defines a patient's acute risk state as opposed to chronic risk status. Acute risk state indicators include current SI, recent psychosocial stressors, active symptoms of depression, and the quality of patients' therapeutic engagement or alliance. These risk factors are fluid and dynamic, which makes them more amenable to intervention. These differ from static and demographic risk factors such as sex, age, and marital status, which correlate more with chronic risk status.

Standardized instruments for suicide risk evaluation can assist the provider's assessment: the Beck Suicide Scale and the Columbia Suicide Severity Rating Scale are two of the most commonly known. However, clinicians often need to use their clinical judgment and cannot rely on rating scales alone. See Table 14–2 for one formulation of common acute and chronic risk factors.

The lethality of a patient's suicidal behavior or suicide attempt does not always correlate with a patient's intent to die, and the two should be considered as separate dimensions (Gjelsvik et al. 2017). Clinicians should maintain a low threshold for placing

TABLE 14–1.   Common medications used for agitation management

Medication	Adult dosage	Uses	Side effects
Haloperidol	0.5–5 mg po/iv/im (up to 15 mg/day)	As needed for psychosis or agitation	EPS QTc prolongation
Olanzapine	5–10 mg po/im (up to 20 mg/day)	As needed for psychosis or agitation when QTc prolongation is to be avoided	Low maximum dosage Expensive
Risperidone	0.5–2 mg po	As needed for psychosis or agitation when QTc prolongation is to be avoided	EPS at higher dosages
Lorazepam	0.5–4 mg po/iv/im		Oversedation Respiratory depression
Benztropine	0.5–2 mg po/im	May substitute for diphenhydramine	Anticholinergic side effects (including delirium in elderly)
Diphenhydramine	25–50 mg po/im	Sedating, with anxiolytic properties	Delirium in elderly Paradoxical activation
Intramuscular Haldol, Ativan, diphenhydramine	5 mg, 2 mg, 50 mg, respectively	Emergent cases when patient is refusing oral	EPS QTc prolongation Oversedation Respiratory depression Delirium in elderly Paradoxical activation
Intramuscular olanzapine/ diphenhydramine	10 mg/50 mg	Emergent cases when patient is refusing oral and QTc prolongation is to be avoided	Do not use intramuscular olanzapine with intramuscular benzodiazepines due to risk of respiratory depression

Note.   EPS=extrapyramidal symptoms, including dystonic reactions.

Source.   Adapted from Winder GS, Glick R: "The Agitated Patient," in *Clinical Manual of Emergency Psychiatry*, 2nd Edition. Edited by Riba M, Ravindranath D, Winder GS. Washington, DC, American Psychiatric Publishing, 2015, pp 153–177. Used with permission. Copyright © 2015 American Psychiatric Publishing.

patients who have acted on their suicidal impulses, either by engaging in parasuicidal behavior or making an attempt, into a higher-risk category regardless of lethality.

Deception in the Suicidal Emergency Department Patient

Dealing with deception is an additional unfortunate but unavoidable aspect of working in the ED. Patients may engage in deception by denying, maximizing, or minimizing their symptoms in ways that can be difficult for clinicians to detect. Nevertheless, clinicians are well advised to avoid relying solely on a patient's self-report as the basis

TABLE 14–2. **Common chronic and acute risk factors for suicide**

Chronic risk factors	Acute risk factors
Often difficult to modify	Often modifiable
Convey statistical risk over time, not immediate risk	Dynamic and fluid, impact the immediate situation
Male gender	Access to means
Older age	Substance intoxication
Prior suicide attempts	Significant psychosocial stressors
Family history of suicide	Loneliness
Chronic nonpsychiatric illness or pain	Hopelessness
Substance abuse disorder or history of impulsive decision making	Physical warning signs of severe depression (irritability, restlessness/akathisia)
	Lack of therapeutic alliance or engagement

Source. Adapted from Simon 2008.

of a determination of suicide risk. Internal inconsistencies within patients' narratives, between their narratives and their examinations, or between their narratives and the information gathered from collateral informants may be indicators of deception. The same may be true for vague narratives with considerable missing or incomplete details. Behavioral assessments of the patient's suicide risk state, such as their verifiable prearrival behaviors or observation of the patient's behaviors while in the ED, can also be compared to the patient's subjective report (Simon 2008).

When possible, procuring collateral information is critical. The Health Insurance Portability and Accountability Act (HIPAA) provides an exception to confidentiality in emergency situations, although written consent for discussion with collateral informants should be obtained if the patient is amenable (U.S. Department of Health and Human Services 2014). Providers should consider contacting family, friends, emergency contacts, and outpatient providers. Prudent clinicians should familiarize themselves with local statutes, because state laws differ in regard to legal thresholds for protecting patient privacy.

Structured and clinically informed assessments of suicide risk state can help to differentiate whether patients' expressions of SI are consistent with their circumstances. When deception is suspected, clinicians may have to give apparent risk factors more or less weight, based upon the context and the physician's observations (Beach et al. 2017). Although physicians can become frustrated when confronted with patients who are deceptive, such behavior often signals unmet needs elsewhere in the patient's life, and efforts should be made to understand and address these if possible.

Treatment

A recent multicenter study of ED suicide prevention has demonstrated that screening alone, without further intervention, does not decrease the risk of death from suicide (Miller et al. 2017). Therefore, suicidal patients in the ED should begin to receive treatment immediately. ED personnel, including psychiatrists, can begin helping patients process their suicidal thoughts, engage in collaborative problem solving to address the issues driving the patient's current crisis, and identify sources of support (Betz and Boudreaux 2016).

Multiple trials of ED interventions with suicidal patients have found these interventions increase the likelihood of a safe outpatient disposition. Creating a "suicide safety plan" is one simple and straightforward intervention. The suicide safety plan asks patients for written descriptions of their triggers for SI, self-soothing tasks to distract from the suicidal thoughts, people whom they could contact in a crisis, their professional supports, and plans for means restriction (Stanley et al. 2016). Suicide safety planning is not the same as "contracting for safety," which has limited supporting evidence and is no longer recommended (Betz et al. 2016).

Suicide safety plans alone have not shown benefit in an ED population; however, when combined with telephonic outreach from the health system after an ED visit, they have the capacity to decrease suicidal behavior (Stanley et al. 2018). Thus, follow-up after leaving the ED is another critical component of care. The multicenter Emergency Department Safety Assessment and Follow-up Evaluation (ED-SAFE) study followed patients discharged from the ED with weekly check-in phone calls until the patient attended an outpatient appointment. The study found a 5% absolute reduction in suicide attempt risk (relative risk reduction of 20%) (Miller et al. 2017).

Availability of rapid follow-up after an ED encounter is also protective against death from suicide (Knesper 2011). Although suicide safety plans and telephonic case management can provide support, these crisis management measures are not replacements for definitive treatment. Some hospital systems can make an immediate referral to an outpatient provider, such that the patient leaves the ED with an outpatient appointment in hand. Other hospital systems have the capacity for bridging follow-up appointments in the ED itself. Some hospital systems are not part of an integrated system but employ case managers to help the ED patient in crisis find outpatient treatment. Some EDs stand alone and may only have access to mental health expertise through a telepsychiatry contract. Given the variety of options and possibilities, ED psychiatrists and consultants should be aware of the options available at the hospitals in which they work.

Disposition

Acute risk formulation is a fluid and dynamic process. Patients receiving treatment in the ED may respond in ways that change their acute risk state. High-risk patients are those in crisis who cannot collaborate with interventions including suicide safety planning, marshaling social supports, or restricting access to means. Low-risk patients are those who have intermittent thoughts of death or suicide but find that these thoughts do not persist for long and can provide multiple reasons as to why they would not kill themselves, are hopeful for improvement in their current state of affairs, and are committed to working with professionals to address their psychiatric problems. Moderate-risk patients fall in between these two categories. Interventions undertaken in the ED may convert a patient who was high risk on arrival into a lower risk category by the end of the ED encounter. The final assessment of the patient's risk should be made after available efforts are exhausted.

If acute risk remains high despite ED treatment, then clinicians should pursue hospitalization. Voluntary hospitalization is preferred if the patient is willing to consent, as in the case of Ms. J described earlier. However, if a patient meets criteria for civil commitment and refuses voluntary hospitalization, then the ED psychiatrist should pursue involuntary hospitalization (see Chapter 17, "Civil Commitment"). Involuntary civil commitment procedures vary from state to state, and ED psychiatrists should be familiar with the process in the state in which they practice.

The ED provider is responsible for the safety of the patient in the ED until a receiving hospital can be identified and the patient transferred. While waiting for transfer, patients should be reassessed periodically. The treating ED team as well as the mental health team should continue to provide indicated treatment interventions while determination of final disposition is ongoing. Once a transfer has been arranged, secure transportation will be required to ensure that the patient arrives to the destination without incident.

Special Populations

Children and Adolescents

Suicide risk assessment in children and adolescents can also be challenging, given that these patients have unique mental health needs (see Chapter 18, "Children and Adolescents"). An age-appropriate approach to the interview has the greatest chance for eliciting truthful information. As with any ED evaluation, the patient's risk for self-injurious behavior in the present crisis should be determined and compared to the patient's baseline risk for self-injurious behavior. If the risk is significantly elevated and cannot be modified through ED intervention, then the patient may require psychiatric hospitalization.

In this population, information from parents or guardians is required. These individuals are responsible for the patient's care and may provide the most useful collateral information for determining the patient's risk for suicidal behavior. In many states, children and adolescents can only be psychiatrically admitted or receive outpatient treatment with the permission of a parent or guardian, even if the patient has the clinical capacity to consent. If parents or guardians disagree with the ED provider's treatment recommendations, they may be endangering the child and a Child Protective Services report may need to be filed.

Patients With a History of Multiple Suicide Attempts

Patients who have a history of multiple low-lethality suicide attempts are particularly challenging for the ED mental health provider. The degree of the patient's intent can be especially difficult to discern. On the one hand, the current crisis may be the time when the patient actually dies from suicide. On the other hand, many reasons exist to avoid unnecessarily hospitalizing these patients, including conserving limited mental health financial resources and inpatient beds and unintentionally "rewarding" nonconstructive behavior/promoting regression. These clinical consequences can exacerbate the underlying mental illness.

Regardless of the difficulties of managing these patients in the ED, they do in fact have serious mental illness. The presence of longstanding affective disorders, drug/

alcohol use disorders, anxiety, and a first suicide attempt at a young age all correlate with repeated attempts (Lopez-Castroman et al. 2011). Moreover, multiple attempters have a more severe clinical profile, such as traumatic childhood backgrounds, increased psychopathology, more SI, and poorer interpersonal functioning, even when controlling for a comorbid personality disorder (Forman et al. 2004).

In these patients, trying to discern the details of the current psychosocial crisis is essential in determining the risk of suicide, because the thoughts of suicide are the result of a psychosocial spiral. Although they presented to the ED with SI, creative interventions may be needed to prompt these patients to talk about the trigger for their worsening thoughts of suicide. Examiners will likely have to try a variety of strategies to get the patient to talk about an undoubtedly upsetting experience. As with all ED cases, contact with current providers or other collateral informants can be essential in determining the details of the current crisis.

Even with patients who repeatedly attempt suicide, each presentation to the ED must be evaluated as a single and separate emergency. Each suicidal crisis needs to be addressed and the risk of death from suicide decreased before the patient can be discharged from the ED. If the patient is too emotionally overwrought to reasonably discuss the details of the crisis that precipitated the SI or to engage in safety planning, then hospitalization may be necessary, despite its clinical disadvantages for these patients.

Homeless Patients

Homeless patients present another challenge because their complaints of SI present the possibility that they are seeking hospitalization to avoid living on the street. As discussed, an assessment of patients' behavior—rather than their self-report—provides a more accurate evaluation of risk. Even if homeless patients are judged to be at sufficiently low risk to be discharged to the community, they may refuse to participate in safety planning or other treatment planning. For these patients, finding safe shelter in a hospital may be worth refusing outpatient psychiatric assistance. Some communities have homeless outreach programs to which homeless patients can be referred. Advising homeless patients that additional resources may be available to them may improve their engagement with treatment planning.

Documentation

ED psychiatrists should carefully document suicide risk assessments and the factors contributing to the patient's acute risk state. These include the presence or absence of the following:

- Active SI
- Plan or intent
- Rehearsal behaviors
- Psychosocial stressors
- Access to means, especially firearms
- Interpersonal factors (thwarted belongingness, perceived burdensomeness, hopelessness; see Chapter 7, "Depressive Disorders")
- Protective factors

Clinicians should document any interventions attempted in the ED and their impact, if any, on the patient's acute risk state. They should also document historical and statistical factors associated with the patient's chronic risk status. Documentation of assessments of patients with an elevated chronic risk of death from suicide should include a discussion of the difference between current condition and baseline state in order to acknowledge that although suicide risk fluctuates over time, certain individuals require closer long-term monitoring and follow-up.

For patients suspected of engaging in deception or pursuing a non–mental health agenda, documentation should be very thorough. The risk assessment should carefully review risk and protective factors, the weight given to each, and the formulation of level of risk. The documentation should reference past records that establish patterns of behavior and cite conversations with collateral informants. Assessments should avoid pejorative language and negative bias and should demonstrate an attempt to understand the patient's actions and needs. Attempts to meet the patient's needs and the patient's response to these offers should also be recorded.

Timely documentation by all ED clinical staff is critical to timely disposition. If a patient is being transferred to an admitting facility, the receiving hospital may request the ED's medical and laboratory evaluations that have established medical stability, suicide risk assessments, and any anticipated needs during hospitalization.

Conclusion

Suicide risk assessment in the ED plays a major role in the assessment and treatment of patients with severe psychiatric illnesses. Assessing a patient's acute versus chronic risk factors for death from suicide in the context of multiple potential complicating factors, including nonpsychiatric illnesses, intoxication, or substance use, and psychosocial factors such as chronic homelessness, poses a rigorous yet critically important challenge for physicians in the ED. Fortunately, a number of strategies and tools exist to help physician make their assessments and intervene to reduce risk of death from suicide in order to ensure that this population receives the best care possible.

Key Points

- All suicidal patients should be placed on special precautions and should receive a general medical evaluation.

- Emergency department (ED) evaluations should differentiate carefully between acute risk and chronic risk.

- Critical data to obtain in the ED assessment include active suicide ideation, active plan or intent to die, rehearsal behaviors, access to means, recent psychosocial stressors, active symptoms of depression, and quality of patients' therapeutic engagement or alliance.

- Obtain collateral information wherever possible.

- Intoxication can influence risk for suicide significantly; some patients may need to be maintained in a safe space until no longer under the influence of substances.

- Suicide screening alone is insufficient. A suicide safety plan or other forms of collaborative problem solving, as well as rapid follow-up after leaving the ED, should be implemented.

- If unable to modify a patient's high risk of death from suicide in the ED, then consider hospitalization. Each ED admission must be evaluated as a separate emergency regardless of past history.

References

Australasian College for Emergency Medicine: The Australasian Triage Scale. Emerg Med (Fremantle) 14(3):335–336, 2002 12549430

Beach SR, Taylor JB, Kontos N: Teaching psychiatric trainees to "think dirty": uncovering hidden motivations and deception. Psychosomatics 58(5):474–482, 2017 28602447

Betz ME, Boudreaux ED: Managing suicidal patients in the emergency department. Ann Emerg Med 67(2):276–282, 2016 26443554

Betz ME, Wintersteen M, Boudreaux ED, et al: Reducing suicide risk: challenges and opportunities in the emergency department. Ann Emerg Med 68(6):758–765, 2016 27451339

Centers for Disease Control and Prevention: FastStats. Atlanta, GA, Centers for Disease Control and Prevention, November 26, 2018. Available at: https://www.cdc.gov/nchs/fastats/deaths.htm. 2019. Accessed February 9, 2019.

Centers for Disease Control and Prevention: Fatal Injury Reports, National, Regional and State, 1981–2017. Atlanta, GA, Centers for Disease Control and Prevention, 2019. Available at: https://webappa.cdc.gov/sasweb/ncipc/mortrate.html. Accessed February 9, 2019.

Coburn VA, Mycyk MB: Physical and chemical restraints. Emerg Med Clin North Am 27(4):655–667, ix, 2009 19932399

Da Cruz D, Pearson A, Saini P, et al: Emergency department contact prior to suicide in mental health patients (EMJ). Emerg Med J 28(6):467–471, 2011 20660941

Derlet RW, Richards JR: Overcrowding in the nation's emergency departments: complex causes and disturbing effects. Ann Emerg Med 35(1):63–68, 2000 10613941

Forman EM, Berk MS, Henriques GR, et al: History of multiple suicide attempts as a behavioral marker of severe psychopathology. Am J Psychiatry 161(3):437–443, 2004 14992968

Gjelsvik B, Heyerdahl F, Holmes J, et al: Is there a relationship between suicidal intent and lethality in deliberate self-poisoning? Suicide Life Threat Behav 47(2):205–216, 2017 27416812

Holloman GH Jr, Zeller SL: Overview of Project BETA: best practices in evaluation and treatment of agitation. West J Emerg Med 13(1):1–2, 2012 22461914

The Joint Commission: Detecting and treating suicide ideation in all settings. Sentinel Event Alert 56, February 24, 2016. Available at: https://www.jointcommission.org/assets/1/18/SEA_56_Suicide.pdf. Accessed November 12, 2018 26915165

The Joint Commission: 2019 National Patient Safety Goals. Oakbrook Terrace, IL, The Joint Commission, 2019. Available at: http://www.jointcommission.org/standards_information/npsgs.aspx. Accessed February 9, 2019.

Knesper DJ: Continuity of Care for Suicide Prevention and Research. Washington, DC, Suicide Prevention Resource Center, 2011. Available at: http://www.sprc.org/resources-programs/continuity-care-suicide-prevention-research. Accessed November 13, 2018.

Lopez-Castroman J, Perez-Rodriguez MdeL, Jaussent I, et al: Distinguishing the relevant features of frequent suicide attempters. J Psychiatr Res 45(5):619–625, 2011 21055768

McHugh M, Tanabe P, McClelland M, et al: More patients are triaged using the Emergency Severity Index than any other triage acuity system in the United States. Acad Emerg Med 19(1):106–109, 2012 22211429

Miller IW, Camargo CA Jr, Arias SA, et al: Suicide prevention in an emergency department population: the ED-SAFE study. JAMA Psychiatry 74(6):563–570, 2017 28456130

Miller WR, Rollnick S: Motivational Interviewing: Preparing People for Change, 2nd Edition. New York, Guilford, 2002

Pisani AR, Murrie DC, Silverman MM: Reformulating suicide risk formulation: from prediction to prevention. Acad Psychiatry 40(4):623–629, 2016 26667005

Quinn DK, Geppert CM, Maggiore WA: The Emergency Medical Treatment and Active Labor Act of 1985 and the practice of psychiatry. Psychiatr Serv 53(10):1301–1307, 2002 12364679

Shah SJ, Fiorito M, McNamara RM: A screening tool to medically clear psychiatric patients in the emergency department. J Emerg Med 43(5):871–875, 2012 20347248

Simon RI: Behavioral risk assessment of the guarded suicidal patient. Suicide Life Threat Behav 38(5):517–522, 2008 19014304

Sood TR, Mcstay CM: Evaluation of the psychiatric patient. Emerg Med Clin North Am 27(4):669–683, ix, 2009 19932400

Stanley B, Chaudhury SR, Chesin M, et al: An emergency department intervention and follow-up to reduce suicide risk in the VA: acceptability and effectiveness. Psychiatr Serv 67(6):680–683, 2016 26828397

Stanley B, Brown GK, Brenner LA, et al: Comparison of the safety planning intervention with follow-up vs usual care of suicidal patients treated in the emergency department. JAMA Psychiatry 75(9):894–900, 2018 29998307

U.S. Department of Health and Human Services: Bulletin: HIPAA Privacy in Emergency Situations. Washington, DC, U.S. Department of Health and Human Services, Office for Civil Rights, November 2014. Available at: https://www.hhs.gov/sites/default/files/ocr/privacy/hipaa/understanding/special/emergency/hipaa-privacy-emergency-situations.pdf. Accessed February 9, 2019.

CHAPTER 15

Outpatient Treatment of the Suicidal Patient

James C. West, M.D.

Derrick A. Hamaoka, M.D.

Robert J. Ursano, M.D.

Managing suicidal ideation in the outpatient setting is common in psychiatric practice. Many patients experience intermittent but chronic suicidal ideation as part of their illness. Patients at risk of death from suicide may require inpatient hospitalization in their most acute presentations, but most will continue treatment as outpatients once the acute crisis has passed. Suicidal ideation can develop in many psychiatric disorders treated in the outpatient setting.

Effective outpatient treatment of the patient at risk of death from suicide is based on attention to several important elements of care. Screening and risk assessment are imperative to identify patients at elevated risk. For those at increased risk of death from suicide, establishing and sustaining what can be a fragile therapeutic alliance is an essential aspect of treatment. In addition, in the past decade, researchers have increasingly investigated the effectiveness of specific psychotherapies and other interventions to address suicidal ideation and suicide risk in outpatients. This chapter reviews the role of therapeutic alliance in the management of outpatients with suicidal ideation and reviews specific interventions in the outpatient setting.

Disclaimer: The views expressed are those of the authors and do not necessarily reflect the views of the Department of Defense, the Uniformed Services University, the Department of Health and Human Services or the United States Public Health Service. This work was prepared by a military or civilian employee of the U.S. Government as part of the individual's official duties and therefore is in the public domain and does not possess copyright protection (public domain information may be freely distributed and copied; however, as a courtesy it is requested that the Uniformed Services University and the author be given an appropriate acknowledgment).

Case Example

Charles is a 42-year-old man who recently started treatment for major depressive disorder. His symptoms from the beginning included recurrent thoughts of death as an escape from his current troubles. Previously a successful manager, he lost his job 6 months prior and had difficulty finding similar work. His wife of 15 years continued to have a successful career, leaving him feeling worthless because he was not able to contribute financially to the family. At the start of his treatment he denied suicidal ideation, and he denied a plan or intent to act. He had no past history of psychiatric treatment or suicide attempts. Six weeks into treatment, he was feeling better and responding to antidepressant medication and cognitive-behavioral therapy (CBT). It was at this time that his wife told him she had recently had an extramarital affair. This news sent Charles into an emotional tailspin. He became acutely suicidal and was hospitalized for 5 days.

Therapeutic Alliance

The *therapeutic alliance*, also called the *working alliance* or *working relationship*, is a core component of outpatient treatment and is a particular focus for the treatment of the patient at risk of death from suicide. This is true for patients who develop or disclose suicidal ideation in the course of treatment as well as those who come into treatment following hospitalization for suicidal ideation or attempt. The therapeutic alliance has been defined many ways, but most definitions incorporate the central concept of a bond between patient and therapist based on an interpersonal relationship and shared goals of treatment (Horvath et al. 2011).

The therapeutic alliance is the intentionally and explicitly negotiated agreement between patient and therapist to collaborate in the treatment task (Plakun 2009). This implies a shared responsibility between patient and therapist to remain in treatment and also implies that the patient will stay alive to do so. The therapist has the additional responsibility of accepting and containing transference from the patient and specifically recognizing suicidal ideation or attempt as a rupture of the therapeutic relationship. A patient's attempt at suicide may also reflect hostility directed toward the therapy; if so, the therapist should offer appropriate interpretation. In this context, one further goal of treatment is for therapist and patient to repair the alliance after a suicide attempt (Plakun 2009).

The bond between therapist and patient allows for the experience of negative feelings and reactions within therapy while taking the steps needed to maintain patient safety. Experiencing negative emotions and externalizing behavior within a therapeutic relationship focused on rebuilding trust and confidence can enable the suicidal patient to recover. However, this alliance is not one in which the therapist attempts to exert control over the patient's desires to die from suicide (Dunster-Page et al. 2017). Such a stance would be countertherapeutic and usually activates the patient's needs for independence and control. The elements that go into forming a therapeutic alliance are reviewed in Table 15–1.

Several techniques promote developing a therapeutic alliance with the suicidal patient (Michel and Jobes 2011; see Table 15–2). The first of these is *narrative interviewing*. The goal of narrative interviewing is to encourage patients to describe in their own words the circumstances that led up to the suicidal act. Although the patient may freely associate a comprehensive narrative from an open-ended question, therapists

---

TABLE 15–1. **Elements of therapeutic alliance in suicide risk management**

Explicit and negotiated agreement between patient and therapist

Patient commitment to remain in the treatment relationship

Therapist commitment to accept transference and negative emotions and interpret

Promoting and acknowledging attachment between patient and therapist

Rebuilding of trust

TABLE 15–2. **Building the therapeutic alliance: techniques**

---

1. Establishing the initial relationship, narrative interviewing: "Help me understand what was happening when you took the overdose."
2. Mentalizing and validation: "What you just described sounds incredibly painful. I appreciate that you are able to share that with me."
3. Framing in interpersonal terms: "Is there any reason I should be worried about you?"

---

may have to provide additional prompting for some patients to add detail or fill gaps in the narrative.

This approach contrasts with that of a typical diagnostic interview in which the therapist tries to delineate particular symptoms in order to confirm a specific diagnosis. Clearly delineating symptoms of specific illnesses usually is also necessary but is secondary to gaining understanding of the events and state of mind of the patient. Suicidal patients commonly believe that they are experiencing a state of mental pain to which no other person could possibly relate. Engaging with the patient's narrative creates the space to contradict that belief (Michel et al. 2002).

Mentalizing and validation are additional techniques that promote the therapeutic alliance with the suicidal patient (Michel and Jobes 2011). Suicidal patients often view themselves as alone in an unimaginably painful emotional state. *Mentalizing* on the part of the therapist involves listening and appreciating patients' state of mind and conveying that appreciation to patients in such a way that they do not see themselves as alone or misunderstood. *Validation* as a therapeutic technique goes beyond understanding the patient's experience. Through validation, the therapist conveys acceptance of the patient's experience without trying to change it immediately. This can be particularly challenging for therapists in an emergency setting or early in a therapeutic relationship. Therapists in these circumstances tend to focus on setting up barriers to death from suicide. However, if patients do not feel understood and accepted, therapists risk substantially damaging any subsequent therapeutic alliance.

In-session techniques that potentially enhance the therapeutic alliance include framing the interaction in highly interpersonal terms. A question such as, "Is there any reason I should be worried about you or worried about your safety?" is an example of this. Such questions overtly recognize the dyad of patient and therapist and promote patients' consideration of the implication that the therapist is committed to staying in the treatment relationship.

The interpersonal theory of suicide posits that three primary elements lead to a patient's suicide attempt: thwarted belongingness, perceived burdensomeness, and the acquired capacity for self-harm. Viewing the therapeutic alliance from this theoretical perspective (Van Orden et al. 2010), the establishment of the relationship with a therapist fundamentally undermines the patient's sense of thwarted belongingness. A suicide attempt requires that the patient act against the attachment, however tenuous, between patient and therapist. Indeed, alliance-based interventions for suicidal thoughts and behaviors leverage this concept in the unstated expectation that the therapist can only be of use to the patient so long as the patient stays in therapy and therefore stays alive (Plakun 2009).

Suicidal patients may experience significantly more negative reactions to therapy, such as missing sessions or acting out. The therapeutic alliance can moderate these elements and sustain a positive treatment outcome (Perry et al. 2013). However, early in treatment, this alliance may not be a robust predictor of improvement in suicidal ideation (Bryan et al. 2012). A recent study of suicide behaviors in U.S. Army soldiers identified several factors contributing to an increased risk of suicide attempt among those with suicidal ideation, including recent onset of ideation, presence of a recently conceived suicide plan, low controllability of suicidal thoughts, risk-taking behaviors, and failure to answer questions about characteristics of suicidal thoughts (Naifeh et al. 2019).

No-Harm Contracts

Safety planning is an important part of developing treatment plans for patients with suicidal ideation in the outpatient setting. One aspect of safety planning is the "no-harm contract." In this discussion and exchange, the patient makes various agreements about safety with the therapist, such as to not attempt suicide for a defined period of time or to contact the therapist if suicidal ideation or impulses arise (Garvey et al. 2009). The concept behind "contracting for safety" is based on the existence of a strong therapeutic relationship in which the patient feels "bound" by a promise to the therapist. The critical element, which is often overlooked when psychiatrists and other mental health professionals engage in safety contracts with patients, is the development of trust, mutual respect, and engagement between the provider and the patient.

Regardless, compared to more intensive crisis planning, safety contracts are inferior in preventing subsequent attempts in patients who have attempted suicide (Bryan et al. 2017). In fact, no evidence has demonstrated that suicide contracts mitigate the risk of death from suicide. Therefore, no-harm contracts are not a valid substitute for thorough assessment of risk of death from suicide. Use of a no-harm contract without a strong therapeutic alliance may give therapists a false sense of security while at the same time making the patient feel controlled, which can actually disrupt the development of the therapeutic relationship.

Safety Planning

Collaborative safety planning is an essential element of outpatient therapy with patients who have a history of suicidal thoughts and behaviors and, in contrast to safety contracts, has been shown to be more effective in preventing subsequent self-harm. When working with patients at risk of death from suicide, therapists should strive to avoid addressing safety planning from a defensive mindset. For example, therapists

TABLE 15–3.	Safety planning steps

1. Identify warning signs for increased risk—isolating, self-shame, desire to use substances
2. Prepare and practice internal coping strategies—distracting activities, workouts, mindfulness exercises
3. List people and social settings that provide distraction—peers, family, church groups
4. List people to contact for help—peers, family
5. List professionals or other agencies that can offer help—therapist, emergency departments, help lines
6. Create a safe environment—remove or restrict access to firearms, remove excess medications, eliminate drugs of abuse

who focus too heavily on obtaining information from a checklist may find that patients do not feel heard and understood. Defensive postures can undermine the therapeutic relationship and hamper effective safety planning.

Working collaboratively with the suicidal patient to develop a safety plan is a more preferable approach. Effective safety planning incorporates strategies of means restriction and problem solving and seeks to improve coping skills and enhance social supports for the patient at risk of death from suicide (Brodsky et al. 2018). Establishment of safety plans is a central tenet in most treatment guidelines. In clinical practice, substantial variation exists in the creation and application of such plans. However, the need for explicit, detailed, and perhaps even practiced plans for those at higher risk is uniformly recognized. Safety plans should be established for all patients regardless of their risk level. Practicing the safety plan can be an important part of increasing a patient's sense of assurance that the work being done with the therapist is practical, that therapy goals are achievable, and that the therapist cares about the patient's safety.

Collaboration with the patient is key in the development of an effective safety plan. Prefabricated or "coached" safety plans are not likely to be of benefit to the patient and often will not be used. Actions the patient can take to create a safer living environment, such as restricting access to firearms and substances of abuse, are one component of a safety plan. Stanley and Brown (2012) delineated general elements and techniques for collaborative development of a safety plan, and these are summarized in Table 15–3.

The best safety plans incorporate self-reflection and self-efficacy. Elements of self-reflection include how to recognize warning signs such as increased anxiety, increased irritability, or increased interpersonal conflict. Specifically defining with the patient what these feelings states mean for them, rather than generically naming them, is the core of the process. Often, the next step in the safety plan asks the patient to initiate practiced calming exercises such as deep breathing or centering.

Secondary strategies include distraction, such as listening to music, taking a walk, or some other engaging activity. Writing down thoughts and feelings is another method patients can use to engage cognitive thinking while allowing time for an emotional crisis to pass. These actions promote the other key element of self-efficacy: feelings of mastery or competence, that is, "I can do it" or "I am able to…." If self-care actions are not sufficient to mitigate thoughts of self-harm, patients should have a list of people to whom they can reach out for emotional support. The phone numbers and e-mails of these individuals can be added to a cell phone or reviewed in the patient's phone as part of the process.

Safety plans are more effective if developed and shared with important others in the patient's life, especially with those whom the patient identifies as emotional supports. Safety plans should be practiced within sessions, including use of roleplaying. Practice allows the patient and therapist to evaluate the feasibility of these collaboratively developed steps, modify them as needed, and in the process further enhance the therapeutic alliance. An increasing number of smartphone and web-based applications are available to assist patients and therapists in safety planning, but at present evidence to support their use is very limited.

> At Charles' first outpatient session after his hospitalization, his psychiatrist encouraged him to speak freely about the events, thoughts, and emotions that led up to his suicidal crisis. She then validated Charles' feelings of being emotionally overwhelmed and exhausted with life. She also took the opportunity to strengthen their therapeutic alliance by asking him about how he perceived their treatment relationship and told him she was hopeful to have the opportunity to help him in crisis in the future. Together they reviewed the interim safety plan Charles had developed while at the hospital and made some minor changes to include transferring his pistol from a lockbox in the house to storage at a local gun range. They also agreed to add his name to a high-risk list maintained in the clinic to ensure that he would not be lost to follow-up and so that on-call providers would quickly respond if Charles contacted them in crisis.

Outpatient Psychotherapy

Many psychotherapy approaches to working in the outpatient setting with patients with suicidal thoughts and behaviors are available. Some, such as CBT, are an adaptation or specific application of common psychotherapeutic techniques. Others, such as collaborative assessment and management of suicidality (CAMS), are distinct treatments developed to address patients with suicidal thoughts and behaviors.

CBT, as a psychotherapy for patients with suicidal ideation and behaviors, is the technique best supported by research evidence. CBT interventions appear to significantly reduce repetition of self-harm and suicidal ideation at 6 and 12 months after treatment (Hawton et al. 2016). Cognitive therapy targets the "suicidal mode," which has been postulated to consist of an interconnection of cognitive, affective, motivational, physiological, and behavioral schemas activated by internal and external events in such a way that the patient contemplates or engages in suicidal behavior. Cognitive interventions include working with the patient to develop a conceptualization of suicide as the result of core beliefs and automatic thoughts, to improve problem solving, and ultimately to work toward restructuring distorted core beliefs (Berk et al. 2004).

Dialectic behavioral therapy (DBT; Linehan 1993), developed in the 1990s as a treatment for borderline personality disorder, is perhaps the form of psychotherapy most extensively studied for its capacity to reduce self-harm in patients with and without borderline personality disorder. DBT incorporates components of individual therapy, group skills training, and telephonic consultation to help patients improve distress tolerance and learn to regulate painful emotions. A key treatment goal of DBT is reduction of self-harm, including suicide attempts and nonsuicidal self-injury. In randomized trials, DBT appears to reduce the frequency but not the overall recurrence of self-harm (Hawton et al. 2016).

CAMS is a not a specific psychotherapy but rather a psychotherapeutic framework that systematically addresses both patients' suicidal thinking and their reasons for living. This intervention offers therapists a method of identifying, measuring, and addressing suicide risk factors. Randomized controlled trials of CAMS, compared to enhanced care as usual, show decreased suicidal ideation, although not always at a significant level, most likely due to a need for larger trials (Comtois et al. 2011; Jobes et al. 2017).

Acceptance and Commitment Therapy (ACT) is a form of psychotherapy that targets avoidance of unwanted thoughts and emotions, encouraging patients to "accept" mental events as transient and to sustain their focus on actions important to their values. Limited studies of the efficacy of ACT in the treatment of suicidal patients are available. A systematic review of studies of ACT for suicidal ideation and self-harm showed no significant benefit (Tighe et al. 2018). However, one randomized controlled trial of ACT showed significant improvement in suicidal ideation compared to progressive relaxation training at 3 months (Ducasse et al. 2018).

Attempted Suicide Short Intervention Program (ASSIP) targets patients who have recently attempted suicide and incorporates elements of narrative interviewing and video playback of sessions for self-confrontation. At the core of ASSIP is the use of narrative interviewing to encourage patients to tell the story of how they reached the point of attempting suicide, including the process of planning and the attempt. Patient and therapist then watch a recording of the narrative together and process automatic thoughts, emotional reactions, and decision making. Afterward, the therapist follows up with the patient by mail periodically over the next 24 months. A recent small study of ASSIP in outpatients reported an 80% reduction in subsequent suicide attempts (Gysin-Maillart et al. 2016). Although ASSIP appears to be a very promising intervention in suicidal patients, more research is necessary.

Regardless of the specific psychotherapeutic technique employed, several factors contribute to improvement in outpatient treatment. Internalizing action-oriented techniques such as reaching out to loved ones and introspective techniques such as challenging negative automatic thoughts seem to be key factors for improvement in suicidal patients in therapy (Schembari et al. 2016). Patients also identify the relationship with the therapist, including a perception of being heard and validated, as a significant contributor to their recovery.

> Subsequent psychotherapy focused on deconstructing the thoughts and feelings leading up to Charles' suicidal crisis. Using a cognitive model, Charles was able to identify several thought distortions, including catastrophizing about the breakup of his marriage and self-shaming over his responsibility in his wife's affair. Charles was able to recognize these patterns and consider acceptable alternatives, with improved mood and no further suicidal ideation. After 4 weeks of therapy targeting his suicidal ideation, his risk diminished, and both Charles and his psychiatrist agreed his name could be taken off the clinic's high-risk list.

Follow-Up Care After Hospitalization for Suicidal Ideation or Attempt

Increasing evidence points to the 12 months after psychiatric hospitalization as a suicidal crisis period, a time of increased risk of death from suicide. The Army Study to Assess Risk and Resilience in Servicemembers (Army STARRS) study demonstrated a concentration of risk for suicide attempt and patient death from suicide within the year following hospitalization for any psychiatric diagnosis, with 5% of the highest-risk hospitalizations accounting for 50% of patient deaths from suicide in one sample (Kessler et al. 2015).

Several interventions have been proposed to reduce the risk of subsequent suicide attempts after hospitalization. Caring contacts, in which a mental health worker makes periodic contact with the patient after hospitalization, show some promise in reducing subsequent risk of death from suicide (Brown and Green 2014). Different studies have used regular telephone, in-person, or mail contacts delivered over 1–5 years after a patient's suicidal crisis. In some studies, patients who received such contacts show fewer deaths from suicide.

Text messaging has been explored as a method of reducing suicide attempts among high-risk outpatients. In one study, patients who received text messages twice weekly for 6 months showed a significant decrease in suicide attempts and increase in help-seeking behaviors (Kodama et al. 2016). However, a study of American military personnel examining use of monthly text messages in patients with suicidal ideation showed no significant reduction in ideation after 12 months and no reduction in subsequent hospital admissions or emergency department visits (Comtois et al. 2019). The reason for these inconsistent findings on the efficacy of caring contacts is unclear. The possible efficacy of this low-cost intervention may be enhanced by an increased understanding of how to use such caring contacts, with which patients, by which treatment providers, and when the contacts might be most beneficial. Regardless, most treatment guidelines and current U.S. quality benchmarks promote an in-person contact within 7 days of hospital discharge.

Clinical Practice Guidelines

A number of clinical practice guidelines and other clinical resources are available (Brodsky et al. 2018; International Association for Suicide Prevention 2018; National Action Alliance for Suicide Prevention 2018; U.S. Department of Veterans Affairs 2013). These guidelines are applicable exclusively to the outpatient setting and have applicability across multiple clinical settings. Most provide guidance and "best practices" to mitigate suicidal behavior. Some focus on the individual patient and mitigation strategies, whereas others expand their scope to suggest how health care systems can help mitigate risk. Guidelines for Medicare encourage primary care physicians to develop screening, referral, and treatment programs for depression (Centers for Medicare and Medicaid Services 2011). These may also offer opportunities for identifying those at risk of death from suicide.

The role of mental health treatment providers and how their actions play a significant part in managing patients at high risk of death from suicide are central to most of the clinical guidelines. Screening instruments in the outpatient setting deserve mention given their frequent use and reference in available guidelines. No evidence that routine screening in the general population reduces rates of suicide attempts or mortality is available; the evidence for their use in evaluation of risk in those with greater risk is equivocal. Regardless, screening continues to be widely administered across a multitude of settings. Screening measures assist in the clinical setting by revealing areas of focus for appointments. Screening instruments also may highlight patterns that help track and document clinical status over time.

Numerous screening instruments are available. The most useful instruments are those that are easy to administer, have acceptable reliability and accuracy, and are cost effective. Screening instruments meeting these criteria include but are not limited to the Ask Suicide-Screening Questions (ASQ) from the National Institute of Mental Health; the Columbia Suicide Severity Rating Scale (C-SSRS); the Patient Health Questionnaire–9 (PHQ-9) Depression Scale; and the Suicide Behavior Questionnaire–Revised (SBQ-R). In addition to these screening tools, assessment instruments may provide additional clinical data in the event that a patient screens positive for increased suicide risk. Clinical practicality and use follow the same principles as screening instruments (e.g., efficient, reliable, valid, and cost effective). These include, for example, the C-SSRS and the Reasons for Living inventory.

Some clinical practice guidelines recommend assigning categories based on the severity and acuity of risk factors. Categories vary, but most use categories of high risk (need for immediate clinical attention), moderate risk, and low risk (acknowledges presence of risk but does not require higher level of care). Interventions are recommended based on such stratification. As an example, patients considered to be in the high-risk category would typically be referred for inpatient hospitalization.

Clinical practice guidelines have also proposed the maintenance of a registry or list of patients at greatest self-harm risk (Labouliere et al. 2018; U.S. Air Force Medical Operations Agency 2014). These lists have appeal to large, high-volume clinics where patients at high risk could be identified and followed over time. Increased visibility across clinic providers and support staff can be of benefit for cross-coverage and additional attention should these patients call or miss appointments. Entry criteria onto "high-risk" lists vary and ultimately depend on the provider's clinical judgment. Common patient characteristics for inclusion on a high-risk list are patients with the greatest clinical need, patients with a significant increase in risk factors, and patients at higher need during transitions in care.

The use of such lists is often associated with recommended or mandated courses of action. Caring for a patient on the list would justify more frequent and closer interval appointments. Patients missing appointments may also trigger activation of certain protocols, such as contact with a patient or their next of kin should they miss an appointment without prior notice. Although these classification lists can be helpful to a busy practice, the goal of inclusion for a higher level of intervention is for patients to eventually achieve a level of stability and safety to have themselves removed from such a list. Removal criteria are varied and may include clinical stability for a given period of time, reduction or mitigation of high-risk factors, and clinician judgment.

Conclusion

Treatment and management of suicidal thoughts and behaviors in the outpatient setting requires developing and sustaining the therapeutic alliance between patient and therapist, a significant contributor to the treatment response. Safety planning is a key component of all treatment plans for outpatients at risk of death from suicide and is most effective when conducted as a collaborative process. A number of psychotherapeutic approaches to the treatment of suicidal thoughts and behaviors are available, and evidence indicates they are reasonably effective. These concepts are found in many available clinical practice guidelines that can serve as guidelines and reminders for the therapist.

Key Points

- The therapeutic alliance is a core component of treating outpatients at risk of death from suicide.

- Effective safety planning requires more than "no-harm contracts" with suicidal patients and includes elements of recognizing warning signs, identifying coping strategies and external supports, and taking measures to create a safe environment.

- Many psychotherapies have been proposed for treatment of suicidal ideation and self-harm. Of these, cognitive-behavioral therapy has the greatest evidence of benefit.

- Treatment guidelines for care of the suicidal patient recommend best practices such as screening, risk stratification, and maintaining "high-risk" lists.

References

Berk MS, Henriques GR, Warman DM, et al: A cognitive therapy intervention for suicide attempters: an overview of the treatment and case examples. Cogn Behav Pract 11(3):265–277, 2004

Brodsky BS, Spruch-Feiner A, Stanley B: The zero suicide model: applying evidence-based suicide prevention practices to clinical care. Front Psychiatry 9:33, 2018 29527178

Brown GK, Green KL: A review of evidence-based follow-up care for suicide prevention: where do we go from here? Am J Prev Med 47(3 suppl 2):S209–S215, 2014 25145741

Bryan CJ, Corso KA, Corso ML, et al: Therapeutic alliance and change in suicidal ideation during treatment in integrated primary care settings. Arch Suicide Res 16(4):316–323, 2012 23137221

Bryan CJ, Mintz J, Clemans TA, et al: Effect of crisis response planning vs. contracts for safety on suicide risk in U.S. Army soldiers: a randomized clinical trial. J Affect Disord 212:64–72, 2017 28142085

Centers for Medicare and Medicaid Services: Decision Memo for Screening for Depression in Adults (CAG-00425N). Baltimore, MD, Centers for Medicare and Medicaid Services, October 4, 2011. Available at: https://www.cms.gov/medicare-coverage-database/details/nca-decision-memo.aspx?NCAId=251. Accessed February 25, 2019.

Comtois KA, Jobes DA, S O'Connor S, et al: Collaborative assessment and management of suicidality (CAMS): feasibility trial for next-day appointment services. Depress Anxiety 28(11):963–972, 2011 21948348

Comtois KA, Kerbrat AH, DeCou CR, et al: Effect of augmenting standard care for military personnel with brief caring text messages for suicide prevention: a randomized clinical trial. JAMA Psychiatry 2019 30758491 Epub ahead of print

Ducasse D, Jaussent I, Arpon-Brand V, et al: Acceptance and Commitment Therapy for the management of suicidal patients: a randomized controlled trial. Psychother Psychosom 87(4):211–222, 2018 29874680

Dunster-Page C, Haddock G, Wainwright L, et al: The relationship between therapeutic alliance and patient's suicidal thoughts, self-harming behaviours and suicide attempts: a systematic review. J Affect Disord 223:165–174, 2017 28755624

Garvey KA, Penn JV, Campbell AL, et al: Contracting for safety with patients: clinical practice and forensic implications. J Am Acad Psychiatry Law 37(3):363–370, 2009 19767501

Gysin-Maillart A, Schwab S, Soravia L, et al: A novel brief therapy for patients who attempt suicide: a 24-months follow-up randomized controlled study of the Attempted Suicide Short Intervention Program (ASSIP). PLoS Med 13(3):e1001968, 2016 26930055

Hawton K, Witt KG, Taylor Salisbury TL, et al: Psychosocial interventions for self-harm in adults. Cochrane Database Syst Rev (5):CD012189, 2016 27168519

Horvath AO, Del Re AC, Flückiger C, et al: Alliance in individual psychotherapy. Psychotherapy (Chic) 48(1):9–16, 2011 21401269

International Association for Suicide Prevention: IASP Guidelines for Suicide Prevention. Washington, DC, International Association for Suicide Prevention, 2018. Available at: https://www.iasp.info/suicide_guidelines.php. Accessed February 25, 2019.

Jobes DA, Comtois KA, Gutierrez PM, et al: A randomized controlled trial of the collaborative assessment and management of suicidality versus enhanced care as usual with suicidal soldiers. Psychiatry 80(4):339–356, 2017 29466107

Kessler RC, Warner CH, Ivany C, et al: Predicting suicides after psychiatric hospitalization in US Army soldiers: the Army Study To Assess Risk and Resilience in Servicemembers (Army STARRS). JAMA Psychiatry 72(1):49–57, 2015 25390793

Kodama T, Syouji H, Takaki S, et al: Text messaging for psychiatric outpatients: effect on help-seeking and self-harming behaviors. J Psychosoc Nurs Ment Health Serv 54(4):31–37, 2016 27042926

Labouliere CD, Vasan P, Kramer A, et al: "Zero suicide": a model for reducing suicide in United States behavioral healthcare. Suicidologi 23(1):22–30, 2018 29970972

Linehan M: Cognitive Behavior Treatment of Borderline Personality Disorder. New York, Guilford, 1993

Michel K, Jobes DA: Building Therapeutic Alliance With the Suicidal Patient. Washington, DC, American Psychological Association, 2011

Michel K, Maltsberger JT, Jobes DA, et al: Discovering the truth in attempted suicide. Am J Psychother 56(3):424–437, 2002 12400207

Naifeh JA, Mash HBH, Stein MB, et al: The Army Study to Assess Risk and Resilience in Servicemembers (Army STARRS): progress toward understanding suicide among soldiers. Mol Psychiatry 24(1):34–48, 2019 30104726

National Action Alliance for Suicide Prevention: Recommended Standard Care for People With Suicide Risk: Making Health Care Suicide Safe. Waltham, MA, Education Development Center, 2018. Available at: https://theactionalliance.org/sites/default/files/action_alliance_recommended_standard_care_final.pdf. Accessed February 25, 2019.

Perry JC, Bond M, Presniak MD: Alliance, reactions to treatment, and counter-transference in the process of recovery from suicidal phenomena in long-term dynamic psychotherapy. Psychother Res 23(5):592–605, 2013 23937543

Plakun EM: A view from Riggs: treatment resistance and patient authority—XI. An alliance-based intervention for suicide. J Am Acad Psychoanal Dyn Psychiatry 37(3):539–560, 2009 19764850

Schembari BC, Jobes DA, Horgan RJ: Successful treatment of suicidal risk. Crisis 37(3):218–223, 2016 26831214

Stanley B, Brown GK: Safety planning intervention: a brief intervention to mitigate suicide risk. Cogn Behav Pract 19(2):256–264, 2012

Tighe J, Nicholas J, Shand F, et al: Efficacy of Acceptance and Commitment Therapy in reducing suicidal ideation and deliberate self-harm: systematic review. JMIR Ment Health 5(2):e10732, 2018 29941419

U.S. Air Force Medical Operations Agency: Air Force Guide for Suicide Risk Assessment, Management, and Treatment. Lackland, TX, U.S. Air Force Medical Operations Agency, 2014. Available at: https://www.usuhs.edu/sites/default/files/media/mps/pdf/mholloway-afguidesuiciderisk.pdf. Accessed February 25, 2019.

U.S. Department of Veterans Affairs: U.S. Department of Defense: VA/DoD Clinical Practice Guideline for Assessment and Management of Risk for Suicide. Washington, DC, U.S. Department of Veterans Affairs, U.S. Department of Defense, 2013. Available at: https://www.healthquality.va.gov/guidelines/MH/srb/VADODCP_SuicideRisk_Full.pdf. Accessed February 25, 2019.

Van Orden KA, Witte TK, Cukrowicz KC, et al: The interpersonal theory of suicide. Psychol Rev 117(2):575–600, 2010 20438238

CHAPTER 16

Inpatient Treatment

Richard L. Frierson, M.D.

The vast majority of psychiatric treatment typically occurs in the outpatient setting. The development of inpatient psychiatric treatment was guided in part by the need to prevent persons who were viewed as a danger to themselves from dying from suicide or engaging in serious self-harm behaviors. Inpatient 24-hour observation was believed to be superior to routine outpatient treatment in suicide prevention. In order to maximize patient autonomy, psychiatric treatment should normally occur in the least restrictive setting possible, provided that the treatment setting is likely to be efficacious while ensuring patient safety (*Lake v. Cameron* 1966). However, when patients are at significant suicide risk due to the severity of their mental illness, a lack of insight, or inadequate outpatient resources (including family or other support systems), inpatient hospitalization has become the standard of care (American Psychiatric Association 2003).

Inpatient psychiatric treatment in the United States is facing multiple challenges in the twenty-first century, most notably a significant shortage of available public and private inpatient psychiatric beds. Deinstitutionalization and cuts to state public funding for mental health services have shifted some of the burden of behavioral health treatment to emergency departments (Medford-Davis and Beall 2017). In some jurisdictions, patients are held in an emergency department for days without adequate treatment or a hospital room (see Chapter 14, "Emergency Services"). This crisis has recently come to the attention of the court system, which may force increased state funding for inpatient beds in the future (Appelbaum 2015).

Alternatively, patients who need inpatient treatment but for whom beds cannot be found are sometimes released back to the community, with disastrous consequences (Bursiek 2018). Because of inpatient bed shortages, patients who are actually hospitalized may have more severe mental illness and may be at increased risk for inpatient suicide. In addition to its impact on general hospital emergency departments, the current shortage of psychiatric beds has also resulted in a greater probability of jail detention for minor charges among persons diagnosed with severe mental illness (Yoon et al. 2013). Jails are often poorly equipped to handle persons with severe mental illness, including those at risk of suicide (see Chapter 21, "Jails and Prisons"). Finally, this critical decline in psychiatric beds may have contributed to the recent increase in the overall suicide rate in the United States (Bastiampillai et al. 2016).

This chapter reviews inpatient treatment of suicidal patients, including the decision-making process for hospitalizing patients with suicide risk, the incidence and epidemiology of suicide in the inpatient setting, the risk factors for inpatient suicide, and the principles of risk management. Specific strategies in risk management, including observation and staffing levels, are reviewed as well as newly proposed environmental requirements from the Centers for Medicare and Medicaid Services (CMS) through The Joint Commission (formerly the Joint Commission for the Accreditation of Healthcare Organizations). Finally, through presentation of a malpractice case involving an inpatient suicide death, the interaction between patient and environment, including inpatient unit design, is discussed.

Making the Decision to Hospitalize

The decision to hospitalize a patient can only be made after a thorough evaluation of the patient's clinical condition, including the presence or absence of a psychiatric disorder, the severity of current symptoms (including hopelessness and impulsivity), past suicide attempts and their severity, overall functioning, and the availability of outpatient support systems. The clinician should also explore activities that give the patient a reason to live. In situations with a high potential for dangerousness to self or others, inpatient treatment may be warranted even if additional history is not available or the patient is unable to meaningfully participate in a psychiatric examination due to agitation, psychosis, or other factors.

The decision to hospitalize must also include an examination of the possible negative effects of hospitalization, including disruption of employment, financial hardship caused by hospitalization, and other psychosocial stress (e.g., inability to care for a dependent child or adult due to hospitalization). It should also include an evaluation of the patient's ability to provide self-care and to manage a crisis and seek appropriate help (e.g., family members, emergency care). Thus, the degree of suicide risk should be balanced with these various elements when making a decision about treatment settings. Guidelines for decision making can be found in Table 16–1.

Once the decision to hospitalize a potentially suicidal patient is made, the psychiatrist must next decide whether the hospitalization should occur on a voluntary or involuntary basis. Voluntary admission is always preferred, because it upholds the principle of patient autonomy, but the psychiatrist must consider civil commitment if a patient refuses admission. All states permit civil commitment for patients who present a danger to themselves, and most states allow for civil commitment of persons deemed "gravely disabled" (Kapoor 2018; see Chapter 17, "Civil Commitment"). Finally, if the psychiatrist is concerned about possible elopement or if the patient has a history of elopement from psychiatric facilities, hospitalization should occur on a secured unit. A significant number of inpatient suicides have occurred immediately following elopement (Madsen et al. 2017).

TABLE 16–1. **Guidelines for selecting a treatment setting for patients at risk for suicide or suicidal behaviors**

Admission generally indicated

After a suicide attempt or aborted suicide attempt if

Patient is psychotic

Attempt was violent, near lethal, or premeditated

Precautions were taken to avoid rescue or discovery

Persistent plan or intent is present

Distress is increased or patient regrets surviving

Patient is male, older than age 45 years, especially with new onset of psychiatric illness or suicidal thinking

Patient has limited family or social support, including lack of stable living situation

Current impulsive behavior, severe agitation, poor judgment, or refusal of help is evident

Patient has change in mental status with a metabolic, toxic, infectious, or other etiology requiring further workup in a structured setting

In the presence of suicidal ideation with

Specific plan with high lethality

High suicidal intent

Admission may be necessary

After a suicide attempt or aborted suicide attempt, except in circumstances for which admission is generally indicated, such as in the presence of suicidal ideation with

Psychosis

Major psychiatric disorder

Past attempts, particularly if medically serious

Possibly contributing medical condition (e.g., acute neurological disorder, cancer, infection)

Lack of response to or inability to cooperate with partial hospital or outpatient treatment

Need for supervised setting for medication trial or electroconvulsive therapy

Need for skilled observation, clinical tests, or diagnostic assessments that require a structured setting

Limited family or social support, including lack of stable living situation

Lack of an ongoing clinician–patient relationship or lack of access to timely outpatient follow-up

In the absence of suicide attempts or reported suicidal ideation/plan/intent, but evidence from the psychiatric evaluation or history from others suggests a high level of suicide risk and a recent acute increase in risk

Release from emergency department with follow-up recommendations may be possible

After a suicide attempt or in the presence of suicidal ideation/plan when

Suicidal thoughts and behaviors are a reaction to precipitating events (e.g., exam failure, relationship difficulties), particularly if the patient's view of situation has changed since coming to emergency department

Plan/method and intent have low lethality

Patient has stable and supportive living situation

Patient is able to cooperate with recommendations for follow-up, with treater contacted if patient is currently in treatment

TABLE 16–1.   **Guidelines for selecting a treatment setting for patients at risk for suicide or suicidal behaviors (continued)**

Outpatient treatment may be more beneficial than hospitalization

Patient has chronic suicidal ideation or self-injury without prior medically serious attempts, if a safe and supportive living situation is available, and outpatient psychiatric care is ongoing

Source.   Adapted from Jacobs DJ, Baldessarini RJ, Conwell Y: *Practice Guideline for the Assessment and Treatment of Patients With Suicidal Behaviors.* Arlington, VA, American Psychiatric Association, 2010. Available at: http://psychiatryonline.org/pb/assets/raw/sitewide/practice_guidelines/guidelines/suicide.pdf Accessed September 8, 2018. Used with permission. Copyright © 2010 American Psychiatric Association.

Incidence of Inpatient Suicide

The inpatient setting allows for the implementation of constant observation, seclusion, or physical or pharmacological restraint, which are all modalities designed to prevent a patient from acting on suicidal impulses. However, inpatient suicides occur at a surprising rate, accounting for between 5% and 6% of all suicides in the United States (Busch et al. 2003). Psychiatric inpatients have a suicide rate that is 13 times higher than the annual global age-standardization suicide rate (Madsen et al. 2017). The estimated number of hospital inpatient suicides per year in the United States ranges from 48.5 to 64.9, which is far below the previously widely cited figure of 1,500 per year (Williams et al. 2018). Additionally, the prevalence of inpatient suicide attempts is 10-fold that of inpatient deaths from suicide, and many attempts involve serious injury (Brunenberg and Buijhl 1998).

The Joint Commission considers inpatient suicide a *sentinel event*, defined as a patient safety event that results in any of the following: death, permanent harm, or severe temporary harm with intervention required to sustain life. Inpatient suicide was the second most common sentinel event reported between 1995 and 2005, and 1,100 voluntary reports of suicides occurred in health care settings in the United States between 2010 and 2014 (Knoll 2012; Stempniak 2016). More importantly, about 21% of The Joint Commission's accredited behavioral health care organizations and 5% of its accredited hospitals are noncompliant with The Joint Commission's recommended practices to identify patients at risk of suicide. Inpatient suicide is not unique to the United States; a study in the United Kingdom found that nurses, on average, were confronted with a death from suicide of one of their patients suicide every 2.5 years (Nijman et al. 2005).

Epidemiology and Risk Factors for Inpatient Suicide

Out of all types of suicide, inpatient suicide should be viewed as the most avoidable and preventable due to the proximity of patients to hospital personnel, including mental health professionals. For that reason, courts and juries in malpractice claims attribute a greater responsibility to inpatient facilities to prevent suicides. Whereas about one in four outpatient suicides will result in a malpractice claim, about one in two inpatient suicides will result in a claim (Knoll 2012).

Identifying risk factors for inpatient suicide is difficult because suicide, although the tenth leading cause of death in the United States, is a rare event occurring at a base rate of 13.5/100,000 population (Centers for Disease Control and Prevention 2017). Studies attempting to secure robust risk estimates on the more restricted and smaller population of inpatients are even more difficult. Additionally, the evidence-based suicide risk factors used for suicide risk assessment in the outpatient setting are not correlated with inpatient suicide. For example, outpatient risk factors such as age, sex, marital status, unemployment, and lower educational level are not necessarily risk factors in inpatient settings (Busch et al. 2003).

Similarly, whereas depression is the most common diagnosis in outpatient suicide, schizophrenia and psychotic disorders are just as likely as mood disorders to be found in patients who died from suicide in the hospital (Spiessl et al. 2002). In a 9-year review of all inpatient suicides in Germany, identifiable risk factors included history of being a victim of assault, personality disorder, previous suicide attempt, psycho-pharmacological treatment resistance, suicidal thoughts on admission, schizophrenia, depression, female sex, and length of stay (Neuner et al. 2008). However, a systematic review and meta-analysis demonstrated that the most established risk factors for inpatient suicide are depressive symptoms during admission, a diagnosis of a mood disorder or schizophrenia spectrum disorder, and a history of deliberate self-harm (Large et al. 2011). Additionally, meta-analyses have identified a family history of suicide or mental illness, high levels of hopelessness, feelings of worthlessness or guilt, prescribed antidepressants, and longer length of hospitalization as inpatient suicide risk factors (Madsen et al. 2017).

Many studies have found that inpatient suicide is most likely to occur outside of the hospital when a patient is on leave or has absconded from an inpatient psychiatric unit (Madsen et al. 2017). Among suicides that occur inside the confines of a psychiatric unit, the vast majority occur by hanging. In one large study, hanging accounted for 73% of all suicides that occurred on the inpatient unit; most occurred in a private area (e.g., bedroom, bathroom) using a door corner as an anchor point (Meehan et al. 2006). More than 90% of inpatient suicides took place in private spaces, such as the bathroom, bedroom, closet, and shower. In a multiyear review of suicide attempts and completions at U.S. Department of Veterans Affairs (VA) inpatient facilities, hanging accounted for 76% of deaths from suicide, with most using a door, door handle, or wardrobe/locker as an anchor point and sheets, bedding, or clothes as a ligature (Mills et al. 2008). In one review, case fatality after attempted suicide by hanging was 70%, but the majority (80%–90%) of those who reached medical treatment alive survived (Gunnell et al. 2005).

The risk of inpatient suicide is highest in recently admitted patients, with as many as one-quarter of inpatient suicides occurring during the first week of admission (Madsen et al. 2017). This is particularly true when a readmission to a psychiatric hospital has occurred within 30 days of the last discharge (Madsen et al. 2012). Inpatient suicides occur even while patients are under observation. In a 6-year study in England and Wales, 16% (*n*=113) of all inpatient suicides (*N*=715) occurred while patients were under observation (Flynn et al. 2017). Of the suicides that occurred while patients were under observation, 96% of the patients were under intermittent observation and 4% were under constant observation. In 65% of these cases, the patient died on the inpatient ward; in 35%, the patient had absconded from the hospital while on observation. Finally, most occurred when less-senior staff (e.g., student nurses or health care assistants) or staff members who were unfamiliar with the patient (e.g., pool nurses, staff agency nurses) were performing the observations.

Inpatient Treatment and Suicide Risk Management

The first goal of inpatient treatment is patient safety. Because the risk of suicide is greatest in the first week of hospitalization, patients should be placed on an appropriate level of observation. Many hospitals have developed written policies regarding mandatory observation levels for newly admitted patients with suicidal ideation. Patients at high suicide risk should be placed on direct intensive psychiatric observation (i.e., one-to-one observation) for at least the first 24–48 hours. Observers performing this level of observation should be freed of other clinical duties. Patients at mild to moderate risk may be placed on continuous observation where one observer is responsible for watching two or three patients. Although some hospitals use "15-minute check" schedules, 15 minutes is more than enough time for a patient to die from hanging, and many hospital suicides have occurred while patients were under this observation level. Camera monitoring of patients also is not recommended because observers can become bored or distracted or be called away to other tasks.

The observation of psychiatric patients as an intervention to mitigate risk of suicide requires a complex, sustained interaction between the patient, observer, psychiatrist, nurse, other treatment team members, and the psychiatric unit environment. Staff members who are directly responsible for observing a patient should be active members of the patient's treatment team (Janofsky 2009) and should be trained in cardiopulmonary resuscitation (CPR) and suicide prevention, including means restriction. Interdisciplinary collaboration is also needed when making the decision to discontinue direct observation and institute some form of intermittent observation. The observer and nursing staff supervisors should have direct and open communication regarding any unusual changes in an observed patient's behavior. Finally, psychiatrists and other staff should conduct a suicide risk assessment before decreasing levels of observation. Once an observation level has been decreased or discontinued, the onset of new stressors during hospitalization (e.g., the ending of a romantic relationship, loss of employment due to hospitalization) should lead to reassessment for the need to maintain or increase levels of observation.

After the management of safety issues, the main goal of inpatient treatment is to establish a therapeutic alliance and to initiate appropriate biological and psychosocial therapeutic interventions. The provision of a supportive inpatient environment can also help relieve stressors, strengthen and develop coping skills, and instill hope for the future. In inpatient settings, treatment is administered using a team approach, typically with a psychiatrist leading a group consisting of nurses, social workers, psychologists, and other mental health workers (e.g., activity therapists, mental health technicians), with each member providing input. Communication in team meetings can be improved by adding to the agenda a specific discussion of patients identified as a potential suicide risk. Psychiatrists should remain aware at all times that although a collaborative approach is used in patient treatment, treating psychiatrists ultimately bear the responsibility for critical decisions.

- Inpatient suicide is one of the leading sentinel events reported to The Joint Commission. Most inpatient suicides occur via hanging in private areas (bedroom or bathroom) using a door or door handle and a ligature made from sheets, bedding, or clothes.

- Potentially suicidal patients should be placed on an appropriate observation level immediately after admission and a suicide risk assessment should be completed.

- Prior to discharge, a safety plan should be developed that focuses on means restriction, using outpatient supports, and developing a contingency plan.

- Periodic environmental risk assessments of inpatient units should be conducted to identify potential hazards that could be used in a suicide attempt, and policies should be developed outlining appropriate and coordinated responses to medical emergencies such as suicide attempts.

References

American Psychiatric Association: Practice guideline for the assessment and treatment of patients with suicidal behaviors. Am J Psychiatry 160(11 suppl):1–60, 2003 14649920

Appelbaum PS: "Boarding" psychiatric patients in emergency rooms: one court says "no more." Psychiatr Serv 66(7):668–670, 2015 26130151

Bastiampillai T, Sharfstein SS, Allison S: Increase in US suicide rates and the critical decline in psychiatric beds. JAMA 316(24):2591–2592, 2016 27812693

Boyer CA, McAlpine DD, Pottick KJ, et al: Identifying risk factors and key strategies in linkage to outpatient psychiatric care. Am J Psychiatry 157(10):1592–1598, 2000 11007712

Brunenberg W, Buijhl R: Suicide en suicidepreventie: in het psychiatrisch ziekenhuis [Suicide and suicide prevention in the psychiatric hospital]. Maandblad Geestelijke Volksgezondheid [Monthly Journal of Mental Health] 53:13–26, 1998

Bursiek A: Virginia's mental health care system is "chaotic" and must be addressed, says Sen. Deeds. The Virginian-Pilot, January 14, 2018. Available at: https://pilotonline.com/news/government/politics/virginia/article_a39eb6a3-50c9-5c7e-a907-dd4e0c4e890b.html. Accessed October 26, 2018.

Busch KA, Fawcett J, Jacobs DG: Clinical correlates of inpatient suicide. J Clin Psychiatry 64(1):14–19, 2003 12590618

Centers for Disease Control and Prevention: Deaths: final data for 2015. National Vital Statistics Reports 66(6), November 27, 2017. Available at: https://www.cdc.gov/nchs/data/nvsr/nvsr66/nvsr66_06.pdf. Accessed October 30, 2018.

Centers for Medicare and Medicaid Services: Clarification of ligature risk policy (memo). Quality, Safety and Oversight—General Information, December 8, 2017. Available at: https://www.cms.gov/Medicare/Provider-Enrollment-and-Certification/SurveyCertificationGenInfo/Policy-and-Memos-to-States-and-Regions-Items/Survey-and-Cert-Letter-18-06.html?DLPage=1andDLEntries=10andDLSort=2andDLSortDir=descending. Accessed September 29, 2018.

Fink M, Kellner CH, McCall WV: The role of ECT in suicide prevention. J ECT 30(1):5–9, 2014 24091903

Flynn S, Nyathi T, Tham SG, et al: Suicide by mental health in-patients under observation. Psychol Med 47(13):2238–2245, 2017 28397618

Gunnell D, Bennewith O, Hawton K, et al: The epidemiology and prevention of suicide by hanging: a systematic review. Int J Epidemiol 34(2):433–442, 2005 15659471

Janofsky JS: Reducing inpatient suicide risk: using human factors analysis to improve observation practices. J Am Acad Psychiatry Law 37(1):15–24, 2009 19297628

The Joint Commission: Special Report: Suicide Prevention in Health Care Settings. November 2017 Perspectives Preview, October 25, 2017. Available at: https://www.jointcommission.org/issues/article.aspx?Article=GtNpk0ErgGF%2B7J9WOTTkXANZSEPXa1%2BKH0/4kGHCiio%3D. Accessed September 9, 2018.

Jordan JT, McNiel DE: Characteristics of a suicide attempt predict who makes another attempt after hospital discharge: a decision-tree investigation. Psychiatry Res 268:317–322, 2018 30096659

Kapoor R: Civil commitment, in Textbook of Forensic Psychiatry, 3rd Edition. Edited by Gold LH, Frierson RL. Washington, DC, American Psychiatric Association Publishing, 2018

Knoll JL 4th: Inpatient suicide: identifying vulnerability in the hospital setting. Psychiatric Times, May 22, 2012. Available at: http://www.psychiatrictimes.com/suicide/inpatient-suicide-identifying-vulnerability-hospital-setting. Accessed September 9, 2018.

Lake v Cameron, 2364 F.2d 657, 124 U.S.App. D.C. 264 (1966)

Large M, Smith G, Sharma S, et al: Systematic review and meta-analysis of the clinical factors associated with the suicide of psychiatric in-patients. Acta Psychiatr Scand 124(1):18–29, 2011 21261599

Linehan MM, Armstrong HE, Suarez A, et al: Cognitive-behavioral treatment of chronically parasuicidal borderline patients. Arch Gen Psychiatry 48(12):1060–1064, 1991 1845222

Madsen T, Agerbo E, Mortensen PB, et al: Predictors of psychiatric inpatient suicide: a national prospective register-based study. J Clin Psychiatry 73(2):144–151, 2012 21903026

Madsen T, Erlangsen A, Nordentoft M: Risk estimates and risk factors related to psychiatric in-patient suicide: an overview. Int J Environ Res Public Health 14(3):253, 2017 28257103

Medford-Davis LN, Beall RC: The changing health policy environment and behavioral health services delivery. Psychiatr Clin North Am 40(3):533–540, 2017 28800807

Meehan J, Kapur N, Hunt IM, et al: Suicide in mental health in-patients and within 3 months of discharge. National clinical survey. Br J Psychiatry 188:129–134, 2006 16449699

Mills PD, DeRosier JM, Ballot BA, et al: Inpatient suicide and suicide attempts in Veterans Affairs hospitals. Jt Comm J Qual Patient Saf 34(8):482–488, 2008 18714751

Neuner T, Schmid R, Wolfersdorf M, et al: Predicting inpatient suicides and suicide attempts by using clinical routine data? Gen Hosp Psychiatry 30(4):324–330, 2008 18585535

Nijman H, Bowers L, Oud N, et al: Psychiatric nurses' experiences with inpatient aggression. Aggress Behav 31(3):217–227, 2005

Sarchiapone M, Mandelli L, Iosue M, et al: Controlling access to suicide means. Int J Environ Res Public Health 8(12):4550–4562, 2011 22408588

Sharfstein SS, Dickerson FB, Oldham JM: Introduction, in Textbook of Hospital Psychiatry. Edited by Sharfstein SS, Dickerson FB, Oldham JM. Washington, DC, American Psychiatric Publishing, 2008

Spicer RS, Miller TR: Suicide acts in 8 states: incidence and case fatality rates by demographics and method. Am J Public Health 90(12):1885–1891, 2000 11111261

Spiessl H, Hübner-Liebermann B, Cording C: Suicidal behaviour of psychiatric in-patients. Acta Psychiatr Scand 106(2):134–138, 2002 12121211

Stempniak M: Joint Commission shines spotlight on suicide in hospitals and other settings, with 8 steps to detect growing concern. Hosp Health Netw February 24, 2016

Williams SC, Schmaltz SP, Castro GM, et al: Incidence and method of suicide in hospitals in the United States. Jt Comm J Qual Patient Saf 44(11):643–650, 2018 30190221

Yoon J, Domino ME, Norton EC, et al: The impact of changes in psychiatric bed supply on jail use by persons with severe mental illness. J Ment Health Policy Econ 16(2):81–92, 2013 23999205

CHAPTER 17

Civil Commitment

Annette Hanson, M.D.

Most patients with suicidal ideation and behavior will be treated on an outpatient basis. Nevertheless, patients at high risk of death from suicide may require inpatient hospitalization to immediately mitigate acute risk. A voluntary hospitalization is one in which a competent patient agrees to be admitted for inpatient treatment. If a patient is at high risk of death from suicide and refuses to consider inpatient treatment, psychiatrists may need to initiate an involuntary admission process—that is, a civil commitment. All states have civil commitment statutes that require the individual to be a danger to him- or herself or others as a result of mental illness in order to meet the criteria for involuntary hospitalization (Treatment Advocacy Center 2014). A majority of states also allow civil commitment of persons with mental illness who demonstrate grave disability or lack of decisional capacity (Treatment Advocacy Center 2014). This chapter reviews the issues that arise when considering and referring a patient for civil commitment to decrease the risk of death from suicide.

Civil Commitment and the Clinician's Dilemma

The decision to deprive a patient of freedom is easily the most agonizing clinical dilemma faced by psychiatrists. At some point in a psychiatric career, most doctors will have at least one sleepless night over a decision to release a high-risk patient from an emergency department (ED) or an inpatient unit. A careful risk assessment and treatment plan can mitigate risk of death from suicide, often just by keeping someone safe until an acute crisis has been resolved. One study of American Psychiatric Association members revealed that 62% of surveyed psychiatrists had had direct experience with involuntary commitment in the preceding 24 months, although these patients represented less than 0.03% of their entire patient caseload (Brooks 2007).

The decision-making process is further complicated by the fact that a patient could easily conceal pertinent data, deny or minimize symptoms, or withhold contact information for collateral historians with relevant information. More than any other clinical decision, the decision to involuntarily admit a patient relies upon an authentic trusting relationship between doctor and patient and the patient's willingness to provide accurate information about his or her thoughts and feelings. A capricious or cavalier approach to civil commitment risks damage to that therapeutic alliance and could undermine the patient's willingness to seek treatment or be truthful about his or her mental state in the future (Miller and Hanson 2016). Furthermore, inpatient psychiatric resources have become increasingly limited, making it important to use such resources wisely and to avoid unnecessary commitments.

Willingness to involuntarily admit a patient depends upon the clinician's individual risk tolerance and personal experience with patients' deaths from suicide. Self-doubt is a common reaction in the aftermath of a patient's death, and a past tragic outcome can powerfully influence future behavior. Personal distress over a patient death is not alleviated by the fact that the decision to discharge or release the patient was made reasonably after a sound risk assessment. The axiom "once bitten, twice shy" becomes particularly apt in this situation. Willingness to commit a patient also increases after high-profile tragic events such as a mass shooting (Fisher and Grisso 2010).

The risk-benefit analysis of a civil commitment decision is also influenced by the fact that psychiatrists can assess only the *risk* of death from suicide; death from suicide itself cannot be predicted (Large 2018). Although relatively few patients with suicidal ideation will go on to make an attempt or die from suicide, a thorough suicide risk assessment and appropriate treatment plan can help avoid a patient's death from suicide, which can be devastating not only to the patient but also the patient's family and the physician. Traditional psychiatric training emphasizes suicide risk assessment and prevention but does little to prepare a clinician for the sequelae of a patient's death (see Chapter 31, "Teaching Suicide Risk Assessment in Psychiatric Residency Training"). Feelings of guilt, shame, anxiety, and bereavement may go unrecognized and unaddressed. Clinicians themselves may be reluctant to raise the issue in discussion with others out of concerns regarding personal liability or fear of judgment by colleagues (see Chapter 32, "Psychiatrist Reactions to Patient Suicide and the Clinician's Role").

Ultimately, consultation with understanding colleagues and peer support can mitigate this psychological fallout while providing constructive case review and advice. Institutional mortality reviews also provide feedback regarding any needed corrective actions and can be conducted under the protection of state discovery rules. Social connection and professional support are crucial during the period of professional and personal vulnerability that physicians often experience after a patient suicide.

Process of Civil Commitment

Since the creation of the first psychiatric hospital in the United States, the goal of civil commitment has gradually shifted from care and treatment to preventive detention. Based upon the principle of *parens patriae* (literally translated as "the parent of the country"), civil commitment laws allowed the states to intervene *in loco parentis* ("in the place of the parent") on behalf of people with mental illness who were unable to care for themselves. Later laws granted states the legal right to exercise police powers to admit patients based upon their perceived dangerousness to themselves or others (Testa and West 2010).

Most civil commitments are based upon the risk of danger to self rather than danger to others; however, in rare cases these risks are conflated. Between 2000 and 2013, an in-depth review of 63 mass shooters revealed that nearly half had expressed suicidal intent prior to their offenses (Silver et al. 2018). Similarly, a study done by the Violence Policy Center (2015) revealed that during the first 6 months of 2014, eleven murder-suicides took place every week in the United States. Fortunately, in spite of the media attention given to these events, the average clinician will never evaluate or treat a patient who later becomes a mass shooter.

Proponents of involuntary treatment often claim that tragedies such as suicides and mass shootings could have been prevented if more inpatient beds were available, if doctors were more liberal about seeking involuntary hospitalization, or if each state had a mechanism for coercing care for potentially dangerous patients in the community. Critics of involuntary treatment point out that mental illness is rarely the sole or primary factor for violence, even when coupled with suicide. The vast majority of people with mental illness are not dangerous, but the link between certain untreated psychiatric illnesses and violence cannot be completely discounted.

More commonly, psychiatrists treat patients who are experiencing the stress of a recent trauma, a significant loss or change in life circumstances, or the disabling effects of a serious mental illness such as schizophrenia. Being able to frankly discuss the patient's sense of hopelessness or despair is essential to recovery and adaptation and may be enough to obviate the need for inpatient treatment. When the patient's decompensation becomes sufficiently severe, the nonjudgmental atmosphere of a psychiatrist's outpatient office may not provide the safe holding environment that the patient requires. In that case, if the patient refuses a voluntary inpatient admission, involuntary admission may become necessary.

Emergency Detention

All states allow police to transport people to the hospital against their will under certain conditions. This process is known as an *emergency hold* or *emergency petition*, although in some states it may be referred to by the name of the law or the number of the statute. For example, the Florida emergency evaluation procedure is known as the Baker Act, while in California it is known as a "5150 hold." Most patients brought to EDs every year are not admitted, and no nationwide data are routinely kept regarding the number of people brought in on emergency detention orders. The length of time a patient can be held on an order without other judicial oversight varies tremendously from state to state, from as little as a matter of hours to as long as 10 days (Hedman et al. 2016).

In the case of a patient already in treatment, the emergency detention order process is started when a psychiatrist files a petition documenting the clinical assessment that the patient is both mentally ill and dangerous. The petition is given to the police department in the appropriate jurisdiction, and the police then attempt to locate the patient for transport to the nearest emergency evaluation facility, usually the ED of a local hospital. If the patient presented to the ED or was brought to the ED by family, friends, or law enforcement and is assessed to be at high risk, inpatient treatment may also be recommended. In such cases, the ED physician typically begins the emergency detention process.

If the potentially suicidal patient is an outpatient or not in an ED, involuntary admission becomes more complicated. Ideally, the patient is located swiftly and transported voluntarily. Sadly, in some cases the interaction between a suicidal or violent patient and a police officer results in a deadly confrontation. The term "suicide by cop" was coined to describe situations in which suicidal persons with weapons directly confront police officers with the intended effect of provoking the officer to kill them. One study of 707 officer-involved shootings collected over 1 year from 90 North American police departments determined that as many as 36% were intentionally provoked confrontations that could be classified as suicide by cop (Mohandie et al. 2009). In these cases, individuals were almost always armed with a weapon, usually a gun, and in half the cases the weapon was discharged at the police officer. In other cases, the individual feigned possession of a weapon but the risk of danger to others in the vicinity caused the officer to react. The mental health history of many of these subjects was unknown; however, 16% had a known history of previous suicide attempts.

Even when the police contact is nonviolent, an emergency detention order carries collateral social consequences. Police policy may require that the patient be placed in handcuffs in transit. Although physical restraint may be necessary if the patient is overtly violent or resists transport, this practice may be viewed as punitive and risks public humiliation and stigma if done in front of friends or neighbors. Even if patients are released after evaluation in an ED, they have been separated from family and have lost time from work. The incident may also lead to internal law enforcement documentation that the individual has a mental illness, which many individuals experience as stigmatizing and humiliating.

If an emergency evaluation determines that the patient requires admission, the patient must be offered an opportunity to be admitted voluntarily. Due process protections require that the patient be treated in an environment that represents the "least restrictive alternative," meaning that efforts must be made to preserve the patient's physical freedom if possible (*Lake v. Cameron* 1967). Documentation that the patient has refused or been nonadherent with outpatient care can support a decision that no less-restrictive alternative is appropriate. Documented nonadherence with prescribed psychiatric or somatic medication can provide evidence that the patient has been unwilling or unable to cooperate with voluntary care. When possible, clinicians should document the patient's own verbatim statements rather than a mere clinical conclusion.

Certain patients may be unable to sign a voluntary admission agreement because of impaired decision-making capacity or may be barred from voluntary admission as a matter of law. States are required to ascertain that voluntarily admitted patients are mentally competent to sign admission forms (*Zinermon v. Burch* 1990). Juveniles must be signed in by a parent or guardian, and some states do not allow an adult under guardianship to consent to psychiatric admission. Some states allow patients who possess decision-making capacity to be admitted involuntarily if the patient is merely unwilling to sign in voluntarily. This option is important because certain conditions, such as anorexia nervosa, may not cause cognitive impairment even when the patient is acutely ill. An assessment of decision-making capacity should include the ability to understand relevant information about the proposed treatment, the ability to appreciate the situation and its consequences, the ability to hypothesize and weigh alternatives, and the ability to communicate a decision (Appelbaum 2007).

Temporary Detention and Civil Commitment: Due Process

Superficially, loose criteria for emergency detention orders and for involuntary admission may seem like an arbitrary or improper use of the state's police powers. However, these laws are intended to set a low standard for temporary observation and evaluation during emergencies.

If a patient on emergency hold is assessed as meeting commitment criteria, the patient is certified for involuntary admission until a hearing regarding full civil commitment can be held. The time interval between when the patient is certified and when the patient is taken to a commitment hearing is known as the *observation period* but is also referred to as *temporary detention*. The length of the allowed observation period varies by jurisdiction but is generally limited to as little as few days or as long as 2 weeks (Treatment Advocacy Center 2014). During this time a patient may sign in voluntarily or may be discharged if assessed as no longer needing inpatient care. Patients who no longer meet commitment criteria and are not willing to be admitted voluntarily must be discharged.

After a period of observation or temporary detention, additional due process protections take effect. Patients held on temporary detention as involuntarily admitted inpatients are required to be informed about their rights, which include a right to a hearing by a neutral factfinder, a right to counsel, a right to confront and cross-examine witnesses, and a right to periodic review of commitment (*Fasulo v. Arafeh* 1977; *Lessard v. Schmidt* 1972). The party seeking commitment, which at this point is the hospital that admitted the patient for observation, must also prove that the patient is mentally ill and dangerous by, at minimum, "clear and convincing evidence," a higher and stricter evidentiary standard than that used in deciding most civil legal issues (*Addington v. Texas* 1979; Parry 2018).

The challenge for many clinicians is determining which facts constitute a "danger to self or others." Each state accepts an overt act of violence against oneself or others as evidence of dangerousness. Some also include a broader definition of dangerousness that may encompass involuntary admission for patients who are not overtly suicidal or homicidal. A person being determined as "gravely disabled" or unable to provide for basic needs such as food, clothing, shelter, or medical treatment might be explicitly defined by statute. This is also sometimes known as the "need for treatment" standard. Some variation of grave disability criteria exists in 49 states, 45 through legislation and 4 through court decisions (Treatment Advocacy Center 2014).

As commitment criteria have evolved over time, some states, such as Montana and Wisconsin, also have incorporated a broader standard specifically for patients who have required repeated hospitalization due to noncompliance and lack of insight (Montana Code Annotated 2017; Wisconsin Statute Annotated 1999–2000). Sometimes called the "risk of deterioration" standard, these laws are designed to capture a very small segment of people with mental illness who have demonstrated a high risk of dangerousness during relapse.

Regardless of the statutory grounds, many psychiatrists do not have an accurate understanding of their commitment standards. One survey of psychiatrists revealed that, in states that have a gravely disabled statute, 70.7% were aware that grave disability was grounds for commitment; conversely, in states with no gravely disabled commitment statute, the majority (61.5%) of respondents erroneously believed that grave disability could result in commitment (Brooks 2007). The variation in state standards, and clinician misunderstanding of those standards, may explain why in many cases an obviously ill person may not meet civil commitment criteria.

Civil commitment procedures have common elements in addition to minor jurisdictional variation. The challenge for clinicians and policymakers is to craft procedures that protect patients from arbitrary detention and loss of freedom while ensuring that people with serious mental illness do not suffer the consequences of delayed treatment. New programs and alternatives to involuntary treatment have been created in an attempt to balance these interests. The federal 21st Century Cures Act (2016) contained provisions to improve access to care and reduce civil commitment by appropriating money to implement and expand jail diversion programs, mental health courts, crisis response programs, assertive community outreach teams, and assisted outpatient treatment (AOT).

Assisted Outpatient Treatment

All but four states now have AOT laws, also known as involuntary outpatient treatment (IOT) or outpatient commitment. AOT is a court-mandated treatment plan that requires qualified patients to comply with mental health care if, without treatment, they would be unable to care for themselves or would be a danger to themselves or others. Outpatient commitment may be used as a condition of release from a hospital or as an alternative to inpatient civil commitment. Qualification criteria vary between states but generally require past evidence of dangerousness to self or others while ill or at least one previous civil commitment.

Presently AOT is not regularly used in half of the states where it is a legal option for treatment. When it is used, the program's jurisdiction is usually limited to a small geographic area such as a city or county. Implementation of AOT has been limited by insufficient funding and lack of community services (Meldrum et al. 2016).

AOT outcome studies have been mixed, but some have shown clinical efficacy as measured by decreased number of hospitalizations, medication adherence, and improved abstinence from drugs of abuse if the commitment order is sustained over time and accompanied by adequate intensive community services. Results are difficult to generalize due to the variation in outpatient commitment criteria and procedures among states and the type and range of services offered through the treatment plan. Noncompliance with AOT plans also limits generalizability due to patient nonadherence and dropout. The effect of AOT on suicide rates is unknown because no outcome study has looked at mortality rates among participants. With regard to danger to others, a pooled meta-analysis of outpatient commitment studies showed that 238 outpatient commitment orders were needed to prevent one arrest (Kisely et al. 2011). The increased sensitivity needed to potentially prevent one act of violence means that a much larger number of nonviolent people with mental illness would also be affected.

The 21st Century Cures Act (2016) provided states with a financial incentive to increase use of AOT in the name of public safety. Although thousands of papers have been published about AOT, few were controlled trials, and none has examined the effect on overall rates of violent crime or suicide. Following an intensive review of the evidence, the American Psychiatric Association (2015) endorsed the use of AOT but cautioned that it should not be considered as a primary tool to prevent acts of violence.

Substance Use Disorders and Civil Commitment

The latest trend in involuntary treatment policy involves the adoption of civil commitment laws specifically for the treatment of substance use disorders. Given that drug and alcohol abuse is strongly associated with suicide and violence, one would expect that substance abuse commitment policies would be promoted under the state's police powers doctrine to protect the public. Instead, due to the current opioid epidemic, the laws are being adopted on a *parens patriae* basis (i.e., to assist those who cannot assist themselves) to prevent opioid overdose deaths.

In 2012, thirty-two states and the District of Columbia had statutory provisions for civil commitment of people with substance use disorders (Christopher et al. 2015). The procedures may be found in either existing civil commitment procedures, where substance use disorders are included within the definition of mental illness, or through a separate substance abuse treatment statute. The frequencies with which states use these statutes vary greatly; some states have committed thousands of patients whereas other states commit few or none.

The clinical efficacy of substance abuse commitment laws is unproven, as is the effect on criminal recidivism and suicide prevention. To date, only one small descriptive study examined the characteristics and outcomes of patients petitioned for commitment. Lamoureux et al. (2017) reviewed the cases of 28 patients petitioned for substance abuse commitment from a medical unit and examined legal and emergency department records over a 24-month follow-up period. Of the 28 subjects, 68% of the requests for commitment either were denied by the court or hearings were not sought by the county that received the petition. Many of those who were committed had a history of violent felonies. Regardless of eventual commitment status, patients who were held for a hearing were less likely to be convicted of crimes after hospitalization. No study has examined effects on suicide rates.

Civil Commitment and Psychiatric Testimony

Few experiences are as anxiety provoking as giving expert testimony in a civil commitment hearing. A psychiatrist may have to discuss personal and sensitive patient information in front of people who are unknown to the patient. If the psychiatrist has been treating the patient on an outpatient basis or has been assigned to treat the patient on an involuntary inpatient basis, the psychiatrist's testimony could undermine the patient's trust and compromise the therapeutic relationship long after the hearing has ended. Cross-examination by a patient's attorney can be uncomfortable and intimidating. A hospital may or may not have legal counsel available to help the doctor prepare for testimony, and the hearing officer or judge may not be experienced or knowledgeable regarding the clinical issues involved in the case.

Preparation is always the key to providing competent testimony. In addition to a recent patient assessment, the testifying psychiatrist should review all documentation provided by the ED and be familiar with factual information documented in the patient's chart. Time and date information is relevant to ensure that all due-process protections were carried out within statutory time limits. Descriptive information regarding the patient's behavior and symptoms can be gathered from family members or others, such as police officers, who sought the emergency detention order. Family members may be allowed to testify as well, so patients should be prepared for this possibility and the potential for interpersonal conflict as a result.

In order to be qualified to testify, psychiatrists must establish their expertise through training and experience. An up-to-date curriculum vitae is a straightforward means of qualification, and a resident in training should not be deterred if this document appears scanty or insufficient. Academic publications or credentials are not necessary to establish one's expertise as a psychiatrist; standard residency training provides enough education and experience to meet qualification requirements.

Testimony is designed to elicit general categories of information relevant to the state's commitment standards: the presence of mental illness, the patient's inability to recognize a need for treatment or to comply with treatment, and general information regarding dangerousness or impairment. A testifying psychiatrist should be able to directly state the pertinent statutory language and to connect the clinical facts of the case to that statute. Writing out answers to anticipated questions is helpful for residents in training and those who have little experience with commitment hearings.

One of the more challenging aspects of testimony is having to explain psychiatric diagnoses to magistrates or judges. Some judges, such as administrative law judges, may preside over commitment hearings only occasionally in addition to hearing other legal matters, such as employment and disability cases or other regulatory issues. The judge may have heard of DSM-5 (American Psychiatric Association 2013) but may not understand the medical terms or jargon within it. For example, the testifying psychiatrist may be required to explain the difference between substance intoxication and a substance-induced psychosis, or why delirium is a medical condition even though it is also a psychiatric diagnosis. Of course, most clinicians are also not familiar with legal terminology. Knowing the statutory definition of "mental disorder" for the purpose of civil commitment can help the clinician translate information for the judge.

Testimony about dangerousness is more straightforward and typically is based upon statements or behaviors exhibited by the patient immediately prior to admission or while under observation during temporary detention. Attempts to harm self or others may occur on the inpatient unit between the time the patient was admitted and the time of the hearing. Inability to care for self or grave disability can be illustrated by a patient's medical history and laboratory findings. Evidence of malnutrition or dehydration or a failure to adhere regularly to life-sustaining medication such as insulin can support an opinion of danger to self.

To a certain extent, dangerousness also depends upon the environmental context and therefore is related to testimony regarding the least restrictive treatment setting. A patient could be gravely disabled if released to a living situation that does not provide nursing support or assistance with activities of daily living but nondangerous if released to an assisted living or day program. A cross-examination will typically query testifying physicians as to whether they have considered these alternative discharge options. Of course, if none of these resources is available to the patient, this should be stated on the record.

Finally, clinicians should be mindful of general principles common to all testifying experiences. The doctor should maintain a calm and nondefensive demeanor even in the face of intimidating cross-examination. Clinicians should also avoid speculating about situations where information is missing or answering questions that are beyond the scope of one's training. Testimony should be descriptive and include specific examples, but responses should be concise and to the point of the question. Clinicians should be sure to listen fully to the question before answering and ask for clarification when the question is ambiguous or confusing.

Following these guidelines will minimize the risk that a dangerous or gravely ill patient is released on a technical issue or a misinterpretation of the law.

Conclusion

People with mental illness often bear the consequences of unproven policies and laws based on unfounded public fear, especially the fear that people with mental illness are inevitably dangerous. In addition to reinforcing stigma, these laws undermine community reintegration and legitimize the liability concerns of clinicians who work with patients at risk of dying from suicide. However, involuntary treatment is a necessary intervention for people with serious mental illness who lack insight and the ability to care for themselves or are dangerous to themselves or others due to their symptoms. Loss of freedom and involuntary treatment may be traumatic for people with serious mental illness, but it is life saving for some patients. It also provides an opportunity for patients to reengage with society, family, and other loved ones.

Ultimately, suicide deaths will be reduced through timely access to voluntary mental health services and efforts to educate the public regarding effective treatments for clinical depression and other psychiatric conditions. Early intervention and peer support can also reinforce the hope and trust that patients need to survive.

Key Points

- People with mental illness, including those with suicidal ideation, are rarely violent, but on rare occasions suicidal individuals may pose a risk to others.

- Civil commitment processes vary between states but generally consist of an emergency detention for evaluation followed by a period of observation or temporary detention before a civil commitment hearing.

- All civil commitment laws require the presence of a mental disorder, although the statutory definition of "mental disorder" may vary between states and does not rely solely upon criteria from DSM-5.

- The criteria for civil commitment in all states require evidence of danger to self or others but may also include a "grave disability" or "need for care" standard.

- Assisted outpatient treatment improves adherence with mental health care but has not been studied with regard to suicide prevention.

- Civil commitment for the treatment of substance use disorders may be allowed in some states, but the efficacy of this intervention for suicide prevention is unknown.

- Testimony for a civil commitment hearing will be most effective if the psychiatrist has a sound grasp of the clinical history and facts of the case, understands the appropriate commitment standard, and can testify succinctly while avoiding medical jargon.

References

21st Century Cures Act, Pub.L. No. H.R. 34 (2016). Available at: https://www.congress.gov/114/bills/hr34/BILLS-114hr34enr.pdf. Accessed August 16, 2018.

Addington v Texas, 441 U.S. 418, 99 S.Ct. 1804 (1979)

American Psychiatric Association: Diagnostic and Statistical Manual of Mental Disorders, 5th Edition. Arlington, VA, American Psychiatric Association, 2013

American Psychiatric Association: Resource Document on Involuntary Outpatient and Related Programs of Assisted Outpatient Treatment. Arlington, VA, American Psychiatric Association, October 2015. Available at: https://www.psychiatry.org/File%20Library/Psychiatrists/Directories/Library-and-Archive/resource_documents/resource-2015-involuntary-outpatient-commitment.pdf. Accessed August 25, 2018.

Appelbaum PS: Clinical practice: assessment of patients' competence to consent to treatment. N Engl J Med 357(18):1834–1840, 2007 17978292

Brooks RA: Psychiatrists' opinions about involuntary civil commitment: results of a national survey. J Am Acad Psychiatry Law 35(2):219–228, 2007 17592168

Christopher PP, Pinals DA, Stayton T, et al: Nature and utilization of civil commitment for substance abuse in the United States. J Am Acad Psychiatry Law 43(3):313–320, 2015 26438809

Fasulo v Arafeh, 173 Conn. 473, 378 A.2d 553 (1977)

Fisher WH, Grisso T: Commentary: civil commitment statutes—40 years of circumvention. J Am Acad Psychiatry Law 38(3):365–368, 2010 20852222

Hedman LC, Petrila J, Fisher WH, et al: State laws on emergency holds for mental health stabilization. Psychiatr Serv 67(5):529–535, 2016 26927575

Kisely S, Campbell L, Preston N: Compulsory community and involuntary outpatient treatment for people with severe mental disorders. Cochrane Database Syst Rev (2):CD004408, 2011 21328267

Lake v Cameron, 267 F.Supp. 155 (D.D.C. 1967)

Lamoureux IC, Schutt PE, Rasmussen KG: Petitioning for involuntary commitment for chemical dependency by medical services. J Am Acad Psychiatry Law 45(3):332–338, 2017 28939731

Large MM: The role of prediction in suicide prevention. Dialogues Clin Neurosci 20(3):197–205, 2018 30581289

Lessard v Schmidt, 349 F.Supp. 1078 (1972)

Meldrum ML, Kelly EL, Calderon R, et al: Implementation status of assisted outpatient treatment programs: a national survey. Psychiatr Serv 67(6):630–635, 2016 26828396

Miller D, Hanson A: Committed: The Battle Over Involuntary Psychiatric Care. Baltimore, MD, Johns Hopkins University Press, 2016

Mohandie K, Meloy JR, Collins PI: Suicide by cop among officer-involved shooting cases. J Forensic Sci 54(2):456–462, 2009 19220654

Montana Code Annotated, § 53.21.126, Trial or hearing on petition. (2017) Available at: https://leg.mt.gov/bills/mca/title_0530/chapter_0210/part_0010/section_0260/0530-0210-0010-0260.html. Accessed March 31, 2019.

Parry J: Involuntary inpatient commitments of adults, in Treatise on Health Care Law. Edited by MacDonald MG, Kaufman RM, Capron AM, et al. New York, Matthew Bender and Co, 2018

Silver J, Simons A, Craun S: A Study of the Pre-Attack Behaviors of Active Shooters in the United States Between 2000–2013. Washington, DC, Federal Bureau of Investigation, U.S. Department of Justice, 2018. Available at: https://www.fbi.gov/file-repository/pre-attack-behaviors-of-active-shooters-in-us-2000-2013.pdf/view. Accessed July 22, 2018.

Testa M, West SG: Civil commitment in the United States. Psychiatry (Edgmont Pa) 7(10):30–40, 2010 22778709

Treatment Advocacy Center: Mental Health Commitment Laws: A Survey of the States (website). Arlington, VA, Treatment Advocacy Center, February 2014. Available at: https://www.treatmentadvocacycenter.org/mental-health-commitment-laws. Accessed March 24, 2019.

Violence Policy Center: American Roulette: Murder-Suicide in the United States. Washington, DC, Violence Policy Center, 2015. Available at: http://www.vpc.org/studies/amroul2015.pdf. Accessed July 22, 2018.

Wisconsin Statute Annotated, §51.20(1)(a)2e, Petition for examination. (1999–2000) Available at: https://docs.legis.wisconsin.gov/statutes/statutes/51/20/1/a. Accessed March 31, 2019.

Zinermon v Burch, 494 U.S. 113, 110 S. Ct. 975 (1990)

PART IV

Special Populations

CHAPTER 18

Children and Adolescents

Cheryl D. Wills, M.D.

Parents hope their children mature to become happy, successful individuals. However, at times, children experience seemingly untenable situations that, when not mitigated in a timely manner, can lead to a variety of unhealthful emotions, mental disorders, pervasive hopelessness, and in extreme cases, death from suicide. This chapter examines the phenomenology of suicide in children and adolescents, suicide prevention, treatment approaches for youths who contemplate or attempt suicide, and strategies to reduce sensationalism and contagion, or copycat behavior, after a suicide attempt or suicide death.

Definitions

The spectrum of suicide behaviors has its own nomenclature, and the following definitions are used in this chapter. *Nonsuicidal self-injurious behavior* occurs when a person intentionally engages in self-harm but without the desire to die. *Suicide ideation* refers to thoughts about suicide. Suicide ideation with plan exists when a person has identified at least one way to end her life. *Suicide plan with intent* refers to contemplating how to end one's life. A *suicide attempt* occurs when a person follows through with the suicide plan. Last, *dying from suicide* or *suicide death* refers to intentionally ending one's life.

Epidemiology

Since 2010, suicide has been the second leading cause of death in the United States for youth ages 10–17; suicide is the eleventh leading cause of death in children ages 5–11 (Centers for Disease Control and Prevention 2018). Youth suicide rates, although lower than those for adults, have been increasing, as have the percentage of pediatric hospital visits for suicide attempts. Plemmons et al. (2018) determined that the number of hospital admissions for suicide attempts in 31 hospitals increased from 6,392 in 2008 to 25,085 in 2015. Attempts were more common in females (64%), 15- to 17-year-olds (50%), and youths who were at least 12 years old (94.2%) (Plemmons et al. 2018). These results, unfortunately, are consistent with findings in other U.S. studies of suicide behavior in youths.

Contributing Factors

Genetics

More than a dozen studies have identified an association between a suicide death in a family member and suicide ideation in surviving youth (Evans et al. 2005). Also, suicide ideation in a family member can be associated with suicide behavior in a youth (Evans et al. 2005). Evans et al. (2005) suggested that the greater range of suicide behavior in the latter group may be related to the larger number of family members who attempt suicide than those who die from suicide. Serotonin activity in the brain, which has been associated with suicide behavior in adults, is influenced by genetic factors but has not been studied in children and adolescents.

Mental Disorders

Up to 30% of youths in the United States contemplate or attempt suicide (Evans et al. 2005). In one clinical study, U.S. youths who attempted suicide by ingestion were more likely to have mental disorders than youths who did not attempt suicide (77.5% vs. 2%; Ghanem et al. 2013). Youths at highest risk for suicide behavior include those who have psychosis with command hallucinations, mood disorders, anxiety disorders, substance use disorders, and impulse-control disorders. (See "Special Populations" section for information about autism spectrum disorder [ASD].)

Eating disorders are also a risk factor for suicide. A survey of the parents of 7- to 18-year-olds with bulimia showed that 43% of these youths had attempted suicide (Mayes et al. 2014b). By comparison, 20% of the individuals who had anorexia nervosa had experienced suicide ideation and 3% had attempted suicide (Mayes et al. 2014b).

Youths who are impulsive, have poor problem-solving skills, or have high reward dependence are at increased risk for attempting suicide (Ghanem et al. 2013). Youths who engage in antisocial behavior and those who have low self-esteem are also at increased risk (Evans et al. 2005). Hopelessness is also a highly predictive determinant for suicide behavior (Soole et al. 2015). Finally, a history of past suicide thoughts or attempts increases the risk for future suicide behavior (Christiansen and Stenager 2012).

Social Determinants

Adverse childhood events such as family instability—including having a caretaker who has a debilitating physical or mental disorder, is unemployed, abandons the family, is incarcerated, or dies—can increase the risk for suicide phenomena in youths (Dube et al. 2001). Chronic exposure to violence; physical, sexual, or emotional abuse; a recent loss; repeated self-destructive behavior; institutional confinement; homelessness; guilt; and other stressors can increase a youth's risk for developing a mental disorder followed by suicide behavior (Christiansen and Stenager 2012; Evans et al. 2005). Academic and behavior problems in school also are indirectly associated with an increase in suicide phenomena (Evans et al. 2005).

Sleep

Sleep deprivation can affect a youth's judgment, emotions, behavior, and suicide risk. An anonymous survey of 67,615 U.S. high school students determined that 17.6% of students (11,912) obtained less than 6 hours of sleep on school nights (Weaver et al. 2018). These adolescents, when compared with students who slept 8 hours on school nights, were three times as likely to feel sad and hopeless and four times more likely to attempt suicide (Weaver et al. 2018). One study has also identified a small but significant temporal relationship between sleep disturbance and deaths from suicide in 140 adolescents (Goldstein et al. 2008).

Suicide Risk Assessment

The suicide risk assessment is essential in evaluating a child or teen's risk of suicide and implementing appropriate steps to mitigate risks. Psychiatrists should elicit information about the youth's past and history of suicide behavior. Details about the antecedents, triggers, intent, severity, and outcomes of past self-harm events are important. The assessment should include the rationale for and intensity of thoughts about dying, recent suicide behaviors, and the existence of a plan, intent, implementation capacity, and anticipated consequences. Data obtained in the risk assessment should guide the crafting of a crisis intervention plan.

Using a standardized suicide risk assessment tool that has been normed in children or adolescents can improve the consistency of the evaluation. However, the clinician should be cognizant of unique risk factors that may not be included on a standardized checklist. For example, a youth who is on break from school when interviewed may appear to be at lower suicide risk if school is a key stressor. In these circumstances, the suicide risk may significantly increase as soon as classes resume. Neurodevelopmental factors, cultural identity, and psychosocial stressors should also be considered when evaluating a youth's risk for suicide.

An assessment of the youth's past mental health history as well as an inventory or screening for existing symptoms of mental disorder are important parts of the risk determination. Younger children who die from suicide are less likely to have a mental disorder. Nevertheless, psychiatrists should assess all potentially suicidal children and teens for the presence of mental disorders, because mitigation of risk will require treatment for mental disorders and will inform the determination of the most suitable treatment interventions. The youth's capacity for problem solving will depend on the youth's mental state. For example, youths who are overwhelmed by auditory hallucinations that order them to end their lives may be less capable of refraining from making a suicide attempt than youths with depression who believe that a medication adjustment and psychotherapy can help them feel better.

Youths and their caretakers should be interviewed separately. Interviewing youths alone is more likely to result in the disclosure of information that they do not want their parents to know. The mental health evaluator should also ascertain how the youth is functioning in a variety of systems: home, school, work, athletics, religious, extended family, and health care. Evaluators should determine whether the suicide behavior may be aggravated or mitigated by involvement with certain individuals, in certain settings, or in one or more activities. The clinician should inquire as to what would compel the youth to engage in suicide behavior and explore the likelihood of the trigger occurring and ways to mitigate this. Compiling lists of the youth's aggravating and protective factors can expedite identifying ways to mitigate the suicide risk.

The safety of the child or teen is paramount. Access to means such as firearms, other weapons, medications, and other items that can be used to inflict self-harm should also be explored. Health care professionals, parents, and, when possible, the youth should collaborate to prioritize the youth's safety. This could include restricting the youth's access to instruments of self-harm but may require inpatient hospitalization in some cases. Identifying a suitable placement can mitigate the suicide risk until the youth can receive appropriate mental health care. Sometimes placement with an informed and responsible relative or family friend may suffice. Again, however, hospitalization may be the least restrictive alternative when risk factors cannot be mitigated adequately with community interventions and lethal means restriction.

Case Example

Fifteen-year-old Jessica Lee argued with her father and threatened to end her life by ingesting pills. She tells the emergency department psychiatrist that she will end her life if she goes home with her father. He says that he can arrange for Jessica to live with her aunt until they are able to work through the crisis. All parties, including Jessica's outpatient psychiatrist, support the plan, so Jessica is sent home with her aunt, who has removed all medications and weapons from Jessica's reach.

Special Populations

Children

Rates of suicide among children ages 5–12 years have been increasing. Data from the Centers for Disease Control and Prevention show that one child died from suicide every 13 days between 1999 and 2012 (Centers for Disease Control and Prevention 2016). The rate increased to one child every 3.4 days in the following 3 years (Centers for Disease Control and Prevention 2016). Also, the suicide rate in 11- and 12-year-olds increased 54% between 2010 and 2016 (Centers for Disease Control and Prevention 2016). These data do not reflect the likelihood that suicide deaths in children are underreported unless evidence irrefutably points to suicide as the method of death because, relative to all causes of death in this age group, few children intentionally end their lives.

Historically, suicide deaths had been more common among boys and white children. These demographic patterns were consistent from 1993 until 2012, when 553 (84%) of the 657 children ages 5–11 years who died from suicide were white boys (Bridge et al. 2015). However, the demographic pattern in regard to race changed after 2012 as the rate of suicide deaths in 5- to 11-year-olds increased among black children and decreased among white youths (Sheftall et al. 2016). The suicide rate among 5- to 12-year-old girls has been increasing more rapidly than that in boys (see Chapter 23,

"Suicide and Gender"). When compared to adolescents and adults, 5- to 11-year-olds, regardless of race, were less likely to have used firearms to end their lives (Bridge et al. 2015; Sheftall et al. 2016; Soole et al. 2015).

Sheftall et al. (2016) reviewed youth suicides in 17 states and concluded that decedents aged 5–13 years were more likely to have been male, black, and have relationship problems with family and friends. They were also less likely to leave a suicide note, less likely to have depression, and more likely to die at home from hanging, strangulation, or suffocation (Sheftall et al. 2016). Additionally, children's deaths from suicide were most often preceded by parent–child conflict (Soole et al. 2015).

Sexual- and Gender-Minority Youth

Sexual- and gender-minority youths are at higher risk for emotional and physical victimization, sexual assault, and homelessness (Haas et al. 2011; Taliaferro and Muehlenkamp 2017; see Chapter 23). They are more likely to develop mental disorders, including substance use disorders and depression, and are two to seven times more likely to attempt suicide (Lucassen et al. 2017; Taliaferro and Muehlenkamp 2017). Sexual orientation independently predicts suicide attempts in sexual-minority male youths more than in sexual-minority females (Haas et al. 2011). These youths, who experience conflict with their caretakers and rejection by friends, are at higher risk for self-destructive behavior, including suicide phenomena (Taliaferro and Muehlenkamp 2017). Acceptance by parents, having an adult mentor, and feeling safe in school can have a protective effect (Evans et al. 2005; Taliaferro and Muehlenkamp 2017).

Autism Spectrum Disorder

ASD increases the risk for depression in youths, starting at age 10 (Rai et al. 2018). Among youths who have both ASD and depression, 14% have experienced suicide behaviors (Mayes et al. 2013). This rate is 28 times that of youths with ASD who do not have depression, although lower than in depressed youths without ASD (Mayes et al. 2013). Youths with ASD and suicide behaviors were more likely to be black or Latinx, male, and of lower socioeconomic status (Mayes et al. 2013).

Chronic Health Conditions

Youths who have chronic medical disorders are at risk for developing mental disorders. For example, relative to their healthy siblings, youths who have diabetes are three times as likely to develop a mental disorder within the first 6 months after diagnosis and are at increased risk for suicide attempts (Butwicka et al. 2015). A Danish study determined youths were at risk for suicide behavior after they received medical care in a hospital, especially youths who had many hospital visits for unstable chronic medical conditions such as epilepsy and asthma (Christiansen and Stenager 2012). The risk for suicide behavior peaked immediately after the hospital visit (Christiansen and Stenager 2012).

Retrospective Study of Youth Suicide

Interviewing suicide contemplators and attempters and their caretakers may be helpful in identifying risk factors for suicide. When a youth has died from suicide, a different investigative approach may be needed. The psychological autopsy uses structured interviews and other evaluative methods to gather historical data from the caretakers, relatives, teachers, coaches, peers, health care providers, and others with whom the youth had relationships. The evaluator strives to learn about the youth's psychiatric history and stressors along with his or her history of suicide behavior, while focusing on the events that preceded the death.

Researchers who conducted 42 psychological autopsies on youths younger than age 15 determined that the 33 who left suicide notes had engaged in suicide behavior more often before they died. They used the notes to explain their actions, accept responsibility for their deaths, express love, and state how they wanted their property distributed. None of the note writers described the emotions or indecision they experienced before ending their lives (Freuchen and Grøholt 2015).

Contemporary Factors: Bullying, Electronic Media, and News Reporting

Bullying is a behavior that is experienced by 10%–20% of youths (Mayes et al. 2014a). Those who have mental disorders, physical deformities, or are otherwise nonconforming are at higher risk for being targeted. Electronic or cyberbullying has become more common because the internet facilitates rapid dissemination of negative commentary without direct confrontation.

Digital self-harm or self-cyberbullying occurs when the youths intentionally post disparaging remarks about themselves on social media. Youths who engage in this behavior, often as a preemptive strike, are more likely to have experienced bullying, cyberbullying, depression, substance use, deviant behavior, or challenges with sexual identity (Patchin and Hinduja 2017). Victims of bullying are at increased risk for engaging in suicide behaviors (van Geel et al. 2014).

In 2017, several youths and adults ended their lives before audiences on Facebook Live. In response, Facebook began to use algorithms to identify content suggestive of suicide behavior (Constine 2017). These data, along with subscriber complaints about inappropriate posting, are reviewed by content monitors who are authorized to ask local first responders to conduct welfare checks on individuals who have posted concerning content (see Chapter 25, "Social Media and the Internet"; Constine 2017).

Youths' electronic media use patterns can offer insights into their emotional health. Researchers found that youths in middle and high school who spent more time on electronic media platforms were more likely to have higher levels of emotional health concerns and suicide behavior (Sampasa-Kanyinga and Lewis 2015; Twenge et al. 2018). They have access to poorly vetted and sensationalized accounts of dangerous activities, including suicide behavior, that can catalyze copycat behavior. This is concerning because the risk of suicide attempts increases in youths whose friends have attempted suicide (Evans et al. 2005).

News Media

How suicide is portrayed in the news media can influence vulnerable populations, including youths. A meta-analysis of 55 studies regarding media reports of suicide determined that copycat suicides are 5.27 times more likely to occur when the news

TABLE 18–1.   **Firearms suicide rate per 100,000**

	United States	World Health Organization 23 populous, high-income countries
5–14 years old	0.2	0.0
15–24 years old	4.7	0.4

Source.   Grinshteyn and Hemenway 2016.

media reports about the death of a public figure (Stack 2005). In contrast, news reports that focused on the negative effects of suicide reduced the likelihood of copycat behavior by 99% (Stack 2005).

The World Health Organization (WHO) and other organizations have published guidelines for best practices in media reporting on suicides, but few news outlets in the United States or elsewhere have complied consistently with these guidelines, although some have done a better job than others (Young et al. 2017). Researchers examined the 25 most relevant Canadian news articles about suicide prevention from 2008 to 2012 and determined that 16%–60% followed the WHO guidelines (Easson et al. 2014). Notably, educating media professionals in Austria about the media and suicide resulted in a 20% reduction in reporting of suicides by the media (Stack 2003).

Movies and Television

Media programs that use suicide as a theme can also influence suicide behavior in those who might be vulnerable to self-harm. The Netflix series *13 Reasons Why* is an example of this kind of subject matter. One study showed that admissions for suicide behavior in 4- to 18-year-olds in a tertiary hospital were higher than anticipated, based on retrospective data, in the 7-month period after the series became available on Netflix (Cooper et al. 2018). Determining whether this series had a causative effect on increasing suicidal behavior is not possible. Nevertheless, public health concerns regarding suicide suggest that such programming should include a restrictive warning about the nature of the content, age restrictions for viewers, the adverse effects of suicide, and how individuals can access help (de Leo and Vijayakumar 2008; Gentile et al. 2011).

Methods

The suicide rate in U.S. youths is higher than the average rate in other populous high-income countries (Grinshteyn and Hemenway 2016; see Table 18–1).

In the United States, suffocation (46%) is the most common form of suicide in youths younger than 19, followed by firearms (41%), ingestion/poisoning (6%), jumping/falling (2%), and transportation-related deaths (1%) (Centers for Disease Control and Prevention 2016). In Switzerland, where firearms laws are more restrictive, the most common methods of suicide in youths are hanging (26.9%), railway (26.4%), firearms (17.9%), jumping (17.4%), and poisoning (6.8%) (Steck et al. 2018; see Table 18–2).

Access to firearms may explain why the rate of firearm suicide in U.S. youths is more than twice the rate in Swiss youths. Firearms in the home increase youth suicide

TABLE 18–2.   Suicide manner of death, 5–19 years of age

Swiss youths[1]		U.S. youths[2]	
Hanging	26.9%	Suffocation/Hanging	46%
Railway	26.4%	Firearms	41%
Jumping/Falls	17.4%	Poison	6%
Firearms	17.9%	Falls/Jumping	2%
Poisoning	6.8%	Transportation	1%

Source. [1]Steck et al. 2018. [2]Centers for Disease Control and Prevention 2016.

risk, regardless of a youth's mental health history. Firearms can be fired rapidly and with minimal contemplation and are associated with a 90% mortality rate (Elnour and Harrison 2008). All other means are less fatal, thus increasing chances of survival, and evidence demonstrates that most survivors of suicide attempts die of causes other than suicide (Owens et al. 2002).

Suicide Prevention

Protective Factors

Protective determinants of suicide risk render youths less vulnerable to self-destructive behavior by enhancing their capacity to be future oriented when under stress. Youths who seek and comply with mental health care services reduce their risk for suicide attempts and dying from suicide. Having supportive parents or other caretakers who are invested in the youth's emotional well-being also has a protective effect (Breton et al. 2015; Ghanem et al. 2013). In addition, healthful coping skills, including the capacity to delay gratification, cooperate with others, be future oriented, be self-directed, and be able to influence change in one's life can reduce youth suicide behavior (Breton et al. 2015; Ghanem et al. 2013). These factors should be considered when crafting mental health rehabilitation programs for at-risk youth.

Means Restriction

Means restriction has been demonstrated to be an effective method of reducing suicide deaths (Bridge et al. 2015; Grossman et al. 2005). As discussed, firearms are the most lethal and commonly used means of youth suicide in the United States. Where firearms access laws are less rigid, the rate of death from firearm suicide is 10 times higher than in other developed countries (Grinshteyn and Hemenway 2016). Having a firearm in the home increases the risk of a person, especially a youth who may not be able to legally purchase a gun or who cannot afford to purchase a gun, dying from suicide. In Switzerland, 82% of firearms-involved youth suicides involve a gun owned by a household member (Steck et al. 2018). In 2015, 4.6 million, or 7% of children in the United States, lived in a home with at least one unlocked and loaded firearm (Azrael et al. 2018). That number, which has doubled since 2002, has made it easier for youths to access guns in their homes and the homes of their relatives and friends (Azrael et al. 2018).

The protective measures of storing guns unloaded and with gun locks are 70% and 73% effective, respectively (Grossman et al. 2005). The American Academy of Pediatrics advocates that health care professionals counsel patients and parents about safer firearms storage and gun cable locks (Bridge et al. 2015). Unloaded guns and ammunition should be stored separately in locked boxes or gun safes, and their locations never should be disclosed to youths. Parents and caretakers also should be advised of the importance of inquiring about the presence and safe storage of firearms in homes that their children want to visit before permitting them to do so. However, if the child or teen is in crisis, the safest way to prevent a tragic outcome is, at least temporarily, to remove firearms and ammunition from the home.

Child Access Prevention (CAP) laws exist in at least 27 states and Washington, DC, and are intended to promote responsible gun ownership and reduce youth access to guns (Giffords Law Center 2018). These laws, which are not federally enforceable, have varying levels of accountability. The most restrictive CAP laws exist in 14 states and Washington, DC, and can result in criminal liability for the gun owner whose improperly stored firearm is obtained by a youth (Giffords Law Center 2018). These laws have reduced suicides among 14- to 17-year-olds by 8.3% and have significantly reduced firearms-related injuries in minors (Giffords Law Center 2018).

Treatment

A youth who has suicide behavior should be hospitalized when the aggravating circumstances or risk factors cannot be adequately mitigated in a less-restrictive environment. A meta-analysis of various psychotherapy studies determined that dialectical behavior therapy, cognitive-behavioral therapy, and mentalization-based therapy were most beneficial to youths with suicide and self-injurious behavior (Ougrin et al. 2015).

Pharmacotherapy may benefit youths whose symptoms are sufficiently severe or disabling. Use of medication can also improve the capacity of some youths to benefit from psychotherapy. The prescriber must obtain informed consent from the parent or legal guardian before prescribing the medication to the youth. This includes notifying parents about off-label use of certain psychotropic medication in children and adolescents and the potential side effects, including those that are serious and potentially life threatening, such as suicide ideation.

In October 2004, the U.S. Food and Drug Administration issued a black box warning about the possible association between antidepressants and suicide ideation in minors. The warning was revised in May 2007 to include all persons younger than 24 years of age (Bushnell et al. 2016). In response, physicians began to prescribe fewer antidepressants to this population, at lower initial dosages, and with more frequent monitoring. The frequency of prescribing antidepressants to minors increased as additional research became available and the risk-benefit analysis favored cautious prescribing of antidepressants to alleviate youths' emotional suffering and impairment (Bushnell et al. 2016).

Suicide Prevention in Schools and Community-Based Agencies

Community-based suicide prevention training programs informed by best practices can reduce suicide behavior in children and adolescents by facilitating early identification of and mental health treatment referrals for at-risk youths. One example is the American Psychiatric Association Foundation's (2018) Typical or Troubled program, which has been successfully implemented in more than 150 U.S. cities. This program trains teachers, coaches, and school officials to recognize warning signs of mental health problems, to talk with students about mental health, and to make referrals for crisis and other mental health services when needed (American Psychiatric Association Foundation 2018). Suicide prevention and other mental health education training programs can help reduce the stigma of mental disorders by helping people understand that mental disorders, like physical disorders, are a reality of life and that early intervention can reduce emotional suffering and preempt long-term adverse outcomes.

Conclusion

Death from suicide in children and adolescents is a growing public health crisis that can be reduced by increasing access to treatment resources and restricting their access to lethal means, particularly firearms. Suicide prevention research, screening tools, training, and education programs for youths should be informed by demographic changes and the evolving developmental, medical, psychosocial, and cultural needs of youths. Future suicide prevention programs should focus on the assessment, safety, cultural, and treatment needs of specific groups of children, especially youths with chronic medical illness, nonheterosexual and transgendered youth, and nonwhite boys, whose suicide rate has been growing. Future suicide prevention program modules should also include content to educate youths and families about how electronic media can influence suicide behavior. These interventions, along with responsible reporting about suicide prevention by the media, can reduce suicide behavior in youths.

Key Points

- Suicide is the second leading cause of death in U.S. 10- to 17-year-olds.

- The suicide rate in U.S. youths has been increasing, although it has remained stable in other highly developed countries.

- The frequency of deaths from suicide has been increasing in 5- to 11-year-old African American boys and decreasing in 5- to 11-year-old white boys.

- The risk for death from suicide is higher in youths who have chronic medical conditions or autism spectrum disorder or who are sexual or gender minorities.

- Clinicians should ascertain triggers for suicide risk and the youth's degree of hopelessness during every suicide risk assessment.

- Restriction of access to firearms in the home is an effective means to reduce death from suicide in youths.

- Psychiatric disorder, a family history of suicide, stressful life events, and access to firearms are leading risk factors for suicide behavior in youths.

References

American Psychiatric Association Foundation: Typical or Troubled School Mental Health Education Program. Washington, DC, American Psychiatric Association, 2018. Available at: https://apafdn.org/impact/schools/typical-or-troubled. Accessed December 31, 2018.

Azrael D, Cohen J, Salhi C, et al: Firearm storage in gun-owning households with children: results of a 2015 national survey. J Urban Health 95(3):295–304, 2018 29748766

Breton JJ, Labelle R, Berthiaume C, et al: Protective factors against depression and suicidal behaviour in adolescence. Can J Psychiatry 60(2 suppl 1):S5–S15, 2015 25886672

Bridge JA, Asti L, Horowitz LM, et al: Suicide trends among elementary school-aged children in the United States from 1993 to 2012. JAMA Pediatr 169(7):673–677, 2015 25984947

Bushnell GA, Stürmer T, Swanson SA, et al: Dosing of selective serotonin reuptake inhibitors among children and adults before and after the FDA black-box warning. Psychiatr Serv 67(3):302–309, 2016 26567938

Butwicka A, Frisén L, Almqvist C, et al: Risks of psychiatric disorders and suicide attempts in children and adolescents with type 1 diabetes: a population-based cohort study. Diabetes Care 38(3):453–459, 2015 25650362

Centers for Disease Control and Prevention: United States Suicide Injury Deaths and Rates per 100,000 (via WISQARS), 2016. Available at: https://webappa.cdc.gov/sasweb/ncipc/mortrate.html. Accessed January 23, 2018.

Centers for Disease Control and Prevention: 10 Leading Causes of Death by Age Group—United States, 2016. Atlanta, GA, National Center for Injury Prevention and Control, Centers for Disease Control and Prevention, 2018. Available at: https://www.cdc.gov/injury/wisqars/pdf/leading_causes_of_death_by_age_group_2016-508.pdf. Accessed December 27, 2018.

Christiansen E, Stenager E: Risk for attempted suicide in children and youths after contact with somatic hospitals: a Danish register based nested case-control study. J Epidemiol Community Health 66(3):247–253, 2012 20947873

Constine J: Facebook rolls out AI to detect suicidal posts before they're reported. Techcrunch.com, November 2017. Available at: https://techcrunch.com/2017/11/27/facebook-ai-suicide-prevention. Accessed December 31, 2018.

Cooper MT Jr, Bard D, Wallace R, et al: Suicide attempt admissions from a single children's hospital before and after the introduction of Netflix series 13 Reasons Why. J Adolesc Health 63(6):688–693, 2018 30454731

de Leo D, Vijayakumar L: Preventing Suicide: A Resource for Media Professionals. Geneva, Switzerland, World Health Organization, Department of Mental Health and Substance Abuse, 2008

Dube SR, Anda RF, Felitti VJ, et al: Childhood abuse, household dysfunction, and the risk of attempted suicide throughout the life span: findings from the Adverse Childhood Experiences Study. JAMA 286(24):3089–3096, 2001 11754674

Easson A, Agarwal A, Duda S, et al: Portrayal of youth suicide in Canadian news. J Can Acad Child Adolesc Psychiatry 23(3):167–173, 2014 25320610

Elnour AA, Harrison J: Lethality of suicide methods. Inj Prev 14(1):39–45, 2008 18245314

Evans E, Hawton K, Rodham K, et al: The prevalence of suicidal phenomena in adolescents: a systematic review of population-based studies. Suicide Life Threat Behav 35(3):239–250, 2005 16156486

Freuchen A, Grøholt B: Characteristics of suicide notes of children and young adolescents: an examination of the notes from suicide victims 15 years and younger. Clin Child Psychol Psychiatry 20(2):194–206, 2015 24096369

Gentile DA, Maier JA, Hasson MR, et al: Parents' evaluation of media ratings a decade after the television ratings were introduced. Pediatrics 128(1):36–44, 2011 21690115

Ghanem M, Gamaluddin H, Mansour M, et al: Role of impulsivity and other personality dimensions in attempted suicide with self-poisoning among children and adolescents. Arch Suicide Res 17(3):262–274, 2013 23889575

Giffords Law Center: Child Access Prevention. San Francisco, CA, Giffords Law Center to Prevent Gun Violence, 2018. Available at https://lawcenter.giffords.org/gun-laws/policy-areas/child-consumer-safety/child-access-prevention. Accessed December 31, 2018.

Goldstein TR, Bridge JA, Brent DA: Sleep disturbance preceding completed suicide in adolescents. J Consult Clin Psychol 76(1):84–91, 2008 18229986

Grinshteyn E, Hemenway D: Violent death rates: the US compared with other high-income OECD countries, 2010. Am J Med 129(3):266–273, 2016 26551975

Grossman DC, Mueller BA, Riedy C, et al: Gun storage practices and risk of youth suicide and unintentional firearm injuries. JAMA 293(6):707–714, 2005 15701912

Haas AP, Eliason M, Mays VM, et al: Suicide and suicide risk in lesbian, gay, bisexual, and transgender populations: review and recommendations. J Homosex 58(1):10–51, 2011 21213174

Lucassen MF, Stasiak K, Samra R, et al: Sexual minority youth and depressive symptoms or depressive disorder: a systematic review and meta-analysis of population-based studies. Aust N Z J Psychiatry 51(8):774–787, 2017 28565925

Mayes SD, Gorman AA, Hillwig-Garcia J, et al: Suicide ideation and attempts in children with autism. Res Autism Spectr Disord 7(1):109–119, 2013

Mayes SD, Baweja R, Calhoun SL, et al: Suicide ideation and attempts and bullying in children and adolescents: psychiatric and general population samples. Crisis 35(5):301–309, 2014a 25115491

Mayes SD, Fernandez-Mendoza J, Baweja R, et al: Correlates of suicide ideation and attempts in children and adolescents with eating disorders. Eat Disord 22(4):352–366, 2014b 24842006

Ougrin D, Tranah T, Stahl D, et al: Therapeutic interventions for suicide attempts and self-harm in adolescents: systematic review and meta-analysis. J Am Acad Child Adolesc Psychiatry 54(2):97–107, 2015 25617250

Owens D, Horrocks J, House A: Fatal and non-fatal repetition of self-harm: systematic review. Br J Psychiatry 181:193–199, 2002 12204922

Patchin JW, Hinduja S: Digital self-harm among adolescents. J Adolesc Health 61(6):761–766, 2017 28935385

Plemmons G, Hall M, Doupnik S, et al: Hospitalization for suicide ideation or attempt: 2008–2015. Pediatrics 141(6):e20172426, 2018 29769243

Rai D, Culpin I, Heuvelman H, et al: Association of autistic traits with depression from childhood to age 18 years. JAMA Psychiatry 75(8):835–843, 2018 29898212

Sampasa-Kanyinga H, Lewis RF: Frequent use of social networking sites is associated with poor psychological functioning among children and adolescents. Cyberpsychol Behav Soc Netw 18(7):380–385, 2015 26167836

Sheftall AH, Asti L, Horowitz LM, et al: Suicide in elementary school-aged children and early adolescents. Pediatrics 138(4):e20160436, 2016 27647716

Soole R, Kõlves K, De Leo D: Suicide in children: a systematic review. Arch Suicide Res 19(3):285–304, 2015 25517290

Stack S: Media coverage as a risk factor in suicide. J Epidemiol Community Health 57(4):238–240, 2003 12646535

Stack S: Suicide in the media: a quantitative review of studies based on non-fictional stories. Suicide Life Threat Behav 35(2):121–133, 2005 15843330

Steck N, Egger M, Schimmelmann BG, et al: Suicide in adolescents: findings from the Swiss National cohort. Eur Child Adolesc Psychiatry 27(1):47–56, 2018 28664290

Taliaferro LA, Muehlenkamp JJ: Nonsuicidal self-injury and suicidality among sexual minority youth: risk factors and protective connectedness factors. Acad Pediatr 17(7):715–722, 2017 28865597

Twenge JM, Joiner TE, Rogers ML, et al: Increases in depressive symptoms, suicide-related outcomes, and suicide rates among U.S. adolescents after 2010 and links to increased new media screen time. Clin Psychol Sci 6(1):3–17, 2018

van Geel M, Vedder P, Tanilon J: Relationship between peer victimization, cyberbullying, and suicide in children and adolescents: a meta-analysis. JAMA Pediatr 168(5):435–442, 2014 24615300

Weaver MD, Barger LK, Malone SK, et al: Dose-dependent associations between sleep duration and unsafe behaviors among US high school students. JAMA Pediatr 172(12):1187–1189, 2018 30285029

Young R, Subramanian R, Miles S, et al: Social representation of cyberbullying and adolescent suicide: a mixed-method analysis of news stories. Health Commun 32(9):1082–1092, 2017 27566406

CHAPTER 19

College and University Students

Peter Ash, M.D.

College is often thought of as a time of new and expanded opportunities for young adult students, a move to independence and growth, so the suicide of a student is often seen as a tragic denial to make use of those opportunities. The suicide of a college student often garners considerable attention: in Vienna in 1910, Sigmund Freud chaired a symposium that led to one of the early efforts to examine suicide among university students (Slimak 1990). Although many of the principles pertinent to suicide risk assessment and treatment of adults and adolescents detailed elsewhere in this volume are relevant to the assessment and treatment of suicidal college students, the implementation of these principles by college mental health systems has some special features. The nature of college students' stressors and living circumstances, students' involvement with university staff and teachers, and the availability of college counseling services lead to approaches to college students that differ somewhat from those used with adults. Key differences are shown in Table 19–1. For simplicity, in this chapter the terms *college, university,* and *school* are used interchangeably.

Epidemiology

A number of highly publicized suicides of college students has led to a concern that there is an epidemic of college suicides. However, this perception is false. National registries of causes of death do not code for being a college student. Although studies vary somewhat, a comprehensive survey of colleges with counseling centers found the rate of death from suicide among college students in 2014 was about 5 per 100,000 (Gallagher 2015), which was less than half the rate for all 18- to 22-year-olds in the United States in the same year (Centers for Disease Control and Prevention 2018). Among college students, suicide is the second leading cause of death, after accidents (Turner et

TABLE 19–1.   **Key differences between suicidal college students and nonstudent young adults in the general population**

Category	Compared to the general population, college students have
Epidemiology	About half the rate of deaths from suicide
Treatment availability	College counseling centers that are readily available for initial assessment and treatment planning
Community factors	College environments that allow for simpler implementation of prevention strategies, more organized observations, and more leverage in ensuring treatment compliance
Stressors	Particular stressors related to leaving home, living independently, and opportunities for increased substance abuse
Protective factors	Less availability of firearms
	More observation by peers and university staff

al. 2013). Accurate statistics about means of suicide in the college population are difficult to obtain, but available data suggest that hanging is the most common means (27% of cases), followed by firearms (24%) (Schwartz 2011). Of particular importance when considering prevention efforts is that less than 15% of students who died from suicide had presented to college counseling services (Gallagher 2015).

Rates of suicidal ideation among college students are high. A 2018 survey of college students found that 10.5% of males and 12% of females had seriously considered suicide in the previous year, and 1.6% of each sex had made a suicide attempt (American College Health Association 2018). These statistics imply that for every death from suicide, more than 300 students have made a suicide attempt, which obviously complicates ascertaining which students are at especially high risk. Rates of ideation and attempt are considerably higher for those presenting to college counseling services: 7.9% had seriously considered suicide in the past month and 10% had made a previous suicide attempt (Center for Collegiate Mental Health 2018).

Case Example

Jennifer, a 19-year-old college freshman, told her roommate that she was upset that her boyfriend broke up with her; she was feeling terribly lonely and thinking about hurting herself, but "she wanted to handle it herself." Her worried roommate arranged with several friends that each would take turns staying with Jennifer day and night to help keep her safe. This arrangement came to light when an upperclassman residential advisor commented on how tired the roommate looked. When Jennifer was then interviewed by a more senior college administrator, Jennifer said that she had had some outpatient treatment for depression in high school but did not find it helpful, and she declined to release her mental health records to school officials. She also said she did not want the college to tell her parents. The college administration is considering suspending her from school.

Role of the College or University

Colleges and universities are communities with many unique aspects. Unlike K–12 schools, their students are almost all legally adults—albeit young adults—generally living away from home for the first time, with the attendant stresses and opportunities that represents.

College Counseling Centers

Most colleges provide counseling centers for students. Organizations of college counseling centers and journals devoted to their work provide considerable data and research on their patients. Much less information is available regarding students who are evaluated and treated in private practices or non-college-related agencies. The level of services offered by college counseling centers varies widely across such dimensions as nature and amount of staffing, wait times, availability of overnight infirmary services (rare), funding mechanisms, and number of free mental health sessions available to students (with the median being one session). In a 2014 survey of college counseling centers, 11% of students had sought counseling services during the year (Gallagher 2015).

College counselors, in large part because they are employees of the university and work in a university facility, may feel that they have conflicting roles in their duty of care to their patients and their duty to the university to run smoothly and avoid embarrassment. This role conflict can be pronounced when working with a suicidal patient, especially when considering whether the therapist should advise the student to withdraw from school. However, the therapist must keep in mind that the duty to care for the patient trumps the interests of the school.

When working with a suicidal patient, a therapist may often wish to involve parents and school administrators in setting up a safety plan. In such situations, the therapist should recognize that such a release of information often requires the consent of the patient. Although they work in a college setting, the confidentiality of mental health records does not allow clinicians to release protected health information to school administrators or parents without the consent of the student-patient (assuming the student is 18 or older), unless allowed by the Health Insurance Portability and Accountability Act (HIPAA) or state law. HIPAA explicitly says that if state law affords more privacy than HIPAA, then the state law supersedes, so clinicians need to be familiar with the laws in their state (Health Insurance Portability and Accountability Act of 1996). Privacy laws that prevent colleges from notifying parents of a student's distress have been the subject of much criticism, and some consideration has been given to having students grant permission in advance or having a friend alert the family (Brody 2018).

Role of Administrators

College staff and administrators may get drawn into managing a suicidal student, as in the case example where the student's suicidal thinking came to the attention of the resident hall advisor. College administrators may be concerned about incurring legal liability for a student's suicide and that a spate of student suicides may bring adverse publicity to the school. There have been instances of universities summarily suspending allegedly suicidal students, a practice that can lead to a worsening of the student's depression because the student then has to deal not only with the difficulties he or she had as a student but also with separation from college friends and a sense of failing at college. In a number of highly publicized cases, discharged students later sued their schools for violations of their civil rights and settled for considerable amounts (see, for example, Department of the Public Advocate, Division of Mental Health Advocacy

[New Jersey] 2009). College administrators are therefore put in the challenging position of needing to balance the rights and needs of the suicidal student, the needs of other students, and the public profile of the college. Administrators may feel frustrated that school mental health services require a release from the student in order to obtain information that the administration may find helpful in determining whether to allow the student to stay in school.

College administrators also have an interest in their students obtaining effective treatment. A suicidal student may affect the lives of other students, as exemplified in the case example, where a group of friends took on the taxing chore of keeping a fellow student safe. Most colleges have developed protocols that lay out the procedures for responding to and assisting a suicidal student. These often involve referral to the college counseling center and specify the criteria to be used for making administrative decisions about a student remaining in school. In those cases in which a student does not release mental health information, the school can typically require a mental health assessment, much as an employer might require a fitness-for-duty evaluation for an employee whose job performance or the safety of others may be adversely affected by psychiatric problems.

Administrators may worry about the liability of colleges to prevent suicide, but legal cases over the past 15 years have done much to clarify this. The general trend is to find that, although they do have a special relationship with their students, universities have only limited liability for preventing suicide. In a recent closely watched case, the Massachusetts Supreme Judicial Court held that the school's duty is limited to those instances in which the university had actual knowledge of a previous suicide attempt or that the student had a stated plan, but that the university had no duty to seek out such information (*Nguyen v. Massachusetts Institute of Technology* 2018). The Court further held that when a university had information about a student's suicidal ideation and behaviors, the duty only required the university to activate its suicidal student protocol or, if it had no protocol, to assist the student in obtaining care.

Although release of mental health records of adult college students is controlled by the student, information obtained by school administrators is generally considered part of the educational record. Therefore, information given to an administrator about a student's potential suicidal thoughts and behaviors provided by other students, teachers, or dormitory advisors is typically considered under the control of the university. Release of educational records is governed in large part by the federal Family Educational Rights and Privacy Act (FERPA; 1974). The general thrust of FERPA is that an adult student who is not dependent on parents controls the release of his or her own educational records, but an explicit exception for a health or safety emergency allows a college to release information to parents and other appropriate parties. Thus, in the case example, although the suicidal student does not want the administration to contact her parents, the administration may do so if they think it important in developing a plan to ensure student safety.

Primary Prevention Efforts

Identifying Students at Risk

Because less than one-sixth of college students who die from suicide seek treatment first (Gallagher 2015), colleges have developed programs that aim to reduce suicidal thoughts and behaviors in the student population and to reduce the stigma and other barriers to obtaining treatment. Students live in a community where they are observed by roommates, other students, residence hall advisors, and teaching staff. Training these persons to identify students at risk and to facilitate obtaining treatment for troubled students has shown some promise. The federal Garrett Lee Smith Memorial Act of 2004 (GLS), passed after the college-aged son of U.S. Senator Gordon Smith died from suicide, funded suicide prevention efforts for young adults and included a section for funding campus suicide prevention efforts other than direct treatment. GLS funding has been distributed to more than 100 colleges for development of prevention programs, many of which involve training gatekeepers, including other students, resident advisors, and college staff, to identify at-risk students. GLS funding leaves program design and outcome measurement to the individual institution, so drawing definitive conclusions across sites is difficult. Nevertheless, outcome studies, which include other community GLS-funded projects, do find that such efforts have reduced both youth suicide attempts (Godoy Garraza et al. 2015) and deaths from suicide (Walrath et al. 2015).

A number of organizations have assisted colleges in developing prevention approaches. The Jed Campus protocol, developed by The Jed Foundation with input from the American Psychological Association, emphasizes that

> First, support for emotional well-being and prevention of suicide and serious substance misuse must be seen as a campus-wide responsibility. No longer can these issues fall solely, or primarily, to the health and counseling centers. While those offices have an important role to play, it is the responsibility of everyone on campus to promote and protect the mental health of the student body.
> Second, these efforts that promote emotional health, suicide prevention and substance abuse prevention must have support from leaders on campus. (The Jed Foundation 2019)

The American Association of Suicidology (2019), in conjunction with The Jed Foundation, provides specialized training on issues of college suicide and issues accreditation for those who die from suicide. Some universities have developed protocols that mandate participation in short-term treatment for those assessed to be at significant risk. These have resulted in a reduction in suicide rates (Berk and Adrian 2018). Some colleges have created peer counseling programs where students may consult with other students either in person or by telephone. The peer counselors receive training in handling crisis calls, and many students will approach a peer before consulting a mental health professional.

Assessment

For a student who presents to a college counselor or other mental health practitioner, the key to effective intervention is a careful assessment of suicidal risk. Asking about suicidal ideation and a history of attempts of self-harm, depressive feelings and symptoms, relationship problems, substance use, and recent stressors should be a routine part of the initial evaluation of any college student. The transition from living in a family to college living, particularly for students early in their college career, can be stressful, because they are adjusting to living more independently, away from their support network, and relating to a new peer group.

College also presents more opportunities to abuse alcohol and drugs. In surveys over the past 8 years, about 40% of college students reported binge drinking in the past 2 weeks and about 27% felt the need to reduce their alcohol or drug use (Center for Collegiate Mental Health 2018). Alcohol use can both aggravate and be a result of depression, and intoxication increases impulsivity. The causal effects of heavy alcohol use on suicidal thoughts and behaviors in college students are complex and not well quantified, but alcohol and drug use should be assessed in any patient who is suicidal.

College students often experience sleep deprivation because of sharing a dormitory room, socializing or studying late, or other lifestyle changes, and they report high levels of inadequate sleep, with more than 90% reporting feeling tired, dragged out, or sleepy at least 1 day each week (American College Health Association 2018). Lack of sleep has been shown to be a risk factor for suicide (McCall and Black 2013) and so should be assessed and treated (see Chapter 13, "Sleep and Suicide").

As with adults, no studies have identified factors to help clinicians accurately determine which students will die from suicide. Research has therefore focused on identifying risk factors. The risk factors for college suicide are not all that different from those for adolescents and young adults that are commonly cited in the literature and discussed in detail elsewhere in this volume (see Chapters 1, "Suicide Risk Assessment," and 18, "Children and Adolescents"). A history of a previous suicide attempt remains the strongest risk factor for suicide death among college students. Therefore, a history of previous suicidal ideation and attempts should always be a component of a student's assessment. Of the emotional factors, depression, hopelessness, and loneliness are key areas for inquiry.

Assessing Intent in a Recent Attempt

As noted, assessing risk in college students is complicated by the fact that death from suicide is rare when compared with clinical presentations of suicidal ideation and suicide attempts. Clinically, suicidal ideation or recent attempt, especially when coupled with a plan involving lethal means, is most often the trigger to a judgment of imminent danger requiring hospitalization. Additionally, suicidal intent needs to be differentiated from nonsuicidal self-harm, such as repetitive cutting.

The lethality of a suicide attempt should be assessed as well as the severity and pervasiveness of suicidal thinking. *Severity* refers to the continuum from passive thoughts of wanting to die, through an active wish to die, to an active wish with a plan involving lethal means. *Pervasiveness* refers to the intensity and frequency of the suicidal thinking.

One protective factor on college campuses that differentiates students from similarly aged nonstudents is that most colleges do not allow students to bring firearms on school property, so the rate of firearm suicide among college students is only about one-third of that for nonstudent young adults (Schwartz 2011). Currently, 16 states have an outright ban on concealed weapons on campus. In 23 states, the decision to allow concealed weapons on campus is left up to the individual college or university. However, with the addition of Arkansas and Georgia in 2017, 10 states now allow concealed firearms on campus (also Colorado, Idaho, Kansas, Mississippi, Oregon, Texas, Utah, and Wisconsin) (National Conference of State Legislatures 2018). Future research on the rate of deaths from suicide at colleges that allow concealed weapons versus colleges that do not may guide future policy decisions about guns on campus.

Questionnaire Assessments

Various questionnaires and scales have been developed for the assessment of suicidal ideation and behaviors in clinical samples or for screening community samples (see Chapter 1). The developed scales suffer either from limited psychometric data or low specificity. Therefore, at the present time such scales may be used either as an adjunctive measure or as a screening instrument but should not replace an interview by a mental health professional.

Treatment

Treatment encompasses four major components: protection of the patient, continuing assessment of risk, ameliorating risk factors, and enhancing protective factors.

Protection of the patient is the first crucial consideration. The decision about whether to hospitalize a patient who recently made a suicide attempt turns on a careful balancing of the risk and protective factors discussed earlier. Although no randomized studies have determined whether hospitalization actually saves lives, attempters who express a persistent wish to die or have a clearly treatable mental illness, such as major depression with psychotic features or rapid mood cycling with impulsive behavior and irritability, should be admitted and continued in inpatient treatment until they are stabilized. Liability concerns, both for the clinician and the university, may create pressure to hospitalize, but the limited data on the effectiveness of hospitalization of college students and the disruptive effects and stigma of removing a student from their regular educational program warrant caution in moving to hospitalization too quickly (Pistorello et al. 2017).

The decision by a treating clinician to involve parents and university staff, such as dormitory advisors, requires the consent of the patient. Colleges and universities have become somewhat less liability conscious, given the legal trends that limit their liability, and are less prone to move quickly to suspend or expel a student for mental health reasons than was previously the case. College administrators are generally more willing to partner with mental health services in devising a living and educational plan that will benefit the student. The clinician should be convinced that the living situation to which the patient is returning will provide adequate support, monitoring, and supervision of the patient. A plan for follow-up treatment should be devised, which may be more complicated in counseling centers that have limits on the number of sessions a student may use. In such systems, practitioners in the community may need to be involved in follow-up treatment.

As with adults, "no-suicide contracts" in which patients promise to tell another adult if they are feeling suicidal have not been shown to be effective and should not be relied on to protect a patient, although discussions about these agreements may be useful in assessing and fostering the therapeutic alliance (Simon 2004). A written safety plan that suicidal students keep readily accessible to assist them when they feel overwhelmed can be useful, as well as cards with telephone numbers for emergency help. Safety plan templates are available online (see, e.g., Stanley and Brown 2012).

Berk and Adrian (2018) recommended having the patient create a "hope box" containing items and mementos that elicit positive feelings, cue use of coping skills, and serve as reminders of reasons to live (see also Chapter 24, "Self-Injurious Behavior").

Approaches to psychotherapy of suicidal college students are numerous, but no large-scale treatment studies have been conducted specifically with college populations. Smaller-scale studies of dialectical behavior therapy and collaborative assessment and management of suicidal thoughts and behaviors have shown promise in college populations (Jobes and Jennings 2011; Pistorello et al. 2012). Psychotherapeutic interventions for suicidal adolescents and adults are discussed more fully in Chapters 3 ("Cognitive and Behavioral Therapy") and 4 ("Psychodynamic Treatment").

The use of selective serotonin reuptake inhibitors (SSRIs), the mainstay pharmacological treatment for depression, has become more problematic since 2004 when the U.S. Food and Drug Administration (FDA) began requiring a black box warning for SSRIs about the increased frequency of suicidal thoughts and behaviors in children and adolescents receiving antidepressants. In 2007, the FDA recommended that the warning be extended to persons up to age 24, which would include most college students. The FDA based its decision on a pooled analysis that found that reports of suicidal thinking increased from 2% for those receiving placebo to 4% for those receiving the active drug, although no deaths from suicide occurred in the sample (Hammad et al. 2006). Despite the FDA recommendation for increased monitoring and observation when initiating or changing the dosage of antidepressant treatment, data indicate that most psychiatrists and pediatricians did not increase their level of monitoring (Morrato et al. 2008).

Finally, it must be emphasized that any treatment modality employed with suicidal youth should include ongoing, repeated, and documented assessments of suicide risk. When a patient improves, it is important to recognize that prior suicidal thoughts and behaviors are risk factors for recurrence, so the clinician should periodically reassess the patient's risk. In case of an adverse outcome, the patient's chart will be carefully scrutinized to see if the risk assessments met the standard of care, so it is very important that the clinician document in detail what assessments were done and the reasoning process used to arrive at the determination of risk.

> The dean of students met with Jennifer, and they agreed that for the next 2 months she would participate in such treatment as was recommended by the student mental health service, who would inform the dean as to whether she was participating as recommended, but that other details of her treatment would remain confidential.
>
> When Jennifer met with the psychiatrist at the student mental health service, she was very concerned that if she talked about her suicidal feelings she would be hospitalized. She was relieved when the psychiatrist was empathetic with her suicidal feelings and interested in working on a safety plan with her that would not involve hospitalization. She said she had no definite plan to kill herself but had been feeling very isolated living away from home and high school friends and then was devastated when rejected by her boyfriend. She and the therapist discussed her surprise when her roommate and other friends were so concerned about her and ready to help, and how she could turn to them when she was feeling lonely. They discussed how Jennifer might talk to her parents about how she was feeling. Together, the therapist and Jennifer completed a written safety plan that identified triggers to thinking about self-harm, coping strategies she could use, and people to whom she could go when such feelings arose. Jennifer liked the idea of making a "hope box" and identified some items she would put in it, including the safety plan, pictures of close friends back home, and the published memoir of a

diplomat that she had found inspiring and that had reinforced her wish to ultimately join the diplomatic service.

The psychiatrist determined that Jennifer's imminent risk for suicide was low and that medication was not indicated at this time but might be useful if her depressed mood persisted, and they scheduled a follow-up appointment in 3 days.

Conclusion

The differences in approaches to the problem of college student suicide are driven in large part by the systems unique to the college community, including counseling centers, administrative oversight and its impact on student life, and the style of living on a college campus. These systems allow for collaborations both in preventing college suicides and in providing assessment and interventions for those at risk. A wide variety of approaches have been used, and outcome studies have provided useful information for improving future interventions.

Key Points

- College students die from suicide at about half the rate of similarly aged youth in the general population.

- Suicidal ideation is quite common in college students (>10% per year), and suicide attempts occur at a rate of about 1.6% per year. However, fewer than 1 in 300 attempts results in death. Assessing the lethality of suicidal intent is complex but is nevertheless a key to planning intervention.

- Less than one-sixth of college students who die from suicide make use of college counseling services.

- College-wide suicide prevention programs have shown promise in reducing college suicide rates.

- Assessment of a college student's suicide risk is similar to the assessment of other late adolescents and early adults.

- The nature of the college community allows for mobilizing social supports that are somewhat different from those available in other living situations.

- As a result of legal developments over the past 15 years, college and university administrators have become more aware of their limited liability for preventing suicide and so are less prone to suspend or expel a student for mental health reasons.

References

American Association of Suicidology: College and University Suicide Prevention Accreditation Program. Washington, DC, American Association of Suicidology, 2019. Available at: http://www.suicidology.org/training-accreditation/college-university-accreditation-program. Accessed January 29, 2019.

American College Health Association: American College Health Association National College Health Assessment II: Spring 2018 Reference Group Executive Summary. Silver Spring, MD, American College Health Association, 2018. Available at: https://www.acha.org/documents/ncha/NCHA-II_Spring_2018_Reference_Group_Executive_Summary.pdf. Accessed January 30, 2019.

Berk MS, Adrian M: The suicidal student, in Student Mental Health: A Guide for Psychiatrists, Psychologists, and Leaders Serving in Higher Education. Edited by Roberts LW. Washington, DC, American Psychiatric Association Publishing, 2018, pp 321–337

Brody JE: Preventing suicide among college students. The New York Times, July 2, 2018. Available at: https://www.nytimes.com/2018/07/02/well/preventing-suicide-among-college-students.html. Accessed January 29, 2019.

Center for Collegiate Mental Health: 2017 Annual Report (Publ No STA 18–166). University Park, PA, Center for Collegiate Mental Health, Penn State University, 2018. Available at: https://ccmh.psu.edu/files/2018/02/2017_CCMH_Report-1r4m88x.pdf. Accessed November 25, 2018.

Centers for Disease Control and Prevention: WISQARS Fatal Injury Reports, National, Regional and State, 1981–2016 (website). Atlanta, GA, Centers for Disease Control and Prevention, 2018. Available at: https://webappa.cdc.gov/sasweb/ncipc/mortrate.html. Accessed November 2, 2018.

Department of the Public Advocate, Division of Mental Health Advocacy (New Jersey): College Students in Crisis: Preventing Campus Suicides and Protecting Civil Rights. Trenton, NJ, Department of the Public Advocate, Division of Mental Health Advocacy, 2009

Family Educational Rights and Privacy Act (FERPA), 20 U.S.C. § 1232g; 34 CFR Part 99 (1974)

Gallagher RP: National Survey of College Counseling Centers 2014 (Monograph Series No 9V). Arlington, VA, International Association of Counseling Services, 2015. Available at: http://d-scholarship.pitt.edu/28178/1/survey_2014.pdf. Accessed January 29, 2019.

Garrett Lee Smith Memorial Act of 2004, 42 U.S.C. 201 et seq. (2004)

Godoy Garraza L, Walrath C, Goldston DB, et al: Effect of the Garrett Lee Smith Memorial Suicide Prevention Program on suicide attempts among youths. JAMA Psychiatry 72(11):1143–1149, 2015 26465226

Hammad TA, Laughren T, Racoosin J: Suicidality in pediatric patients treated with antidepressant drugs. Arch Gen Psychiatry 63(3):332–339, 2006 16520440

Health Insurance Portability and Accountability Act of 1996 (HIPAA), 42 U.S.C. §1320d (1996)

The Jed Foundation: Jed's Comprehensive Approach (website). New York, Jed Campus, 2019. Available at: https://www.jedcampus.org/our-approach. Accessed January 29, 2019.

Jobes DA, Jennings KW: The collaborative assessment and management of suicidality (CAMS) with suicidal college students, in Understanding and Preventing College Student Suicide. Edited by Lamas D, Lester D. Springfield, IL, Charles C Thomas, 2011, pp 236–254

McCall WV, Black CG: The link between suicide and insomnia: theoretical mechanisms. Curr Psychiatry Rep 15(9):389, 2013 23949486

Morrato EH, Libby AM, Orton HD, et al: Frequency of provider contact after FDA advisory on risk of pediatric suicidality with SSRIs. Am J Psychiatry 165(1):42–50, 2008 17986680

National Conference of State Legislatures: Guns on Campus: Overview (website). Washington, DC, National Conference of State Legislatures, 2018. Available at: http://www.ncsl.org/research/education/guns-on-campus-overview.aspx. Accessed January 29, 2019.

Nguyen v Massachusetts Institute of Technology, Sup. Jud. Ct. Mass., (slip opinion SJC-12329) (2018)

Pistorello J, Fruzzetti AE, Maclane C, et al: Dialectical behavior therapy (DBT) applied to college students: a randomized clinical trial. J Consult Clin Psychol 80(6):982–994, 2012 22730955

Pistorello J, Coyle TN, Locey NS, et al: Treating suicidality in college counseling centers: a response to Polychronis. J Coll Stud Psychother 31(1):30–42, 2017 28752155

Schwartz AJ: Rate, relative risk, and method of suicide by students at 4-year colleges and universities in the United States, 2004–2005 through 2008–2009. Suicide Life Threat Behav 41(4):353–371, 2011 21535095

Simon RI: Assessing and Managing Suicide Risk: Guidelines for Clinically Based Risk Management. Washington, DC, American Psychiatric Publishing, 2004

Slimak RE: Suicide and the American college and university: a review of the literature. Journal of College Student Psychotherapy 4(3–4):5–24, 1990

Stanley B, Brown GK: Safety planning intervention: a brief intervention to mitigate suicide risk. Cogn Behav Pract 19(2):256–264, 2012. Template available at: http://www.sprc.org/sites/default/files/resource-program/Brown_StanleySafetyPlanTemplate.pdf. Accessed January 29, 2019.

Turner JC, Leno EV, Keller A: Causes of mortality among American college students: a pilot study. J Coll Stud Psychother 27(1):31–42, 2013 26322333

Walrath C, Garraza LG, Reid H, et al: Impact of the Garrett Lee Smith youth suicide prevention program on suicide mortality. Am J Public Health 105(5):986–993, 2015 25790418

CHAPTER 20

Suicide in the Elderly Population

Marilyn Price, M.D.

Pamela Howard, M.D., M.B.A.

Suicide has ranked as the tenth leading cause of death in the United States for all ages since 2008 (Hedegaard et al. 2018). The risk of suicide in the elderly is substantial; suicide was the sixteenth leading cause of death for persons over the age of 65 (Centers for Disease Control and Prevention 2018). An average of one older adult (>65 years of age) dies from suicide every 1 hour and 4 minutes (Drapeau and McIntosh 2017). Older adults face many challenges that increase suicide risk, including psychiatric disorders, physical ailments, neurocognitive decline, financial stressors, retirement, advancing age associated with diminished functional capacity, death of partner/spouse, and the loss of social networks. Suicide risk assessment (SRA) using evidence-based risk and protective factors can identify older adults at low, moderate, or high risk to allow for timely and effective intervention.

Epidemiology

Suicide rates increased in nearly every state between 1999 and 2016 (Centers for Disease Control and Prevention 2018). The age-adjusted suicide rate increased between 2000 and 2016 from 10.4 to 13.5 deaths per 100,000 of the population (Hedegaard et al. 2018). Females aged 10–74 and males aged 15–74 showed increases in suicide rates (Hedegaard et al. 2018). In 2017, men died from suicide 3.54 times more often than women (American Foundation for Suicide Prevention 2018). White males accounted for 77.97% of deaths from suicide in 2017, with the highest suicide rate in those of middle age. The second-highest suicide rates in 2017 occurred in adults older than 85 years (American Foundation for Suicide Prevention 2018). Older men and women

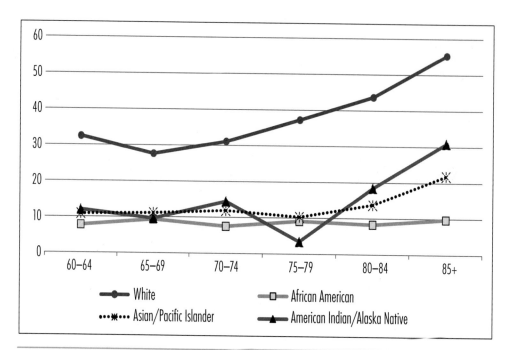

FIGURE 20–1. Male suicide rates by age and race per 100,000 population at risk (2017).

Male suicide rates by age and race from the 2017 WISQARS, in increments of 5 years. These are known suicides, not undetermined-intent deaths. This is the crude rate that calculates adjusting per 100,000 of the population.

Source. Data from Centers for Disease Control and Prevention 2017.

show the highest suicide rate in almost all countries. The suicide rate for white men older than 75 years in the United States was 38.8/100,000 (World Health Organization 2017).

Data from the Centers for Disease Control and Prevention (CDC; 2017) indicated that in 2017, suicide was the fifteenth most common cause of death in males over the age of 65 years. In contrast, suicide was not among the top 20 causes of death for females over the age of 65 in the United States. Firearms were used in 74.3% of deaths from suicide. Suffocation was used in 10% and poisoning in 7.3%.

Figures 20–1 through 20–4 illustrate trends in deaths from suicide among individuals aged 65 and older identified from data derived from the CDC's WISQARS website (Centers for Disease Control and Prevention 2017). This interactive site allows for queries about suicide rates based on variables such as age, sex, and race (Figures 20–1 and 20–2).

Figures 20–3 and 20–4 exhibit the method of suicide by race and sex. The raw number scores are identified and then used for comparison, which enables the visualization of trends. Statistical analysis could not be performed because of the limited number of individuals in some groups. These extrapolations were therefore calculated with the limitations mentioned earlier.

Lifetime suicide attempt prevalence was higher in "young-olds" (aged 65–74 years) compared to "middle-olds" (aged 75–84 years) (Conejero et al. 2018). For males older than 65 years who attempt suicide, 31.6% die from suicide (Bostwick et al. 2016). Explanations for this higher mortality include the frailty of this population, which makes an attempt potentially more lethal, and the use of lethal means (i.e., firearms).

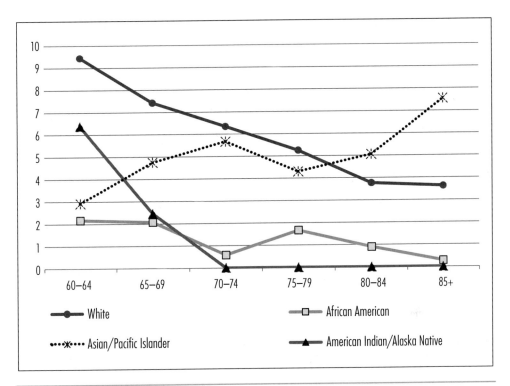

FIGURE 20–2. Female suicide rates by age and race, number of cases per 100,000 (2017).

Source. Data from Centers for Disease Control and Prevention 2017.

Additionally, suicide attempts with more careful planning and less impulsivity are less likely to be discovered.

Malin et al. (2018) summarized the data concerning the rate of deaths from suicide in long-term care facilities. The yearly rate of such deaths in these facilities in the United States varies from 19.7 to 94.9 per 100,000 per year. Nineteen percent of long-term facilities reported at least one episode of suicidal behavior. Residents in long-term care facilities had a 1% prevalence of suicidal ideation, suicide attempts, and deaths from suicide. The common means of suicide for persons in long-term care facilities differs from those of persons living in the community. Suicide by firearm is rare because of the restricted access in long-term care facilities. Instead, more common methods including hanging, jumping from a height, and prescription or over-the-counter drug overdose. Other methods include wrist slashing, asphyxiation, refusal of food or fluids, drowning, and self-poisoning (Malin et al. 2018).

Risk Factors for Suicide in Older Adults

SRA and suicide prevention are dependent on the identification of both evidence-based suicide risk and protective factors (see Chapter 1, "Suicide Risk Assessment"). In addition to considering risk factors, family and care providers must remain alert for warning signs that may signal increased risk of suicidal intent (Conwell and Heisel 2012). When an older person starts giving away possessions or calling to say good-

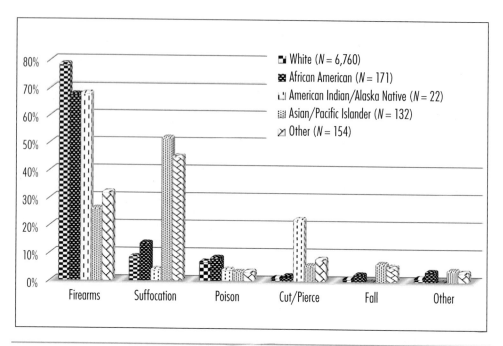

FIGURE 20–3.   Method of suicide by race in males older than 65 years of age, in 2017 (percentiles).

Source.   Data from Centers for Disease Control and Prevention 2017.

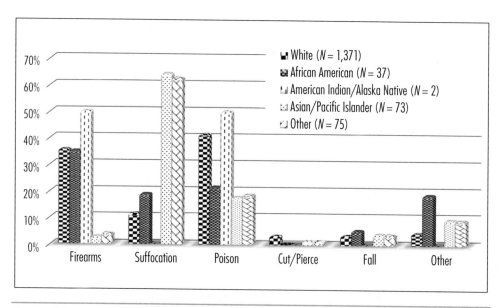

FIGURE 20–4.   Method of suicide by race in females older than 65 years of age, in 2017 (percentiles).

Source.   Data from Centers for Disease Control and Prevention 2017.

bye to friends and family, this should signal an increased risk of death from suicide. When one or more warning signs are present, suicide risk is acutely increased, independent of the presence of long-term or short-term suicide risk factors. Rehearsal behaviors and preparation are also indicative of significant risk (Gold and Joshi 2018).

Elder persons have the same risk and protective factors that apply to all age groups but also have risk factors unique or more frequent in their age group. Commonly identified risk factors include psychiatric illness, declining physical health, social factors, personality factors, and environmental factors. Prior suicide attempts carry the highest risk for future suicide attempts in all populations (Bostwick et al. 2016). Older adults report attempts less often than younger persons, so suicide intent and suicidal behaviors continue to be underrecognized in this population, preventing early intervention. A suicide attempt by an older person may be confused with a medical issue.

Greater than 40% of elder deaths from suicide may be underreported, falling into the category of "silent suicides" (Kiriakidis 2015). Elderly persons may overdose, starve themselves to death, dehydrate themselves intentionally, or have what appears to be an "accident" in attempts to end their lives. A death under these circumstances would not be recognized as a suicide, absent information to suggest suicide intent (Kiriakidis 2015).

Psychiatric Illness

Older individuals who die from suicide have a higher incidence of Axis I diagnoses, including current mood and anxiety disorders (Conwell et al. 2010). Psychiatric illnesses, particularly affective disorder and suicidal ideation, are major risk factors for late-life death from suicide. Late-life depression affects up to 13.3% of the elderly (Van Damme et al. 2018). Psychological autopsy has demonstrated that between 71% and 97% of persons who died from suicide had a mental illness, most commonly depression (Malin et al. 2018).

The presence of a depressive disorder may not be appreciated in older persons because the differential diagnosis includes coexisting medical issues, related psychiatric disorders, adverse pharmacological agents, substance use, infections, or inflammatory diseases. A depressed older person may first present with somatic complaints. Older persons may not feel comfortable discussing emotional issues or may downplay their importance, complicating diagnosis and management of depressive symptoms. Depression and irritability experienced by the elderly may be viewed as just part of natural aging and therefore ignored. Poor quality of life, exacerbation of chronic illnesses, and death from suicide are consequences of untreated late-life depression in the elderly (Van Damme et al. 2018).

Feelings of hopelessness may be prominent with depression. This key psychological variable is a stronger indicator of suicide risk than depression itself. Hopelessness has been identified as a central mediating factor between depression and suicidal behavior and intent in many studies (Abramson et al. 2000). Choi et al. (2016) found hopelessness was significantly associated with suicidal ideation rating in a study of homebound individuals with depression.

Changes in health status, autonomy, and physical and cognitive decline can create the belief that returning to a prior state of functioning is not likely, therefore precipitating feelings of hopelessness. Whereas with a younger patient, a return to prior levels of functioning is possible, for the elderly this may be unrealistic, causing sustained feelings of hopelessness. The caregiver must attempt to find areas for improvement in quality of life for these patients to help abate the feelings of hopelessness. Choi et al. (2016) found that compared to the use of support calls, telehealth problem-solving therapy reduced suicidal ideation in homebound older adults. Older persons who express feelings of hopelessness should be monitored closely.

The presence of anxiety disorders also increases the risk of death from suicide in the elderly. One 15-year study of all deaths from suicide in the United Kingdom found that among older patients (defined as >60 years of age) who had died from suicide, 4.7% had a primary anxiety disorder and 11.9% had a comorbid anxiety disorder. Comparison of younger and older persons who had died from suicide and who also had a history of primary anxiety disorders showed that older persons were more often males and more often lived alone. In addition, older patients were prescribed significantly more psychotropic drugs and received less psychotherapy than younger patients. The researchers concluded that anxiety disorders were present in one of every six patients who died from suicide in the older adult group (Voshaar et al. 2015).

The ratio of deliberate self-harm to death from suicide varies from 200:1 among teenagers to 10:1 in individuals aged 60 and older (Conwell and Thompson 2008). Self-harm behaviors are not as prevalent in the elderly population; however, older people who self-harm have been shown to have an increased suicidal intent (Morgan et al. 2018). A cohort study completed by Morgan et al. (2018) demonstrated that previous mental illness was twice as prevalent in the self-harm cohort and that 20% of the self-harm cohort had previous physical health conditions. Adults with self-harm behaviors, including ingestion of drugs (80.7%) and self-cutting (5.7%), were 20 times more likely to die from unnatural causes in the first year after the self-harm episode. These researchers recommended that clinicians avoid the use of tricyclic antidepressants, which had been prescribed to 11.8% of their self-harm population, due to their higher lethality and increased risk of death from overdose. The use of medications as a means of self-harm brings into question the accuracy of assessing both suicidal behavior and number of deaths from suicide in this population, because a significant number of deaths from suicide in this group are likely categorized as accidental overdose (Morgan et al. 2018).

Drug and alcohol abuse are another risk factor for suicide in the elderly. Alcohol and substance use disorders rank as the second most common psychiatric disorders associated with death from suicide in the elderly. Alcohol use disorders are associated with death from suicide in 35% of elderly men and 18% of women (Malin et al. 2018). Alcohol use disorder, as defined by DSM-5 (American Psychiatric Association 2013) criteria, is highly prevalent in the elderly population according to the results from the National Epidemiological Survey on Alcohol and Related Conditions III (Grant et al. 2015). This survey found that the largest increase in drinking prevalence was among those 65 years of age or older, women, race-ethnic minorities, formerly married persons, and individuals in the lowest education and income categories (Dawson et al. 2015).

Psychological Factors

Maladaptive personality traits can increase the risk of suicidal thoughts and behaviors in the elderly population. Individuals at risk include those who have poor coping mechanisms when faced with life transitions and stressors. Risk factors include being shy or timid, being hostile, having trouble with adjusting to new environments, feeling hopeless, or exhibiting impulsive or aggressive behavior. High neuroticism, obsessional and anxious traits, and rigid coping style also increase risk (Malin et al. 2018). In contrast, protective factors include the presence of good social and coping skills. Persons who show resilience, who can persevere, and who display flexibility are at decreased risk. Protective factors also include having cultural and religious beliefs that oppose death from suicide and being involved in promoting one's health (Malin et al. 2018).

Physical Illness

The presence of physical illness increases the risk of suicidal behavior in the elderly (Oh et al. 2019). The loss or lessening of physical abilities can subsequently lead to a decreased quality of life. An elder person faced with a diagnosis that has a poor prognosis and a progressive course of illness would be at increased risk for developing suicidal thoughts and behaviors while working through the implications and available options. Fässberg et al. (2016) found that suicidal behavior was associated with functional disability as well as with specific medical conditions. These conditions included malignant diseases, neurological disorders, pain, chronic obstructive pulmonary disease, liver disease, male genitourinary disorders, and arthritis. Medical conditions can lessen autonomy and create feelings of frustration and a sense of becoming a burden as disabilities narrow the prospect of independent activities (Fässberg et al. 2016).

Chronic pain can precipitate depressive symptoms in the elderly population. Petrosky et al. (2018) accessed the National Violent Death Reporting System to examine the relationship between death from suicide and chronic pain in 18 states from 2003 to 2014. Of the 123,181 deaths from suicide, 10,789 had evidence of chronic pain. The percentage of those with chronic pain who died from suicide had increased over time from 7.4% in 2003 to 10.2% in 2014. More than half of the individuals with chronic pain who died from suicide used a firearm (53.6%), and 16.2% died from an opioid overdose.

Neurocognitive disorders are prevalent in later life and are associated with neuropsychiatric symptoms such as depression, psychosis, and anxiety. Studies have been mixed on the role of neurocognitive disorder as an independent risk factor for death from suicide (Serafini et al. 2016). Suicide risk in this population has been thought to increase at the time of the diagnosis and during the early stages of these disorders, when patients fear becoming a burden to their families financially and emotionally (Seyfried et al. 2011).

Seyfried et al. (2011) evaluated 294,952 patients in the U.S. Department of Veterans Affairs (VA) health system between fiscal years 2001 and 2005 who were over the age of 60 years and had been diagnosed with dementia using ICD-10 criteria (World Health Organization 1992). The population studied was mostly male. Almost half of those evaluated were white, and the majority were married, limiting the application of the study to other populations. These researchers confirmed that most deaths from suicide occurred in those with a new diagnosis of dementia.

Persons early in the course of their dementia who had accompanying neuropsychiatric symptoms of depression and anxiety in psychiatric treatment were at greatest risk for death from suicide (Morgan et al. 2018). However, death from suicide can also occur many years after the initial diagnosis, with persons with a previous history of attempted suicide at higher risk of dying from suicide (Serafini et al. 2016). The diagnosis of schizophrenia was found to be potentially protective in this population, possibly related to difficulty with executive functioning and planning (Morgan et al. 2018).

Seyfried et al. (2011) also reported that 73% of VA patients with neurocognitive disorder died from suicide using a firearm. The issue of addressing elderly patients' access to firearms is a significant and ongoing challenge in both VA and civilian settings.

Insomnia is a common complaint in older adults associated with increased risk of death from suicide (see Chapter 13, "Sleep and Suicide"). The causes of insomnia can be multifactorial and difficult to manage. Medication management in the elderly could precipitate depression and impair cognition, leading to a further decline in mental functioning, difficulty with mobility, blurred vision, and other side effects. Avoiding the use of sedative and hypnotic medications in this population when at all possible is advisable.

An analysis of medication use patterns in more than 26,000 adults revealed that one-third of U.S. adults may be taking prescription and over-the-counter medications that have the potential to cause depression or increase risk of death from suicide. This is especially concerning for persons who have multiple chronic conditions (Qato et al. 2018). In addition, polypharmacy frequently occurs in older populations, especially those with chronic health conditions. The National Health and Nutrition Examination Survey demonstrated that between 1988 and 2010, the median number of prescription medications used among adults aged 65 and older had doubled from two to four medications. The proportion of older adults taking at least five medications tripled from 12.8% to 39% during this same time period (Charlesworth et al. 2015).

Many medications commonly prescribed in elderly patients, including blood pressure and heart medications, proton pump inhibitors, antacids, hormone replacement medications, and pain medications, can cause depression. Clinicians should be alert to the side effect profile of all medications and check for adverse medication interactions. Providers should coordinate care and medication management, when possible, to cut down on the risk of overmedicating or creating potential adverse drug interactions. The American Geriatrics Society publishes the Beers Criteria, which lists medications that can cause adverse effects in older adults. This can guide clinicians making medication decisions in the elder population (Qato et al. 2018).

Social Factors

Older adult populations often experience both a loss of partnership and autonomy. The loss of a spouse/partner can have a profound impact on quality of life and precipitate depressive symptoms. Social isolation can occur as long-term friends die or move away, resulting in loneliness and poor social integration (Malin et al. 2018).

Placement in an assisted living facility, nursing home, or other residential setting can lead to development or worsening of psychiatric symptoms. Estimates indicate that about 40% of adults aged 65 years and older will need skilled residential nursing care at some point in their lives, significantly altering social status. Assessment is needed to identify those at risk for death from suicide due to this change in living situation, which has likely been precipitated by one or more health-related issues (Malin et al. 2018).

Financial stressors can become overwhelming for elderly adults and can increase the risk of suicidal ideation and behaviors. Home eviction and foreclosure increase risk of death from suicide (Fowler et al. 2015). Cognitive impairment, especially when coupled with social stressors, could impair coping mechanisms. Retirement from work can create a significant social void and social isolation if the person does not find other social activities. Loss of autonomy due to medical conditions could also increase social isolation because prior activities with others may not be possible (Malin et al. 2018).

Environmental Factors

Environmental factors can contribute to or decrease suicide risk. Removal of accessible firearms is a protective measure referred to as *means restriction* (see Chapter 29, "Suicide and Firearms"). Family members may be helpful in securing firearms. Because the ingestion of both prescription and over-the-counter medications is another suicide method used often by older adults, the oversight of medications and assistance with administration of medications in at-risk populations may help decrease the risk of intentional or nonintentional medication misuse.

For persons in long-term care facilities, a move to a new room or introduction of new residents can be stressful. Additionally, some nursing homes have high staff turnovers, and new staff may not recognize or appreciate changes in behavior of elderly residents unknown to them. Residents may not bond with staff, creating further isolation and more opportunities to attempt suicide. The residents are less likely to share that they are depressed or having suicidal ideation with new staff members. Of these factors, the training of staff at facilities to identify risk factors in this population is essential (Malin et al. 2018).

Management of Suicide Risk

The CDC has used a social ecological model to provide a framework encompassing societal, community, relationship, and individual intervention strategies to decrease suicide risk factors (Stone et al. 2017). At the societal level, suicide prevention needs to be discussed as a public health issue, and public service messages can educate the public. Attention to financial supports, access to care, and access to counseling would help decrease the stress experienced by older persons.

At the community level, residential and community settings that serve this population, including religious and civil organizations, could host talks and provide information regarding suicide risk and prevention. This would allow a dialogue with populations at risk for suicidal thoughts and behaviors. Targeting friends, family, caregivers, and others who have relationships with older adults to provide information about suicide in the elderly is critical to promoting awareness of this problem.

At the individual level, the first step in reducing risk is performing an SRA and considering warning signs. The National Guidelines for Seniors' Mental Health for the Assessment of Suicide Risk and Prevention of Suicide, developed by the Canadian Coalition for Seniors' Mental Health, can be helpful in assessing and treating persons at risk of death from suicide. The use of these guidelines can assist in decision making regarding the level of care required, ranging from outpatient management to voluntary or involuntary hospitalization (Malin et al. 2018).

Older persons may downplay significant changes in their lives, requiring that clinicians have a low threshold for further investigation of any significant changes. One validated tool for assessing suicidal ideation in the elderly is the Geriatric Suicide Ideation Scale (Heisel et al. 2016). Heisel and Flett (2006) followed volunteers over a 2-year period and reported strong test reliability and internal consistency.

Evaluating and treating psychiatric diagnoses of mood or psychotic disorders is imperative in managing suicide risk in this population. Elderly patients often do not seek psychiatric care. Nevertheless, some studies have shown that, on average, up to 45% of elderly patients were seen by their primary care provider in the last month before death (Luoma et al. 2002). This makes the primary care specialist an important partner in suicide prevention. However, depression is frequently not identified in the primary care setting.

A collaborative care approach can be effective in older persons. The Improving Mood–Promoting Access to Collaborative Treatment for Late-Life Depression trial for depression in primary care settings found that tailored collaborative care and personalized treatment for older patients significantly reduced both depressive symptoms and suicidal ideation among the intervention group compared to the usual-care group throughout the 24-month follow-up period (Unützer et al. 2002). The Prevention of Suicide in Primary Care Elderly: Collaborative Trial (PROSPECT) assigned participants to either the PROSPECT intervention or usual care. The intervention was the assignment of care managers who were social workers, nurses, and psychologists to help physicians recognize depression, offer algorithm-based interventions, monitor depressive symptoms and side effects, and provide follow-up. Individuals with symptoms of depression in the intervention group had a 2.2 times greater decline in suicidal ideation over a 24-month period compared to those in the usual-care group, although the decline was not statistically significant (Alexopoulos et al. 2009).

Managing suicide risk in elderly individuals involves limiting polypharmacy and medications that could precipitate or worsen psychiatric symptoms. Safe storage of medications reduces the risk of easy access. Substance use disorders must also be identified and managed. The primary care setting is also the likeliest place where these problems would be identified and treatment interventions initiated. Screening should also be completed to rule out neurocognitive disorders and manage cognitive impairment. Elderly patients should be afforded as much autonomy as possible while ensuring they understand the necessity for the planned interventions. This approach will help with compliance. If concerns about suicidal behaviors arise, firearms should be removed and steps should be taken to manage medications and limit other potential methods of self-harm. Inpatient hospitalization, although often a last resort in this population, should be considered when suicide risk is very elevated (see Chapter 17, "Civil Commitment").

Conclusion

Late-middle-aged and older adults are at significant risk of death from suicide. "Baby Boomers" have traditionally higher rates of death from suicide than earlier or subsequent birth cohorts (Conwell et al. 2011), which suggest that as this group ages, deaths from suicide in the elderly population are likely to increase. Older adults are less likely to vocalize symptoms of depression or report suicidal thoughts. Depression can first present with somatic complaints, so diagnosis is often delayed. Clinicians should appreciate the risk factors unique to elderly individuals and repeat SRAs, especially in the event of a recent stressor or life change.

Key Points

- The rates of death from suicide increase with age; white males age 65 and older are demographically at highest risk of death from suicide.

- Risk factors for suicide in the elderly include mental illness, physical illness, family stressors including loss of spouse/partner, environmental and financial stressors, and social factors.

- Many deaths from suicide in elderly persons are misclassified. Deaths from intentional drug ingestion and volitional decrease in nutrition are often listed as death from natural causes.

- Frailty and means of suicide are factors impacting the lethality of suicide in the elderly. Firearms are the number-one means of suicide deaths in this population.

- The presence of firearms in the home significantly increases the likelihood of successful death from suicide.

- Changes in an elderly person's physical, mental, psychological, environmental, or social status should prompt a treatment provider to conduct or update suicide risk assessment.

- Treatment interventions to mitigate risk should be based on a suicide risk assessment that identifies evidence-based risk factors and protective factors.

References

Abramson LY, Alloy LB, Hogan ME, et al: The hopelessness theory of suicidality, in Suicide Science: Expanding the Boundaries. Edited by Joiner TE, Rudd MD. Boston, MA, Kluwer Academic, 2000, pp 17–32

Alexopoulos GS, Reynolds CF 3rd, Bruce ML, et al: Reducing suicidal ideation and depression in older primary care patients: 24-month outcomes of the PROSPECT study. Am J Psychiatry 166(8):882–890, 2009 19528195

American Foundation for Suicide Prevention: Suicide Statistics (website). New York, American Foundation for Suicide Prevention, 2018. Available at: https://afsp.org/about-suicide/suicide-statistics. Accessed September 28, 2018.

American Psychiatric Association: Diagnostic and Statistical Manual of Mental Disorders, 5th Edition. Arlington, VA, American Psychiatric Association, 2013

Bostwick JM, Pabbati C, Geske JR, et al: Suicide attempt as a risk factor for completed suicide: even more lethal than we knew. Am J Psychiatry 173(11):1094–1100, 2016 27523496

Centers for Disease Control and Prevention: Leading causes of death by age group, United States. Web-based Inquiry Statistics Query and Reporting System (WISQARS): Leading Cause of Death Reports 1981–2017. Atlanta, GA, Centers for Disease Control and Prevention, 2017. Available at: https://webappa.cdc.gov/sasweb/ncipc/leadcause.html. Accessed April 7, 2019.

Centers for Disease Control and Prevention: Suicide rising across the U.S. Vital Signs, June 2018. Available at: https://www.cdc.gov/vitalsigns/suicide/modules/June-Vital-Signs-Transcript-6.4.18.pdf. Accessed October 13, 2018.

Charlesworth CJ, Smit E, Lee DS, et al: Polypharmacy among adults aged 65 years and older in the United States: 1988–2010. J Gerontol A Biol Sci Med Sci 70(8):989–995, 2015 25733718

Choi NG, Marti CN, Conwell Y: Effect of problem-solving therapy on depressed low-income homebound older adults' death/suicidal ideation and hopelessness. Suicide Life Threat Behav 46(3):323–336, 2016 26456016

Conejero I, Olié E, Courtet P, et al: Suicide in older adults: current perspectives. Clin Interv Aging 13:691–699, 2018 29719381

Conwell Y, Heisel MJ: The elderly, in Textbook of Suicide Assessment and Management, 2nd Edition. Edited by Hales RE, Simon RI. Washington, DC, American Psychiatric Publishing, 2012, pp 367–387

Conwell Y, Thompson C: Suicidal behavior in elders. Psychiatr Clin North Am 31(2):333–356, 2008 18439452

Conwell Y, Duberstein PR, Hirsch JK, et al: Health status and suicide in the second half of life. Int J Geriatr Psychiatry 25(4):371–379, 2010 19582758

Conwell Y, Van Orden K, Caine ED: Suicide in older adults. Psychiatr Clin North Am 34(2):451–468, ix, 2011 21536168

Dawson DA, Goldstein RB, Saha TD, et al: Changes in alcohol consumption: United States, 2001–2002 to 2012–2013. Drug Alcohol Depend 148:56–61, 2015 25620731

Drapeau CW, McIntosh J: U.S.A. Suicide: 2016 Official Data. Washington, DC, American Association of Suicidology, 2017. Available at: http://www.suicidology.org/Portals/14/docs/Resources/FactSheets/2016/2016datapgsv1b.pdf?ver=2018-01-15-211057-387. Accessed April 9, 2019.

Fässberg MM, Cheung G, Canetto SS, et al: A systematic review of physical illness, functional disability, and suicidal behaviour among older adults. Aging Ment Health 20(2):166–194, 2016 26381843

Fowler KA, Gladden RM, Vagi KJ, et al: Increase in suicides associated with home eviction and foreclosure during the US housing crisis: findings from 16 National Violent Death Reporting System States, 2005–2010. Am J Public Health 105(2):311–316, 2015 25033148

Gold LH, Joshi KG: Suicide risk assessment, in American Psychiatric Association Publishing Textbook of Forensic Psychiatry, 3rd Edition. Edited by Gold LH, Frierson RL. Washington, DC, American Psychiatric Association Publishing, 2018, pp 403–420

Grant BF, Goldstein RB, Saha TD, et al: Epidemiology of DSM-5 alcohol use disorder: results from the National Epidemiologic Survey on Alcohol and Related Conditions III. JAMA Psychiatry 72(8):757–766, 2015 26039070

Hedegaard H, Curtin SC, Warner M: Suicide rates in the United States continue to increase. NCHS Data Brief 309(309):1–8, 2018 30312151

Heisel MJ, Flett GL: The development and initial validation of the geriatric suicide ideation scale. Am J Geriatr Psychiatry 14(9):742–751, 2006 16943171

Heisel MJ, Flett GL, Gordon L, et al: Investigating the psychometric properties of the Geriatric Suicide Ideation Scale (GSIS) among community-residing older adults. Aging Ment Health 20(2):208–221, 2016 26286664

Kiriakidis SP: Elderly suicide: risk factors and preventive strategies. Annals of Gerontology and Geriatric Research 2(2):1028–1033, 2015

Luoma JB, Martin CE, Pearson JL: Contact with mental health and primary care providers before suicide: a review of the evidence. Am J Psychiatry 159(6):909–916, 2002 12042175

Malin MA, Jimenez-Madiedo C, Kohn RL: Suicidal behavior in the elderly and forensic implications, in Geriatric Forensic Psychiatry. Edited by Holzer JC, Kohn R, Ellison JM, et al. New York, Oxford, 2018, pp 283–292

Morgan C, Webb RT, Carr MJ, et al: Self-harm in a primary care cohort of older people: incidence, clinical management, and risk of suicide and other causes of death. Lancet Psychiatry 5(11):905–912, 2018 30337211

Oh KY, Van Dam NT, Doucette JT, et al: Effects of chronic physical disease and systemic inflammation on suicide risk in patients with depression: a hospital-based case-control study. Psychol Med 2019 30606276 Epub ahead of print

Petrosky E, Harpaz R, Fowler KA, et al: Chronic pain among suicide decedents, 2003 to 2014: findings from the National Violent Death Reporting System. Ann Intern Med 169(7):448–455, 2018 30208405

Qato DM, Ozenberger K, Olfson M: Prevalence of prescription medications with depression as a potential adverse effect among adults in the United States. JAMA 319(22):2289–2298, 2018 29896627

Serafini G, Calcagno P, Lester D, et al: Suicide risk in Alzheimer's disease: a systematic review. Curr Alzheimer Res 13(10):1083–1099, 2016 27449996

Seyfried LS, Kales HC, Ignacio RV, et al: Predictors of suicide in patients with dementia. Alzheimers Dement 7(6):567–573, 2011 22055973

Stone D, Holland K, Bartholow B, et al: Preventing Suicide: A Technical Package of Policy, Programs and Practices. Atlanta, GA, National Center for Injury Prevention and Control, Division of Violence, Centers for Disease Control and Prevention, 2017. Available at: https://www.cdc.gov/violenceprevention/pdf/suicideTechnicalPackage.pdf. Accessed April 8, 2019.

Unützer J, Katon W, Callahan CM, et al: Collaborative care management of late-life depression in the primary care setting: a randomized controlled trial. JAMA 288(22):2836–2845, 2002 12472325

Van Damme A, Declercq T, Lemey L, et al: Late-life depression: issues for the general practitioner. Int J Gen Med 11:113–120, 2018 29636629

Voshaar RC, van der Veen DC, Kapur N, et al: Suicide in patients suffering from late-life anxiety disorders; a comparison with younger patients. Int Psychogeriatr 27(7):1197–1205, 2015 25669916

World Health Organization: International Statistical Classification of Diseases and Related Health Problems, 10th Revision. Geneva, Switzerland, World Health Organization, 1992

World Health Organization: Mental Health: Suicide Data (website). Geneva, Switzerland, World Health Organization, 2017. Available at: http://www.who.int/mental_health/prevention/suicide/suicideprevent/en. Accessed April 4, 2019.

CHAPTER 21

Jails and Prisons

Jeffrey L. Metzner, M.D.
Lindsay M. Hayes, M.S.

Local jails, usually administered by city or county officials, are facilities that hold inmates beyond arraignment, generally for 48 hours or more but less than a year. Prisons are state or federally operated correctional facilities in which persons convicted of major crimes or felonies serve sentences that are usually more than 1 year. Six states have combined jail and prisons systems. Despite the clear legal status differences between pretrial detainees in jails and inmates in prisons, the term *inmate* is used throughout this chapter to refer to both.

About 2,246,100 persons were incarcerated in prisons and jails within the United States at year-end 2016. Inmates in state prisons and the federal prison system accounted for almost 70% of the incarcerated population (1,505,400 inmates) housed in about 1,800 different facilities (Stephan 2008). The other 30% (740,700) were held in 2,850 jail jurisdictions (Zeng 2018). Only about 0.07% (<1,000) of the total state prison population was under the age of 18, and 0.5% (3,703) of the total adult jail population was under the age of 18. The total prison population included 111,422 women, which accounted for 7.4% of all prisoners nationwide, as compared with 107,401 women in jail as of December 31, 2016 (14.5% of the total jail population; Carson 2018; Zeng 2018).

At least 15%–30% of prison and jail inmates have psychiatric disorders that result in significant functional disabilities, and another 15%–20% will require some form of psychiatric intervention during their incarceration (Gottfried and Christopher 2017). A very high prevalence rate of substance abuse disorders among prisoners has also been frequently reported (Gunter and Antoniak 2010).

Suicide in Jails and Prisons

From 2000 to 2014, suicide was the leading cause of death in jails, accounting for 25%–35% of all deaths. During the same time, suicide was generally either the fourth or fifth leading cause of death in prisons, following cancer, heart disease, and liver disease.

TABLE 21–1.   Common characteristics of jail suicide victims

More likely to occur within first 24 hours or between 2 and 14 days
Incarceration for violent/personal offense
Close proximity to telephone call, visit, or legal proceeding
Presence of mental illness and prior suicidal behavior

Suicide accounted for 5.9%–7.1% of all prison deaths from 2001 to 2014 (Noonan 2016b). The suicide rate in detention facilities throughout United States has been substantially reduced during the past 28 years, decreasing from 107 county jail suicide deaths per 100,000 inmates in 1986 to 36 suicide deaths per 100,000 inmates in 2006 before rising to 50 per 100,000 inmates in 2014 (Hayes 2012; Noonan 2016a). Suicide rates in State prison dropped from 34 per 100,000 in 1980 to 20 per 100,000 in 2014 (Mumola 2005; Noonan 2016b).

Many deaths from suicide in jails and prisons are preventable. New York experienced a significant drop in the number of jail suicides after the implementation of a statewide comprehensive prevention program (Cox and Lawrence 2010). Researchers reported no deaths from suicide during a 7-year time period in a large county jail in Texas after the development of suicide prevention policies based on the following principles: screening, psychological support, close observation, removal of dangerous items, clear and consistent procedures, and the diagnosis, treatment, and transfer of suicidal inmates to the hospital as necessary (Barker et al. 2014).

Demographics

Research has revealed common characteristics for jail suicide victims based on aggregated jail data. These include average age of 35, white, single, male, violent offenses (particularly sexual assault), substance abuse history, hanging by bedding, and isolated jail housing. Twenty-three percent of deaths from suicide occurred within the first 24 hours, 27% between 2 and 14 days, and 20% between 1 and 4 months (Table 21–1) (Hayes 2012; Mumola 2005). Findings by Daniel and Fleming (2006) and Bonner (2000) relevant to common characteristics of prison suicide victims described in the medical literature are summarized in Table 21–2. However, demographic victim profiles cannot predict suicide risk (Hayes 2012).

Despite these common traits, suicides also occur in jail inmates with a variety of characteristics. For example, jail inmates age 55 or older have the highest rate of death from suicide (58 per 100,000) among adult detainees. Other reported risk factors for suicide include, but are not limited to, first-time nonviolent offenders, the presence of mental illness, substance abuse, past history of suicide attempts, mental health treatment prior to incarceration, receiving "bad news," recent disciplinary action, and manifestation of agitation or anxiety. Studies have found more white inmates, inmates convicted for violent offenses, and inmates with schizophrenia among deaths from suicide and fewer African American inmates (Kovasznay et al. 2004).

An analysis of inmates who died from suicide in the California Department of Corrections and Rehabilitation between 1999 and 2004 (Patterson and Hughes 2008) noted persistent variables, including

TABLE 21–2.   **Common characteristics of prison suicide victims**

Presence of serious mental illness

History of suicide attempts

Older age

Lengthy sentences

Institutional problems involving protective custody and immigration status

Segregated and isolated housing

- Single-cell housing (73%)
- Segregation (46%); within 3 weeks of lockdown (53%)
- Method: hanging (85%)
- Past history of suicidal behavior (62%)
- Preventable or foreseeable, resulting from inadequate assessment (canceled appointments, referrals not completed, past records not reviewed, unsupported diagnosis, inappropriate level of mental health care assignment) (60%)
- Inadequate (or lack of) emergency medical response (27%)
- Mental health history (73%)
- Current mental health caseload (54%)
- Race (African American, 16%; Asian, 3%; Caucasian, 40%; Hispanic, 36%; and other, 5%)
- Gender (male, 94%)

The finding that a disproportionate number of prison suicides occurred in segregation, with most of these deaths occurring within 3 weeks of lockdown, was significant.

Although inmates may become suicidal during certain high-risk periods in a correctional facility, an inmate may become suicidal at any point during his or her incarceration (American Psychiatric Association 2016). Suicide in correctional facilities is also strongly associated with housing assignments. Specifically, an inmate placed in and unable to cope with administrative segregation or other similar specialized housing assignments (especially if single celled) may also be at increased risk of death from suicide as found in the Patterson and Hughes (2008) study.

Case Example 1

John Smith was a 21-year-old male arrested after randomly shooting and seriously injuring five persons in a large shopping mall. While in the county jail, he was initially placed on suicide precautions due to information obtained from the arresting officers that he appeared to be encouraging them to return gunfire in a "suicide by cop" attempt to end his life. During the subsequent 4 months of his incarceration, Mr. Smith was only intermittently compliant with prescribed psychotropic medications for a serious mental disorder associated with auditory hallucinations.

Mr. Smith was later involuntarily hospitalized on the psychiatric unit in the county jail due to increasing depression and suicidal thinking, which he voiced in the context of his almost certain criminal conviction and life sentence. At his hearing, Mr. Smith denied suicidal ideation, and the administrative law judge overturned the petition for involuntary hospitalization.

The mental health staff was therefore required to discharge Mr. Smith from the psychiatric ward immediately. However, mental health staff did not clearly convey to the custody staff their concern regarding Mr. Smith's suicide potential. Mr. Smith was placed in a single cell after custody staff determined that he required segregation for protective custody purposes due to the high-profile nature of his alleged crimes.

A psychiatrist met with Mr. Smith 5 days after his discharge from the mental health unit. Mr. Smith continued to deny suicidal thinking or need for further mental health intervention. The psychiatrist's treatment plan was to follow-up with Mr. Smith at his request on an as-needed basis only. Three weeks later, Mr. Smith was found hanging in his cell. Cardiopulmonary resuscitation (CPR) was unsuccessful.

This case demonstrates the need for effective communication between custody and mental health personnel in the context of suicide prevention efforts. The housing placement for Mr. Smith was not appropriate, nor was the lack of timely and consistent mental health follow-up.

Suicide Prevention Programming

Experience has shown that negative attitudes among correctional staff often impede meaningful suicide prevention efforts. Such attitudes are not simply errors in judgment that contributed to an inmate's death from suicide or a reluctance to thoroughly investigate the death; they reflect a systemic but incorrect belief that inmate deaths from suicide cannot be prevented. Examples of such thinking include the following:

- "If someone really wants to kill themselves, there's generally nothing you can do about it."
- "We didn't consider him suicidal; he was simply being manipulative, and I guess it just went too far."
- "If you tell me you're suicidal, we're going to have to strip you of all your clothes and house you in a bare cell."
- "Suicide prevention is a medical problem…it's a mental health problem…it's not our problem."
- "Statistically speaking, suicide in custody is a rare phenomenon, and rare phenomena are notoriously difficult to predict due to their low base rate."
- "We cannot predict suicide, because social scientists are not fully aware of the causal variables involving suicide."

Comprehensive suicide prevention programming has been advocated nationally by organizations such as the American Correctional Association (2004), American Psychiatric Association (APA; 2016), and National Commission on Correctional Health Care (NCCHC; 2018a, 2018b). These groups have promulgated national correctional standards that are adaptable to individual jail and prison facilities.

The APA and NCCHC standards are the more instructive guidelines and offer recommended elements for a suicide prevention program: identification, training, assessment, monitoring, housing, referral, communication, intervention, notification, reporting, review, and critical incident debriefing (American Psychiatric Association 2016; National Commission on Correctional Health Care 2018a, 2018b). Despite these guidelines, and although most county jail systems experiencing an inmate death from suicide had a written suicide prevention program, according to the most recent national study on jail suicides, the vast majority did not have comprehensive programs that contained most, if not all, of these elements (Hayes 2012). Consistent with these

TABLE 21–3.	Components of a comprehensive suicide prevention policy

Staff training
Intake screening and ongoing assessment
Communication
Housing
Levels of observation and management
Intervention
Reporting
Follow-up/Mortality-morbidity review

national correctional standards, in the following sections we describe eight components of a comprehensive suicide prevention policy as listed in Table 21–3. It is recommended that a suicide prevention committee, consisting of key health care and custody staff, meet on a regular basis to implement and monitor the suicide prevention plan.

Staff Training

An essential component to any suicide prevention program is properly trained correctional officers, who form the backbone of any jail or prison facility. Correctional officers are often the only staff available 24 hours a day and form the primary line of defense in preventing deaths from suicide. All correctional staff members, as well as medical and mental health personnel, should receive between 4 and 8 hours of initial suicide prevention training and 2 hours of annual training. Training should include why correctional environments are conducive to suicidal behavior, staff attitudes about suicide, potential predisposing factors to death from suicide, high-risk suicide periods, warning signs and symptoms, identification of suicide risk despite the denial of suicidal ideation, liability issues, inmate suicide research, recent deaths from suicide or serious suicide attempts within the facility/agency, and details of the facility's/agency's suicide prevention policy (Hayes 2016).

In addition, all staff members who have routine contact with inmates should receive standard first aid and CPR/automated external defibrillator (AED) training. They also should be trained in the location and use of emergency equipment located in each housing unit. In an effort to ensure an efficient emergency response to suicide attempts, mock drills should be incorporated into both initial and refresher training.

Intake Screening and Ongoing Assessment

Screening of inmates when they enter a facility and ongoing assessment are critical to a correctional facility's suicide prevention efforts. Although no single set of risk factors can be used to predict death from suicide, there is little disagreement about the value of screening and assessment in preventing suicide (American Psychiatric Association 2016; Spiers et al. 2006). Screening and assessment are critical because approximately half of all suicide victims communicate their intent some time before death, and any individual with a history of one or more self-harm episodes is at a much greater risk for death from suicide than those without such episodes (Pompili et al. 2016).

Screening for suicide risk may be contained within the medical screening form or as a separate inquiry/form and should include inquiry regarding risk factors as sum-

TABLE 21–4.   **Key points to inquire about in screening for suicide risk**

Past suicidal ideation or suicide attempts

Current ideation

Threat

Plan

Prior mental health treatment and hospitalization

Recent significant loss (e.g., job, relationship, death of family member/close other)

History of suicidal behavior by family member/close other

Lack of forward thinking (expresses hopelessness or helplessness)

Suicide risk during prior confinement

Belief of arresting/transporting officer(s) that inmate is currently at risk

marized in Table 21–4. Staff should ensure that the physical environment provides reasonable privacy to increase the likelihood of an inmate's truthful response. The process should also include procedures for referral to mental health or medical personnel for assessment.

Following the intake process, if staff members hear an inmate verbalize a desire or intent to die from suicide, observe an inmate engaging in self-harm behaviors, or otherwise believe an inmate is at risk for self-harm or death from suicide, referral procedures should be implemented. Such procedures direct staff to take immediate steps to ensure that the inmate is continuously observed until appropriate medical, mental health, and supervisory assistance are obtained. Finally, given the strong association between inmate death from suicide and special-management housing unit placement (e.g., disciplinary or administrative segregation; Kovasznay et al. 2004; Patterson and Hughes 2008), any inmate assigned to such a special housing unit should receive a brief written screening for suicide risk by medical or mental health staff upon admission.

Communication

Certain behavioral signs exhibited by the inmate may be indicative of suicidal behavior. Detection and communication of these signs to appropriate personnel may prevent a death from suicide. The three levels of communication in preventing inmate deaths from suicides are: 1) communication between external entities (e.g., arresting/transporting, family members, court, other inmates) and correctional/health care staff; 2) communication between and among facility staff, including correctional, medical, and mental health staff; and 3) communication between facility staff and the suicidal inmate.

Effective management of suicidal inmates in the facility is based on communication among correctional officers and other professional staff. Communication breakdown between correctional, medical, and mental health personnel is a common factor found in the reviews of many inmate deaths from suicide (Hayes 2007). In both jail and prison systems, communication problems are often caused by lack of respect, personality conflicts, and other boundary issues. Facilities that maintain a strong multidisciplinary approach generally decrease preventable deaths from suicide.

Suicide prevention often begins at the point of arrest. An individual's statements and behavior during arrest, transportation to the jail, and booking are crucial in detecting suicidal behavior. The scene of arrest is often the most volatile and emotional time in the arrest process. Arresting officers should pay close attention to the arrestee during this time; thoughts of suicide or suicidal behavior may be occasioned by the anxiety or hopelessness of the situation, and previous behavior can be confirmed by onlookers such as family and friends. Pertinent information regarding the arrestee's well-being should be obtained by correctional staff from the arresting or transporting officer.

Because inmates can become suicidal at any point during incarceration, including after telephone calls, visits, and legal proceedings (Hayes 2012), correctional officers must maintain awareness, share information, and make appropriate referrals to mental health and medical staff. Facility staff must use various communication skills with the suicidal inmate, including active listening, physically staying with the inmate if they suspect immediate danger, and maintaining contact through conversation, eye contact, and body language. Correctional staff should trust their own judgment and observation and avoid being misled by others (including mental health staff) into ignoring signs of suicidal behavior.

Housing

Housing and other management decisions regarding suicidal inmates are often overly restrictive and not commensurate with the inmate's behavior. When determining the most appropriate housing location for a suicidal inmate, correctional officials (with concurrence from medical or mental health staff) often tend to physically isolate and sometimes restrain the individual. These responses might make management of the inmate more convenient for staff, but they are detrimental to the inmate. This isolation escalates the inmate's sense of alienation and further removes the individual from proper staff supervision. As a result, many otherwise suicidal inmates may be reluctant to share their suicidal ideation for fear of being placed in an environment they perceive as punitive (Hayes 2013).

Housing a suicidal inmate in a general population unit raises a difficult issue when the inmate's security level prohibits such assignment. The solution to this problem generally results in the assignment of suicidal inmates to a housing unit commensurate with their security level. Within a correctional system, this assignment might be a "special housing" unit (e.g., restrictive housing, disciplinary confinement, administrative segregation).

However, to the extent possible, suicidal inmates should be housed in the general population, mental health unit, or medical infirmary, located close to staff. Housing assignments should not be based on decisions that heighten depersonalizing aspects of incarceration; they should be based on the ability to maximize staff interaction with inmates. Furthermore, cancellation of routine privileges (e.g., showers, visits, telephone calls, out-of-cell exercise), removal of clothing (excluding belts and shoelaces), as well as the use of physical restraints (e.g., restraint chairs/boards, leather straps) should be avoided whenever possible. These interventions should be used only as a last resort for periods in which the inmate is physically engaging in self-destructive behavior. Finally, unless exigent circumstances exist, legal proceedings should not be postponed for inmates on suicide precautions.

Suicidal inmates should be housed in suicide-resistant, protrusion-free cells that provide full visibility (Hayes 2006). Each cell door should contain a gauge sheet grade polycarbonate (e.g., Lexan) glass panel large enough to allow staff a full and unobstructed view of the cell interior. Suicide-resistant cells should contain tamper-proof light fixtures and wall/ceiling air vents that are protrusion free. Cells housing suicidal inmates should not contain electrical switches or outlets, bunk holes or gaps between the bunk and wall, towel racks on desks and sinks, radiator vents, or other objects that provide an easy anchoring device for hanging. Finally, each housing unit in the facility should contain emergency equipment, including a first aid kit, Ambu-bag, and rescue tool (to quickly cut through fibrous material). Correctional staff should ensure that such equipment is in working order on a daily basis.

Levels of Supervision

Standard correctional practice requires that "special-management inmates," including those housed in administrative segregation, disciplinary detention, and protective custody, be observed at intervals not exceeding 30 minutes, with inmates with mental illness observed more frequently (American Correctional Association 2003, 2004). Inmates held in clinically ordered "restraints and seclusion" should be observed constantly, with documentation at intervals of not more than 15 minutes (American Psychiatric Association 2016; National Commission on Correctional Health Care 2018a, 2018b).

Consistent with national correctional standards and practices, two levels of supervision are generally recommended for suicidal inmates: close observation and constant observation. *Close observation* is reserved for the inmate who is not actively suicidal but expresses suicidal ideation (e.g., expressing a wish to die, without a plan) or has a recent prior history of self-destructive behavior. An inmate who denies suicidal ideation or does not threaten suicide but demonstrates other concerning behavior (through actions, current circumstances, or recent history) indicating the potential for self-injury should also be placed under close observation. This inmate should be observed by staff at staggered intervals not to exceed every 10–15 minutes. This level of observation is only feasible if the cell is suicide resistant.

Constant observation is reserved for the inmate who is actively suicidal, either by threatening (with a plan) or engaging in self-injury. This inmate should be observed by a staff member on a continuous, uninterrupted basis. Other supervision aids (e.g., closed-circuit television, inmate companions/watchers) can be used as a supplement to, but never as a substitute for, these observation levels. Mental health staff should assess and interact with (i.e., not just observe) suicidal inmates on a daily basis. Reasonable efforts should be made, particularly when considering the discharge of an inmate from suicide precautions, to avoid a cell-side encounter; rather, such assessment should be made in a private and confidential setting.

The daily assessment should focus on current behavior as well as changes in thoughts and behavior during the past 24 hours. For example, if suicidal ideation is denied, then evaluators should ask, "How have your feelings and thoughts changed over the past 24 hours?" and "What are some of the things you have done or can do to change these thoughts and feelings?" Table 21–5 provides a summary of the essential components of these assessments.

An individualized treatment plan (to include follow-up services) should be developed for each inmate who is on suicide precautions longer than 24 hours. The plan should be developed by qualified mental health staff, in conjunction with the inmate and with medical and correctional personnel. The treatment plan should describe signs, symptoms, and the circumstances under which the risk for suicide is likely to

TABLE 21–5.	Essential components of a clinical risk assessment for suicide

History of suicidal intent or suicide attempts

  Is there a history of admitted suicidal intent or suicide attempt?

  Severity of ideation or attempt?

  Recent?

Degree of current suicidal ideation

  Has the person thought about how he or she might end his or her life?

  Did or does the person have a plan?

  Does the person have the means to carry out the plan?

  Was or is the plan reasonable?

  Does the person express feelings of peace/resolution?

  Is the person attending to personal effects?

  Did the person write goodbye letters?

Systematic inquiry into

  Current mood

  Known risk factors—individual and group

  Known protective factors

  Stated intentions about suicide

What has changed since attempt/last assessment?

  Evidence or absence of futuristic thinking

  Evidence of connectedness

  Effect of suicide precautions on denial of suicidal ideation

Is the person's current denial of suicidal ideation being influenced by the restrictive nature of suicide precautions (e.g., restrictive clothing, shower, food, possessions, out-of-cell time)?

If person is removed from suicide precautions, what is the treatment plan?

recur, how recurrence of suicidal thoughts can be avoided, and actions the inmate and staff will take if suicidal ideation reoccurs.

Finally, follow-up care is required to safeguard the continuity of care for suicidal inmates. All inmates discharged from suicide precautions should receive regularly scheduled follow-up assessments by mental health personnel until their release from custody because of the strong correlation between suicide attempts and prior suicidal behavior. Although a nationally accepted schedule for follow-up does not exist, a suggested assessment schedule following discharge from suicide precautions might be 24 hours, 72 hours, 1 week, and for some inmates, periodically until release from custody.

Intervention

The degree and promptness of staff intervention often determines whether the victim will survive a suicide attempt. The planning and preparation for suicide can take several minutes; brain damage from strangulation caused by a suicide attempt can occur within 4 minutes and death often within 5–6 minutes (Gunnell et al. 2005). The quicker the response to a suicide attempt, the likelier that an inmate will survive and without suffering permanent harm.

Facility policy regarding intervention should contain three primary components (National Commission on Correctional Health Care 2018a, 2018b). First, all staff who come into contact with inmates should be trained in standard first aid procedures and CPR/AED. Second, a staff member who discovers an inmate engaging in self-harm should immediately survey the scene to assess the severity of the emergency, alert other staff to call for medical personnel if necessary, and begin standard first aid or CPR as necessary. Third, staff should never presume that the inmate is dead but rather initiate and continue appropriate lifesaving measures until relieved by arriving medical personnel. Finally, in an effort to ensure an efficient emergency response to suicide attempts, medical personnel should ensure that emergency response equipment is in working order on a regular basis, and "mock drills" should be incorporated into both initial and refresher training for all staff.

Reporting

In the event of a suicide attempt or death from suicide, all appropriate correctional officials should be notified through the chain of command. Following the incident, the victim's family should be immediately notified as well as appropriate outside authorities. All staff members who came into contact with the victim prior to the incident should be required to submit a statement including their full knowledge of the inmate and incident.

Follow-Up/Mortality-Morbidity Review

When suicide or suicidal crises occur, staff affected by such a traumatic event should receive appropriate assistance. An inmate death from suicide is extremely stressful for staff who may feel angry, guilty, and even ostracized by fellow personnel and administration officials. After a death from suicide, reasonable guilt is sometimes displayed by the officer, who wonders: "What if I had made my cell check earlier?"

Every death from suicide, as well as each suicide attempt of high lethality (e.g., requiring hospitalization), should be examined through a mortality-morbidity review process. A clinical review through a psychological autopsy is also recommended (Aufderheide 2000; National Commission on Correctional Health Care 2018a, 2018b). The psychological autopsy should not be performed by a clinician involved in the inmate's treatment prior to the suicide.

Ideally, the mortality review should be coordinated by an outside agency to ensure impartiality. The review, separate and apart from other formal investigations that may be required to determine the cause of death, should include information as summarized in Table 21–6. When recommendations are accepted for implementation, a corrective action plan should be created that identifies each recommendation, followed by identified stakeholder(s), status, and deadline for implementation. Finally, the success of a suicide prevention program is not simply measured by the lack of deaths from suicide but rather by sound practices that mirror policies sustained by a fully transparent continuous quality improvement process.

Case Example 2

George Baxter, age 18, enters the reception center at the state department of corrections to serve a 4-year sentence for aggravated robbery. He has a history of mental illness and is taking medication for depression. This is his first prison experience. During the intake screening process at the reception center, Mr. Baxter's behavior and responses to questions from

TABLE 21–6.	Mortality-morbidity review

Critically review the circumstances surrounding the incident.

Critically review procedures relevant to the incident.

Make a synopsis of all relevant training received by involved staff.

Review pertinent medical and mental health services/reports involving the victim.

Consider possible precipitating factors leading to the suicide.

Make recommendations, if any, for changes in policy, training, physical plant, medical or mental health services, and operational procedures.

the nurse are cause for concern. Mr. Baxter appears anxious, expresses helplessness, and is crying during the interview. He has heard stories of violence and intimidation in the state prison system while awaiting transfer from the county jail. Mr. Baxter has made at least three serious prior suicide attempts, and the transporting officer informs the intake nurse that Mr. Baxter was on suicide precautions at the county jail following a hanging attempt a few days earlier. He also has a family history of suicide; his brother died from suicide 6 years earlier, and his mother is currently being treated for depression after a recent drug overdose. After the initial screening process, Mr. Baxter is placed on constant observation in the mental health unit and referred to mental health staff for further assessment.

Mr. Baxter is seen by the reception center psychiatrist the following morning. He denies suicidal ideation and states, "I'm not suicidal. This is all a big mistake." The psychiatrist determines that the constant observation status is "inappropriate," and Mr. Baxter is released from suicide precautions and rehoused with the general population without a cellmate. He is seen by a nurse later that afternoon and appears tearful and scared. He denies any suicidal ideation and requests a cellmate. The nurse tells Mr. Baxter that she will forward his request to the shift supervisor. A few hours later, and approximately 10 hours after his release from suicide precautions, Mr. Baxter is found hanging in his prison cell. Staff were unable to resuscitate him.

A mortality review was subsequently conducted on George Baxter's suicide. The review found that it was uncertain whether the psychiatrist had reviewed Mr. Baxter's medical file, which contained the intake medical screening form. Similarly, it was also unclear whether the transporting officer's observation and the county jail records regarding Mr. Baxter's suicidal behavior were effectively communicated to reception center intake staff. Recommendations offered during the mortality review included the stipulation that inmates placed on constant observation remain on that status as clinically indicated and then be stepped down to close observation for at least another day. Inmates assigned to the mental health unit should not be discharged until their case is reviewed during the weekly treatment team meeting. In addition, a sending agency discharge summary form should be created and completed by the sending agency (e.g., county jail) or transporting personnel prior to the inmate's arrival at the reception center that documents any immediate concerns about the inmate.

Conclusion

Long-term data have indicated falling rates of deaths from suicide in correctional facilities throughout the United States since the 1980s. The growth in the field of correctional mental health services has raised awareness concerning the problem of inmate suicide, which has resulted in the development of effective suicide prevention programs becoming standard operation within this area of practice (Daniel and Fleming 2006; National Commission on Correctional Health Care 2018a, 2018b).

Although lacking the ability to accurately predict if and when an inmate will die from suicide, facility officials and their correctional, medical, and mental health personnel can identify, assess, and successfully manage potentially suicidal behavior. Because inmates can be at risk at any point during confinement, the greatest challenge for those who work in the correctional arena is to view the issue as one that requires a continuum of comprehensive suicide prevention services aimed at the collaborative identification, continued assessment, and safe management of inmates at risk for self-harm.

Key Points

- Inmate death from suicide is a serious public health problem throughout the country.

- Although deaths from suicide in jails share some similarities with those in prisons, they also have distinct differences.

- Negative attitudes impede meaningful suicide prevention efforts.

- Communication breakdown between correctional, medical, and mental health personnel is a common factor found in the reviews of many preventable inmate deaths from suicide.

- Long-term data indicate reduced suicide rates in jails and prisons, and correctional systems that implement and maintain comprehensive suicide prevention programs have effectively reduced the incidence of inmate deaths from suicide.

References

American Correctional Association: Standards for Adult Correctional Institutions Facilities, 4th Edition, Lanham, MD, American Correctional Association, 2003

American Correctional Association: Performance-Based Standards for Adult Local Detention Facilities, 4th Edition. Lanham, MD, American Correctional Association, 2004

American Psychiatric Association: Psychiatric Services in Correctional Facilities, 3rd Edition. Arlington, VA, American Psychiatric Association, 2016

Aufderheide D: Conducting the psychological autopsy in correctional settings. J Correct Health Care 7(1):5–36, 2000

Barker E, Kõlves K, De Leo D: Management of suicidal and self-harming behaviors in prisons: systematic literature review of evidence-based activities. Arch Suicide Res 18(3):227–240, 2014 24611725

Bonner RL: Correctional suicide prevention in the year 2000 and beyond. Suicide Life Threat Behav 30(4):370–376, 2000 11210062

Carson AE: Prisoners in 2016 (NCJ 251149). Washington, DC, Bureau of Justice Statistics, U.S. Department of Justice, 2018

Cox J, Lawrence J: Suicide prevention in correctional settings, in Manual of Forms and Guidelines for Correctional Mental Health. Edited by Ruiz A, Dvoskin J, Scott C, et al. Washington, DC, American Psychiatric Publishing, 2010, pp 121–154

Daniel AE, Fleming J: Suicides in a state correctional system, 1992–2002: a review. J Correct Health Care 12(1):1–12, 2006

Gottfried ED, Christopher SC: Mental disorders among criminal offenders: a review of the literature. J Correct Health Care 23(3):336–346, 2017 28715985

Gunnell D, Bennewith O, Hawton K, et al: The epidemiology and prevention of suicide by hanging: a systematic review. Int J Epidemiol 34(2):433–442, 2005 15659471

Gunter TD, Antoniak SK: Evaluating and treating substance use disorders, in Handbook of Correctional Mental Health, 2nd Edition. Edited by Scott CL. Washington, DC, American Psychiatric Publishing, 2010, pp 167–196

Hayes LM: Suicide prevention and designing safer prison cells, in Preventing Suicide and Other Self-Harm in Prison. Edited by Dear G. New York, Palgrave Macmillan, 2006, pp 167–174

Hayes LM: Reducing inmate suicides through the mortality review process, in Public Health Behind Bars: From Prisons to Communities. Edited by Greifinger R. New York, Springer Science and Business Media, 2007, pp 280–291

Hayes LM: National study of jail suicide: 20 years later. J Correct Health Care 18(3):233–245, 2012 22569904

Hayes LM: Suicide prevention in correctional facilities: reflections and next steps. Int J Law Psychiatry 36(3-4):188–194, 2013 23664363

Hayes LM: Training Curriculum and Program Guide on Suicide Detection and Prevention in Jail and Prison Facilities. Mansfield, MA, National Center on Institutions and Alternatives, 2016

Kovasznay B, Miraglia R, Beer R, et al: Reducing suicides in New York State correctional facilities. Psychiatr Q 75(1):61–70, 2004 14992303

Mumola CJ: Suicide and Homicide in State Prisons and Local Jails (NCJ 210036). Washington, DC, Bureau of Justice Statistics, U.S. Department of Justice, 2005, pp 1–12

National Commission on Correctional Health Care: Standards for Health Services in Jails. Chicago, IL, National Commission on Correctional Health Care, 2018a

National Commission on Correctional Health Care: Standards for Health Services in Prisons. Chicago, IL, National Commission on Correctional Health Care, 2018b

Noonan ME: Mortality in Local Jails, 2000–2014: Statistical Tables (NCJ 250169). Washington, DC, Bureau of Justice Statistics, U.S. Department of Justice, 2016a, pp 1–29

Noonan ME: Mortality in State Prisons, 2001–2014: Statistical Tables (NCJ 250150). Washington, DC, Bureau of Justice Statistics, U.S. Department of Justice, 2016b, pp 1–22

Patterson RF, Hughes K: Review of completed suicides in the California Department of Corrections and Rehabilitation, 1999 to 2004. Psychiatr Serv 59(6):676–682, 2008 18511589

Pompili M, Belvederi Murri M, Patti S, et al: The communication of suicidal intentions: a meta-analysis. Psychol Med 46(11):2239–2253, 2016 27239944

Spiers EM, Pitt SE, Dvoskin JA: Psychiatric intake screening, in Clinical Practice in Correctional Medicine. Edited by Puisis M. Philadelphia, PA, Mosby Elsevier, 2006, pp 285–291

Stephan JJ: Census of State and Federal Correctional Facilities, 2005 (NCJ 222182). Washington, DC, Bureau of Justice Statistics, U.S. Department of Justice, 2008, pp 1–28

Zeng Z: Jail Inmates in 2016 (NCJ 251210). Washington, DC, Bureau of Justice Statistics, U.S. Department of Justice, 2018, pp 1–13

CHAPTER 22

Military Personnel and Veterans

Kaustubh G. Joshi, M.D.

Brian W. Writer, D.O.

Elspeth Cameron Ritchie, M.D., M.P.H.

Suicide is a current health crisis that disproportionately affects U.S. military personnel and veterans. This chapter is intended to serve as a resource to help providers who work with these populations and to complement other chapters in this book that discuss suicide risk assessment, prevention, and treatment. Discussions regarding suicide rates among military personnel are limited to active-duty service members (ADSMs); however, most of the clinical information also applies to guardsmen and reservists, who play an important role our country's defense.

Suicide Rates Among Military Personnel

Suicide rates among ADSMs steadily rose beginning in 2005, several years after Operation Enduring Freedom (OEF, 2001–2014) and Operation Iraqi Freedom (OIF, 2003–2011) began. Suicide was the third leading manner of death, after accidents and illness, among ADSMs from 1998 to 2003, when deaths due to war surpassed the number of deaths due to illness and suicide (Corr 2014). Suicide remained the third leading manner of death until 2011, when the drawdown of forces in Afghanistan began (Corr 2014). Declining war-related deaths led to suicide becoming the second leading manner of death—after accidents—among ADSMs (Corr 2014).

In an attempt to standardize suicide surveillance across all four services, the U.S. Department of Defense (DoD) launched the DoD Suicide Event Report (DoDSER) system in 2008 (Corr 2014). This annual report presents information collected by the services on suicide attempts and deaths (via a secure web-based application), provides official

TABLE 22–1.   Unadjusted suicide mortality rates for active-duty service members (ADSMs) combined across all services[1]

Calendar year (CY)	ADSMs, all services
CY 2011[2]	18.7
CY 2012[2]	22.7
CY 2013[2]	18.7
CY 2014[3]	20.4
CY 2015[3]	20.2
CY 2016[3]	21.1

Note.   [1]Per 100,000 service members.

Source.   [2]Smolenski et al. 2014; [3]Pruitt et al. 2018.

suicide rates, describes risk and contextual factors associated with suicide-related behavior, and details specific characteristics of the suicide-related events to provide comprehensive information about the service members involved (Pruitt et al. 2018).

The most recent DoDSER annual report (calendar year [CY] 2016) revealed that the unadjusted suicide mortality rate for ADSMs combined across all four services remained essentially unchanged since CY 2011 (Pruitt et al. 2018; see Table 22–1 for rates from CY 2011 to 2016). The CY 2016 U.S. general population age-adjusted suicide mortality rate, ages 15–59, was 16.87 per 100,000 (Centers for Disease Control and Prevention 2018). After accounting for the differences in the age and sex distributions between the U.S. general and military populations, the CY 2016 adjusted suicide mortality rate for ADSMs combined across all four services was 17.0 per 100,000 (Pruitt et al. 2018). The adjusted suicide mortality rate for ADSMs was only slightly higher than the U.S. general-population suicide mortality rate.

The Army, Marine Corps, and Navy unadjusted suicide mortality rates were basically unchanged since CY 2011, whereas the Air Force unadjusted suicide mortality rate increased incrementally (Pruitt et al. 2018; see Table 22–2 for service-specific rates from CY 2011 to 2016). The Army has had the highest suicide rate among the four services since CY 2011 (Pruitt et al. 2018).

Prior to the start of OEF, suicide rates among ADSMs were historically lower compared with those in the general population, especially when adjusted for the fact that the military is predominantly young and male (and thus at demographically higher risk for death from suicide) (Bates et al. 2012). General population rates have included unemployed individuals, homeless individuals, and individuals with chronic mental illnesses (Reger et al. 2018). The lower suicide rates among ADSMs were attributed to higher rates of employment (by definition, 100%), better access to health care, the military's "built-in" social support, and the exclusion from initial enlistment/commissioning or the medical discharge of individuals with significant mental illness (Bates et al. 2012). For many years, these differences were cited to explain why suicide rates among ADSMs were lower than rates in the general population; possible explanations for this change include higher rates of mental illness (e.g., posttraumatic stress disorder [PTSD]) and substance use, difficulty readjusting to civilian life, and familiarity with firearms (Reger et al. 2018).

TABLE 22–2. Unadjusted suicide mortality rates for active component of each service[1]

Calendar year (CY)	Air Force	Army	Marine Corps	Navy
CY 2011[2]	12.9	24.8	15.4	15.9
CY 2012[2]	15.0	29.6	24.3	17.8
CY 2013[2]	14.4	23.0	23.1	13.4
CY 2014[3]	19.1	24.6	17.9	16.6
CY 2015[3]	20.5	24.4	21.2	13.1
CY 2016[3]	19.4	26.7	20.1	15.3

Note. [1]Per 100,000 service members.

Source. [2]Smolenski et al. 2014; [3]Pruitt et al. 2018.

Risk Factors Among Military Personnel

Despite the research challenges associated with studying risk factors in this population (e.g., low base rate), identifying risk factors that are either unique to or particularly prevalent among military personnel is an important step in reducing the recent rise in military deaths from suicide (Bates et al. 2012). Those who die from suicide appear to be driven by a combination of factors rather a single factor (Bates et al. 2012).

Certain risk factors have been known for decades, such as a history of suicidal behaviors and a family history of mental illness and suicidal behaviors. The demographic composition of the U.S. military (disproportionately young, male, and white) in itself increases suicide risk in military personnel (Nock et al. 2013). The most common demographic profile for CY 2016 was a non-Hispanic white male, age 20–24 years, rank/grade of E-1 through E-4 (i.e., junior enlisted ranks), and high school educated; this represented almost 19% of all suicide cases (Pruitt et al. 2018).

Although ADSMs are unlikely to have severe and persistent mental illness due to being screened out prior to enlistment or commissioning or being medically discharged during service, they can have or develop mood disorders, anxiety disorders, PTSD, and substance use disorders. For example, 44% of those ADSMs who died from suicide had met the criteria for at least one current or past psychiatric diagnosis (Pruitt et al. 2018). The most frequent diagnoses included mood disorders (22%), substance use disorders (21%), adjustment disorders (21%), and anxiety disorders (19%) (Pruitt et al. 2018). Approximately 30% used alcohol or drugs (including illicit, prescription, and over-the-counter substances) during the suicidal event (Pruitt et al. 2018). Approximately 84% had not been prescribed psychotropic medications within 3 months of their suicide (Pruitt et al. 2018). PTSD, especially combat-related PTSD, is both independently and indirectly associated with suicidal behavior through PTSD-related comorbidities such as depression and substance use disorders (Bates et al. 2012). Furthermore, having a mental disorder alone is not sufficient to explain suicidal behavior because the majority of people with mental disorders never engage in suicidal behavior. Thus, consideration of additional factors that may contribute to death from suicide is important (Nock et al. 2013).

Physical injury (e.g., amputation) and pain are common factors among those who die from suicide and may contribute to suicide risk (Bates et al. 2012). Traumatic brain injury (TBI), regardless of the cause, carries an increased risk of various persistent medical and mental health sequelae. TBIs, including those of mild severity, can both independently and indirectly increase the risk of suicidal behavior (Madsen et al. 2018). Firearms were the most common means of suicide death. The majority (95%) of firearms used were personal possessions, and 59% of those who died from suicide had firearms present in the immediate environment (Pruitt et al. 2018; see Chapter 29, "Suicide and Firearms").

Suicide among military personnel is also associated with psychosocial stressors (Nock et al. 2013). About 40% of individuals who died from suicide had experienced a failed or failing intimate relationship within 3 months of suicide (Pruitt et al. 2018). However, the military is composed largely of young adults who frequently transition between intimate relationships; whether failed relationships truly represent a risk factor or are a general characteristic of this demographic group is unclear (Reger et al. 2018). Within 3 months of death from suicide, approximately 25% had experienced legal or administrative stressors (e.g., citation for driving under the influence, administrative separation, under investigation) and 17% had experienced workplace problems (Pruitt et al. 2018). Most individuals (81%–85%) had not been victims or perpetrators of abuse, assault, or harassment within 12 months of their death from suicide (Pruitt et al. 2018).

Surprisingly, although suicide rates have risen among ADSMs since OEF/OIF, deployment to a war zone itself has not been shown to be associated with deaths from suicide (Reger et al. 2015). One possible explanation behind this finding could be that those who are physically and psychologically healthy are more likely to be deployed multiple times, whereas those who have physical or mental issues are more likely to be medically discharged and thus not deployed to combat zones again.

However, separation from the military has been associated with increased suicide risk regardless of whether service members have deployed (Reger et al. 2015). Suicide rates were elevated for service members who separated with fewer than 4 years of military service or who did not separate with an honorable discharge (Reger et al. 2015). This could be due to a loss of social support when leaving the military or a loss of one's military identity. Transition periods (e.g., going from basic training to less structured advanced individual training, becoming older, or retiring from military service) as well as recently experiencing a life event that results in feelings of humiliation can also increase suicide risk.

Department of Defense Prevention and Management of Suicidal Behaviors

The DoD's prevention and management approaches are mostly similar to those found in the civilian sector; however, military-specific practices and considerations with which providers should familiarize themselves are also available to this population, such as reporting requirements, confidentiality limitations, and command-directed mental health evaluations (CDMHEs). Providers working with military personnel have a responsibility to treat the individual service member *and* to report fitness for duty issues that interfere with military readiness (e.g., deployment, ability to possess a weapon) to that service member's command chain (Bates et al. 2012).

Barriers to service members' engagement in mental health care have included leadership's attitudes and perceptions toward those who seek mental health care and the possibility of negative career repercussions for service members who access care (Tanielian et al. 2016). The federal government has been actively attempting to reduce the stigma associated with mental health treatment. Encouraging service members to voluntarily present for treatment can be effective in reducing and preventing deaths from suicide. Just as in the civilian community, psychotropic medication and therapy (e.g., individual, group) are also the mainstays of treatment.

Service members desire privacy and confidentiality. Although the Health Insurance Portability and Accountability Act of 1996 (HIPAA) applies to the DoD, confidentiality is not absolute in the military. An armed forces exception to confidentiality allows for disclosure to appropriate military command authorities without the service member's consent to ensure the military mission's proper execution. Under this exception, only the disclosure of "minimum necessary" information is allowed (U.S. Department of Defense 2003). This restriction allows a provider to exercise professional judgment in evaluating what information to release.

In addition to this restriction, DoD Instruction (DoDI) 6490.08 places additional limits on disclosure to command authorities by requiring providers to follow a "presumption not to notify a service member's commander" when that service member seeks mental health treatment or substance use treatment unless an exception that requires notification overrides that presumption, such as harm to self, harm to others, harm to mission, or needing inpatient care (U.S. Department of Defense 2011). If disclosure is required, the provider must adhere to the "minimum necessary" requirement. These regulations and instructions provide a balance between confidentiality and required disclosure.

The service member's command chain can be an effective resource in reducing mental health stigma by advocating treatment. Benefits of command chain involvement include providing practical social support, providing important collateral information about the service member's past and current functioning, and temporarily restricting duties while the service member is undergoing treatment (Bates et al. 2012). In the event that the commander determines the need for a mental health evaluation, and the service member either is reluctant to be evaluated or believes the referral to be in response to a complaint against a command, the DoD has established a formal process for the compulsory evaluation of the suspected behavioral health issues (Bates et al. 2012). This formal process is called a *command-directed mental health evaluation*, which is governed by DoDI 6490.04 (U.S. Department of Defense 2013).

CDMHEs are unique in that they have no civilian equivalent (Joshi 2018). They are permissible because commanders need to ensure service members do not have a mental illness that would preclude them from fulfilling their duty requirements (e.g., carrying a weapon, obtaining security clearance). The commander's ability to request these evaluations is not unconditional. Service members are afforded due-process protections because of the potential adverse impact on their military career. For example, in nonemergency situations, the commander must consult with a mental health provider to ensure that the reason for requesting a CDMHE is appropriate and not punitive. If the service member participates in the evaluation, the provider will provide results and recommendations to the commander and the service member in accordance with local mental health clinic policy (Joshi 2018). If the service member declines to participate, the provider notifies the commander; the commander then consults with legal staff to determine future course of action (Joshi 2018). Commanding officers can also implement emergency CDMHEs, in which the service member is brought immediately for an evaluation in the event of concern for imminent harm to self or others.

Similar to the civilian sector, inpatient treatment can be another intervention to lower suicide risk. Should a service member require but refuse such inpatient treatment, involuntary psychiatric hospitalization to a military treatment facility (MTF) can be pursued under DoDI 6490.04 (U.S. Department of Defense 2013). In areas where an MTF is not available, applicable civil commitment laws of the state where the service member is located will govern involuntary psychiatric hospitalization to a community facility. Under no circumstances can a commander order a service member into inpatient or outpatient mental health treatment (Joshi 2018).

Suicide Rates Among Veterans

In an attempt to combat the increasing veteran suicide rate, the U.S. Department of Veterans Affairs (VA; 2018c) initiated an effort in 2016 to conduct the largest, most comprehensive analysis of veteran deaths from suicide. That work, building upon previous VA suicide data reports and Veterans Health Administration (VHA) analyses, provided the first systematic assessment of differences in the rates of death from suicide between veterans who use and do not use VHA services; calculated suicide rates among populations with established and emerging risk factors for death from suicide; and compared veterans with other Americans through 2014 (U.S. Department of Veterans Affairs 2018c).

An expansion of the definition of "veteran," continued analyses of growing databases, and an enhanced sharing of data have contributed to more detailed examinations of veteran subpopulations. To this end, the VA recently released an updated comprehensive report on suicide mortality between 2005 and 2015 (U.S. Department of Veterans Affairs 2018c). This report only focused on 2005–2015 due to data limitations; in addition, data are reported only through 2015 because the source data have a multiyear lag (U.S. Department of Veterans Affairs 2018c).

This updated report included information for suicide deaths among all known veterans of military service (i.e., all veterans who had previously served in the military as opposed to prior reports that only included veterans eligible for full VA care). Findings include 1) direct comparisons of veterans' suicide rates with those of analogous nonveteran populations, 2) calculations of suicide rates among high-risk groups (e.g., veterans diagnosed with mental health and opioid use disorders), and 3) comparisons of veterans with and without recent receipt of VHA services (U.S. Department of Veterans Affairs 2018c). The report's increased scope allowed investigators to discern among groups to a degree not previously possible, such as those who were not eligible for VHA care, those who were eligible for and used VHA care, and those who were eligible for but did not use VHA care (U.S. Department of Veterans Affairs 2018c).

TABLE 22–3.   **Relevant demographic risk factors for veteran suicide**

Younger age (18–34 years)

Older age (>55 years)

Males of any age

White (84% of suicides)

Having served in the Army (40% of suicides)

Source.   U.S. Department of Veterans Affairs 2018c.

This report revealed, among other information, that there are approximately 20 million veterans in the United States, of which about 10% are women, and approximately 45% of veterans are enrolled in VHA services. After adjusting for age, suicide rates increased for veteran and nonveteran populations from 2005 to 2015. In 2015, veterans constituted approximately 8% of the U.S. adult population and accounted for a little more than 14% of all deaths from suicide among U.S. adults. The age-adjusted suicide rate for all veterans was approximately 34 per 100,000 person-years, while the nonveteran rate was approximately 16 per 100,000 person-years (U.S. Department of Veterans Affairs 2018c).

Recent users of VHA services had higher rates of death from suicide as compared to nonveterans, overall veterans, and non-VHA consumers. This result may reflect the relative health burden of each group. Although overall veteran suicide rates have increased from 2005 to 2015 and the absolute rate of death from suicide is higher for recent VHA consumers, the suicide rate of veterans who did not receive care in the VHA rose more rapidly compared with veterans who have used VHA services (U.S. Department of Veterans Affairs 2018c).

Risk Factors Among Veterans

Veteran suicide is associated with the complex interaction of independent yet interrelated risk factors. Independent risk factors (e.g., demographic profile, mental health status, contextual events) increase veteran suicide risk; some of these same factors are also associated with or may mediate other concurrent or emergent risk factors. Continued work with the VA's comprehensive database to identify risk factors and delineate their intricate relationships can assist providers and policymakers in mitigating individual crises and improving population-scale suicide prevention efforts.

Relevant demographic risk factors can be found in Table 22–3. The previously mentioned VA report also revealed that although older veterans represent a larger percentage of deaths from suicide (58%), younger veterans have a higher suicide rate (39 per 100,000). Apparent background contributors to these demographic risks include that the total veteran population comprises more males (approximately 90% or 18 million); more persons of white ethnicity (77%); more Army veterans; and more older veterans. In addition, males are more likely to use firearms to die from suicide. Notably however, in those female veterans who use VHA services, firearm suicide has nearly doubled since 2005 from 23% to 40% (U.S. Department of Veterans Affairs 2018c).

The presence of a psychiatric disorder, such as a mood or substance use disorder, and chronic illness–related pain have been consistently shown to increase suicide risk among both the general population and veterans (Bates et al. 2012). Among veteran VHA users, the prevalence of mental health or substance use diagnoses has increased since 2005 from 33% to 41% (U.S. Department of Veterans Affairs 2018c). The veteran suicide rate of those with a diagnosed mental illness in treatment (61.9 per 100,000) has more than doubled compared with that of veterans without diagnosed or treated mental illness (25.6 per 100,000); the highest rates (120 per 100,000) are found among veterans with bipolar disorders or opioid use disorders (U.S. Department of Veterans Affairs 2018c).

Just as in active military personnel, PTSD (especially combat-related PTSD) is both independently and indirectly associated with suicidal behavior among veterans (Bates et al. 2012). Victims of military sexual trauma are also at increased risk of developing PTSD and other mental health conditions (e.g., substance use disorders) and hence suicidal behavior; the prevalence of PTSD in sexual trauma victims can approach 50% (American Psychiatric Association 2013).

Similar to military personnel, TBI in veterans, regardless of the cause and degree of severity, can both independently and indirectly increase the risk of suicidal behavior (Madsen et al. 2018). Past psychiatric hospitalizations, use of psychotropic medications, and past suicide attempts can increase veteran suicide risk (McCarthy et al. 2015). To assist with identification and management of these interrelated risk amplifiers, the VA has mandated use of standardized suicide risk assessments in outpatient primary care, mental health, and pain clinics.

Relevant contextual suicide risk factors are also significant. These include unstable housing, unstable employment, legal problems, and immediate access to firearms (U.S. Department of Veterans Affairs 2018c). Of these, immediate access to firearms is the most frequently discussed societal concern. The presence of firearms in the home is an independent risk factor for suicide in the general population regardless of sex or age (Bates et al. 2012). Veterans are more likely to possess and use a firearm for suicide compared with the general population (Bates et al. 2012). One theory for this disparity is the relative firearm training that veterans receive while on active duty, especially those deployed to combat zones. In 2015, approximately 67% of veterans who died from suicide used firearms (U.S. Department of Veterans Affairs 2018c). Unstable employment has been directly and indirectly associated with an all-cause increased suicide risk involving interrelated factors such as a negative self-image, mental illness, substance misuse, inability to secure or loss of preexisting housing, and associated obstacles engaging available resources (Bates et al. 2012).

Homelessness is associated with increased rates of all-cause mortality and death from suicide; the suicide rate in homeless veterans is 81 per 100,000 as compared with the domiciled veteran rate of 35.8 (McCarthy et al. 2015). Suicidal behavior sharply accelerates in the 8 weeks prior to onset of homelessness and then decelerates over the next 8 weeks (U.S. Department of Veterans Affairs 2018a).

Nonengagement with available VHA resources is another contextual risk amplifier. Of the 20 million veterans, only about 6 million are VHA consumers; the rate of increase in suicidal behavior has risen most sharply among nonconsumers (U.S. Department of Veterans Affairs 2018c). This finding has prompted the creation of predictive modeling tools and programs to identify and capture veteran nonconsumers into the VA system where individualized interventions are available.

Department of Veterans Affairs Prevention and Management of Suicidal Behaviors

Veteran suicide prevention and management is not composed of a single approach. Although progress toward identifying risk of potential future suicide has been made, the conclusive time frame remains elusive. The VA encourages veterans to use its services and strives to create coordinated support and communication networks across communities in an effort to prevent suicide by mitigating risk factors while enhancing protective factors. Prevention efforts involve a concerted rallying of comprehensive resources to assist veterans before they reach a crisis point.

To this end, the U.S. Department of Veterans Affairs (2018b) has developed the National Strategy for Preventing Veteran Suicide, which aligns with the U.S. Surgeon General's 2012 National Strategy for Suicide Prevention. This strategy attempts to provide a framework for identifying and triaging priorities, organizing efforts, and focusing on veteran suicide prevention via a public health approach. Not all veterans have the same risk for death from suicide; thus, the VA has relied on a prevention framework developed by the National Academy of Medicine that uses a combination of three prevention strategies (universal, selective, and indicated) matched to a veteran's or group of veterans' level of risk (U.S. Department of Veterans Affairs 2018b).

Universal prevention strategies are designed to target all veterans. These strategies include public awareness and education about suicide prevention resources for veterans, promoting responsible coverage of deaths from suicide by the media, and creating barriers or limiting hot spots for suicide, such as bridges and train tracks (U.S. Department of Veterans Affairs 2018b). Promoting and participating in suicide prevention educational efforts throughout the year, including higher visibility outreach during Suicide Prevention Month, is a key universal strategy.

Another particularly important universal strategy is ensuring mass awareness of the Veterans Crisis Line (VCL), which was launched in 2007. Over the years, the VCL developed online and text message capabilities and added call centers (U.S. Department of Veterans Affairs 2018b). VCL is also an important component of selective and indicated strategies, which are discussed later.

Social media campaigns (e.g., #BeThere) and free online suicide prevention trainings (e.g., the VA's Operation S.A.V.E.) have become vital instruments in promoting awareness of veteran deaths from suicide. These programs emphasize the importance of a caring presence, expression of nonjudgmental interest, and responsiveness of supports to those in crisis. Advocating for the VA health care system may lessen the stigma associated with mental health treatment, potentially increasing the use of mental health services. Fostering and sustaining collaboration with the DoD, community health care systems, and non–health care resources (e.g., veteran service organizations) can increase stakeholder understanding of and hence collaborative efficacy of resources.

Selective prevention strategies are designed to reach veteran subgroups that may be at increased suicide risk (U.S. Department of Veterans Affairs 2018b). Selective strategies include outreach targeted to veterans with substance use problems or to female veterans. Another example of a selective strategy is an executive order signed in early 2018 mandating that all new veterans receive mental health care for at least 1 year, thereby enhancing access to care for those transitioning from active duty to the civilian sector (which, as previously mentioned, is a period of increased risk for death from suicide) (U.S. Department of Veterans Affairs 2018b).

Gatekeeper training for intermediaries who may be able to identify high-risk veterans is another selective strategy. Examples of intermediaries include Housing and Urban Development (HUD)-VA Supportive Housing (VASH) personnel who provide veterans with housing assistance; Veterans Justice Outreach personnel who work with veterans entangled in the legal system; and providers in primary care clinics, emergency departments, and specialty clinics (e.g., pain clinic) where veterans with certain suicide risk factors are more likely to be encountered. Education involves periodic suicide-specific training, including identifying risk using screening tools and then making appropriate interventions. Focus on large-scale provider educational efforts to collaboratively develop suicide safety planning has also increased. This intervention has been shown to reduce suicidal behaviors (Stanley et al. 2018).

In an attempt to standardize suicide risk assessments, the VA has adopted a staged process to inform level of risk and areas of needed intervention. A sensitive primary screen (e.g., Patient Health Questionnaire–9), if positive, triggers a secondary screen with increased specificity (e.g., Columbia-Suicide Severity Rating Scale); a positive secondary screen then triggers the VA's new Comprehensive Suicide Risk Assessment (U.S. Department of Veterans Affairs 2018b). Another relatively recent selective strategy includes the Recovery Engagement and Coordination for Health–Veterans Enhanced Treatment (REACH-VET) program, which uses predictive analytics to identify and capture veterans at increased future suicide risk into care. Other selective strategies include firearm locks to reduce immediate access; naloxone rescue kits for veterans receiving opioid pain regimens; and buprenorphine training opportunities to increase numbers of certified prescribers to help respond to the opioid crisis.

Indicated prevention strategies are designed to target individual veterans identified as being high risk for suicidal behaviors, especially those who have made a recent suicide attempt (U.S. Department of Veterans Affairs 2018b). Examples of an indicated strategy are connecting a veteran who expressed suicidal thinking to the VCL or facilitating expedited access to care where additional selective and indicated strategies can be employed.

Most veterans are appropriate for ambulatory-level interventions without direct, ongoing psychiatrist involvement. However, depending on their suicide risk, veterans may need referral to the mental health clinic for additional, specialized treatment. Another indicated strategy is conducting an individualized suicide risk assessment to identify modifiable and nonmodifiable risk factors as well as protective factors. This can inform management planning, including the appropriate level of care (which at times may be court mandated).

Among veterans with suicidal ideation discharged from emergency departments, suicide safety planning with telephone follow-up was shown to reduce suicidal behavior over the proceeding 6 months (Stanley et al. 2018). Indicated strategies for modifiable risk factors include but are not limited to treating mental illness and substance use disorders, addressing active chronic pain for those treated with opioids, and using resources to target unstable housing and lack of health care access.

Another indicated strategy within the VHA system is flagging a patient's electronic medical record for risk of death from suicide. This intervention prompts closer or more frequent follow-up, suggests provision of smaller supplies of medication, and generally increases the awareness of risk by other providers involved in the veteran's care. Indicated strategies become more important in veterans with additional nonmodifiable risk factors (e.g., history of suicidal behavior) or with concurrent lack of protective factors.

Veterans Affairs/Department of Defense Clinical Practice Guidelines and Resources for Providers

Since the 1990s, the VA and DoD, in collaboration with other professional organizations, have been developing clinical practice guidelines for the management of various health conditions in an attempt to improve care by reducing the variation in practice and systematizing "best practices" (available at www.healthquality.va.gov). For mental health services, clinical practice guidelines are available for major depressive disorder, PTSD and acute stress reaction, substance use disorders, and the assessment and management of patients at risk for death from suicide.

The suicide risk assessment and management guideline recommends a framework for the structured assessment of individuals suspected to be at risk for death from suicide and the immediate and long-term management and treatment that should follow once risk has been determined. The guideline does not address risk in children, universal screening for suicidal ideation, or population-level health interventions to reduce the risk of suicide (U.S. Department of Veterans Affairs and U.S. Department of Defense 2013). As with other guidelines, it does not represent the standard of care, is intended for use only as a tool to assist providers, and should not be used to replace clinical judgment.

A vast array of resources is available to help providers who are working with military personnel and veterans. A list of service-specific, DoD, and VA resources is provided in Table 22–4. This list is not exhaustive, and providers are encouraged to contact local DoD or VA facilities to request appropriate additional resources. The appearance of these resources and hyperlinks does not constitute endorsement by these authors. Program names and web addresses change frequently; we encourage readers to search the internet to verify the resource name or hyperlink.

Conclusion

Suicide among military personnel and veterans is a public health crisis. Escalating suicide rates in these populations have garnered increased media attention and public scrutiny, resulting in more research funding to understand the factors that contribute to suicide and provide resources to prevent and manage deaths from suicide. The DoD and VA have taken steps to increase their respective populations' engagement in mental health treatment and to target suicide prevention and management.

TABLE 22–4.   **Service-specific Department of Defense and Department of Veterans Affairs (VA) suicide prevention resources (in alphabetical order)**

Air Force Suicide Prevention Program	www.airforcemedicine.af.mil/SuicidePrevention
	http://static.e-publishing.af.mil/production/1/ afmc/publication/afi90–505_afmcsup/afi90–505_afmcsup.pdf
Army Suicide Prevention Program	www.armyg1.army.mil/hr/suicide
	www.army.mil/e2/downloads/rv7/r2/policydocs/ r600_63.pdf
Center for Deployment Psychology	https://deploymentpsych.org/
Defense Suicide Prevention Office	www.dspo.mil
Marine Corps Suicide Prevention Program	www.usmc-mccs.org/services/support/suicide-prevention
	www.marines.mil/Portals/59/Publications/ MCO%201720.2.pdf
Military Health System Suicide Prevention Resources (Defense Health Agency)	www.health.mil/Military-Health-Topics/ Conditions-and-Treatments/Mental-Health/ Suicide-Prevention/Resources
Military OneSource	www.militaryonesource.mil
National Suicide Prevention Lifeline	https://suicidepreventionlifeline.org/
Navy Suicide Prevention Program	www.public.navy.mil/bupers-npc/support/ 21st_Century_Sailor/suicide_prevention/Pages/ default.aspx
	www.public.navy.mil/surfor/Documents/ 1720_4A.pdf
TRICARE	https://tricare.mil
VA Safety Plan Treatment Manual and Pocket Card	www.mentalhealth.va.gov/docs/ va_safety_planning_manual.pdf
	www.mentalhealth.va.gov/docs/ vasafetyplancolor.pdf
VA Suicide Risk Assessment Guide Reference Manual and Pocket Card	www.mentalhealth.va.gov/docs/ suicide_risk_assessment_reference_guide.pdf
	www.mentalhealth.va.gov/docs/ va029assessmentguide.pdf
VA Traumatic Brain Injury and Suicide: Information and Resources for Clinicians	www.mirecc.va.gov/visn19/docs/ manual_suicide_prevention_strategies_in_TBI.pdf
Veterans Crisis Chat	www.veteranscrisisline.net/get-help/chat
Veterans Crisis Line	www.mentalhealth.va.gov/suicide_prevention
	www.veteranscrisisline.net/about/what-is-vcl

Key Points

- Suicide rates among military personnel and veterans have been increasing.

- Death from suicide in military personnel and veterans is usually due to complex interactions between modifiable and nonmodifiable risk factors.

- Comprehensive and collaborative treatment planning should include addressing safety, addressing underlying mental illness and substance use, leveraging community resources, and addressing access to lethal means.

- Prevention strategies in veteran populations include universal strategies, selective strategies for high-risk populations, and indicated strategies for specific persons known to be at increased suicide risk.

- A broad range of Department of Defense, Department of Veterans Affairs, and other resources are available to help with suicide prevention and management in military personnel and veterans.

References

American Psychiatric Association: Diagnostic and Statistical Manual of Mental Disorders, 5th Edition. Arlington, VA, American Psychiatric Association, 2013

Bates MJ, Bradley JC, Bahraini N, et al: Clinical management of suicide risk with military and veteran personnel, in American Psychiatric Publishing Textbook of Suicide Assessment and Management, 2nd Edition. Edited by Simon RI, Hales RE. Washington, DC, American Psychiatric Publishing, 2012, pp 405–451

Centers for Disease Control and Prevention: Web-based Injury Statistics Query and Reporting System (WISQARS): Fatal Injury Data Tool Visualization (website). Atlanta, GA, Centers for Disease Control and Prevention, 2018. Available at: https://wisqars-viz.cdc.gov. Accessed August 19, 2018.

Corr WP 3rd: Suicides and suicide attempts among active component members of the U.S. Armed Forces, 2010–2012; methods of self-harm vary by major geographic region of assignment. MSMR 21(10):2–5, 2014 25357138

Health Insurance Portability and Accountability Act of 1996 (HIPAA), Publ.L. No 104–191, 110 Stat. 1938 (1996)

Joshi KG: Military forensic psychiatry, in American Psychiatric Association Publishing Textbook of Forensic Psychiatry, 3rd Edition. Edited by Gold LH, Frierson RL. Washington, DC, American Psychiatric Association Publishing, 2018, pp 463–473

Madsen T, Erlangsen A, Orlovska S, et al: Association between traumatic brain injury and risk of suicide. JAMA 320(6):580–588, 2018 30120477

McCarthy JF, Bossarte RM, Katz IR, et al: Predictive modeling and concentration of the risk of suicide: implications for preventive interventions in the US Department of Veterans Affairs. Am J Public Health 105(9):1935–1942, 2015 26066914

Nock MK, Deming CA, Fullerton CS, et al: Suicide among soldiers: a review of psychosocial risk and protective factors. Psychiatry 76(2):97–125, 2013 23631542

Pruitt LD, Smolenski DJ, Bush NE, et al: Department of Defense Suicide Event Report: Calendar Year 2016 Annual Report (Publ No 0-A2345E0). Washington, DC, U.S. Department of Defense, 2018. Available at: http://www.dspo.mil/Prevention/Data-Surveillance/DoDSER-Annual-Reports. Accessed November 27, 2018.

Reger MA, Smolenski DJ, Skopp NA, et al: Risk of suicide among US military service members following Operation Enduring Freedom or Operation Iraqi Freedom deployment and separation from the US military. JAMA Psychiatry 72(6):561–569, 2015 25830941

Reger MA, Pruitt LD, Smolenski DJ: Lessons from the latest US military suicide surveillance data. J Clin Psychiatry 79(1), 2018 29505185

Smolenski DJ, Reger MA, Bush NE, et al: Department of Defense Suicide Event Report: Calendar Year 2013 Annual Report (Publ No 0-D493E45). Washington, DC, U.S. Department of Defense, 2014. Available at http://www.dspo.mil/Prevention/Data-Surveillance/DoDSER-Annual-Reports. Accessed November 27, 2018.

Stanley B, Brown GK, Brenner LA, et al: Comparison of the safety planning intervention with follow-up vs usual care of suicidal patients treated in the emergency department. JAMA Psychiatry 75(9):894–900, 2018 29998307

Tanielian T, Woldetsadik MA, Jaycox LH, et al: Barriers to engaging service members in mental health care within the U.S. military health system. Psychiatr Serv 67(7):718–727, 2016 26975521

U.S. Department of Defense: Regulation 6025.18-R: DoD Health Information Privacy Regulation. Washington, DC, U.S. Department of Defense, 2003

U.S. Department of Defense: Instruction 6490.08: Command Notification Requirements to Dispel Stigma in Providing Mental Health Care to Service Members. Washington, DC, U.S. Department of Defense, 2011

U.S. Department of Defense: Instruction 6490.04: Mental Health Evaluations of Members of the Military Services. Washington, DC, U.S. Department of Defense, 2013

U.S. Department of Veterans Affairs: Homeless Evidence and Research Synthesis (HERS) Roundtable Proceedings: Suicide and Homeless Veterans. Washington, DC, Veterans Health Administration, U.S. Department of Veterans Affairs, 2018a

U.S. Department of Veterans Affairs: National Strategy for Preventing Veteran Suicide 2018–2028. Washington, DC, Office of Mental Health and Suicide Prevention, 2018b

U.S. Department of Veterans Affairs: VA National Suicide Data Report 2005–2015. Washington, DC, Office of Mental Health and Suicide Prevention, 2018c

U.S. Department of Veterans Affairs, U.S. Department of Defense: VA/DoD Clinical Practice Guideline for Assessment and Management of Patients at Risk for Suicide. Washington, DC, U.S. Department of Veterans Affairs and U.S. Department of Defense, 2013

CHAPTER 23

Suicide and Gender

Navneet Sidhu, M.D.

Susan Hatters Friedman, M.D.

Gender plays an important role in suicide risk assessments, and rates of death from suicide vary widely across countries. In the Americas, males die from suicide 3.6 times more frequently than females and similarly in Europe the ratio is 4:1. In all countries except China (Värnik 2012), rates of death from suicide are higher for males than females. Male gender, especially with increasing age, is recognized to confer higher risk. However, with increasing rates of death from suicide among females in recent years (Hedegaard et al. 2018), understanding the identifiable risk factors in preventing female suicide is increasingly important. An improved cultural understanding of gender diversity has highlighted high rates of death from suicide amongst transgender and gender nonconforming individuals.

The Gender Paradox of Suicide

Mental health professionals are familiar with the gender paradox in suicide—that is, the high number of suicide attempts by women relative to deaths from suicide, in contrast to the higher rates of death from suicide in men. Emile Durkheim (1952) famously described suicide as an "essentially male phenomenon" (p. 72). This gendered perception of those at highest risk of death from suicide has resulted in suicide research centering on men. However, women have approximately twice the risk of developing depression throughout their lifetime than do men, and depression is a major risk factor for suicide. In addition, the onset of menstruation, pregnancy, the postpartum state, and the menopausal transition are all periods of increased vulnerability to mental illness (Friedman et al. 2018). Borderline personality disorder, also associated with higher rates of death from suicide, is also more common among women. Eating disorders are more common among women as well, and women with anorexia are at a 50-fold elevation of risk of death from suicide (Vijayakumar 2015).

Although the rate of death from suicide in women is viewed as low, recent data demonstrate growing concerns. According to the National Center for Health Statistics (Hedegaard et al. 2018), the rate of death from suicide increased between 2000 and 2016 for both men and women, with more rapid increases after 2006. For women, the rates of death from suicide rose by 50%, from 4 per 100,000 people in 2000 to 6 per 100,000 in 2016. In men, rates of death from suicide rose by 21% during the same time period, from 17.7 per 100,000 in 2000 to 21.4 in 2016. Rapid increases in rates of death from suicide were noted in women from 2007 to 2016; during this time period, rates of death from suicide rose by 3% per year for women. In males, rates of death from suicide increased 2% per year from 2006 to 2010 and 1% per year from 2010 to 2016.

The National Center for Health Statistics study further noted that the accelerated rates of death from suicide in females were reflected in the narrowing of the male to female suicide ratio from 4.4:1 in 2000 to 3.6:1 in 2016. This study also noted the highest rates of suicide in females were for those aged 45–64 years, both in 2000 (6.2 per 100,000 females) and 2016 (9.9 per 100,000 females). For males, high rates of death from suicide were noted among those aged 75 and over; however, a slight decline was noted between 2000 (42.4 per 100,000 males) and 2016 (39.2 per 100,000 males). The duration of the suicidal process is also much shorter in males than in females: once the process has started, males die from suicide much quicker, and their attempts are much more lethal than those of females (Neeleman et al. 2004).

Another noteworthy gender difference is observed in the *contagion effect* of suicide. This phenomenon is observed in situations such as celebrity suicides or suicides among friends, and adolescents are particularly vulnerable to this effect (see Chapters 18, "Children and Adolescents" and 24, "Self-Injurious Behavior"). Although a full discussion of this phenomenon is outside the scope of this chapter, some gender differences in the contagion effect of suicide have been observed. One study found that adolescent girls were more likely to make a suicide attempt if they knew someone else who had made an attempt, whereas adolescent boys were substantially more likely to make an attempt if they knew someone who had died from suicide rather than someone who had attempted suicide but did not die (Cutler et al. 2001).

Transgender Individuals and Suicide

Societal awareness of marginalization and stigma faced by gender-diverse individuals is increasing. Many transgender individuals experience bullying, employment discrimination, homelessness, and even discriminatory profiling by the police. The National Center for Transgender Equality, a second iteration of the National Transgender Discrimination Survey (NTDS), surveyed 6,450 participants, among whom 41% had attempted suicide as compared with 1.6% of the general population. Suicide risk was increased in those who lost employment due to bias (55%), those harassed and bullied in school (51%), those with low income or who were the victim of physical assault (61%), and those who were sexually assaulted (64%) (Grant et al. 2011). The survey also highlighted higher rates of HIV infection, smoking, depression, and drug and alcohol use in this population.

Family acceptance had a significant protective effect on these health risks, including the risk of death from suicide. Suicide attempts occurred in about one-third of those with accepting families compared with one-half of those without family support. Another significant concern for transgender individuals is barriers to medical care. Almost one-fifth (19%) of transgender individuals report being refused medical care, which can directly impact the risk of suicide and help-seeking behaviors (Grant et al. 2011).

Among nontransgender populations, African Americans, Latinx, and Asians have much lower rates of death from suicide than whites and Native Americans; in transgender populations, African American and Latinx respondents demonstrated dramatically elevated rates of death from suicide in comparison with their rates in the general population. Thus, culture in transgendered persons is also an important consideration when conducting suicide risk assessments. The NTDS survey also noted that—in contrast to the general population, where risk of death from suicide increases with age—in transgender individuals, suicide attempts were highest in the 18- to 24-year age group (Grant et al. 2011).

Some of the risk factors for death from suicide in transgender populations can be mitigated by early intervention. One recent study noted that children who had been socially transitioned (i.e., able to present to others as their chosen gender, wear clothing of their chosen gender, and use their preferred pronouns) had similar rates of depression and only marginally higher rates of anxiety compared with nontransgendered control subjects (Turban 2017). DSM-5 (American Psychiatric Association 2013) has made a significant effort in to destigmatize gender diversity by removing the "gender identity disorder" diagnosis and including the diagnosis "gender dysphoria." The American Psychiatric Association recommends that the ultimate goal should be to categorize the treatment of transgender and gender-nonconforming individuals under endocrine/medical diagnoses (American Psychiatric Association 2013).

Case Example 1: Transgender Female-to-Male Individual

Justin, a 19-year-old transgender male of African American ethnicity, was referred to the consulting psychiatrist after a suicide attempt by intentional overdose. Justin had been born with female biological sex but had always identified as male. He found support for his gender identity among friends, but his family has consistently refused to accept his identification as male. Justin commenced therapy with testosterone injections through his primary care physician a month ago. He has struggled with chronic passive suicidal thoughts since his early adolescence and has a history of self-mutilation motivated by a wish "to feel better." His current suicide attempt was triggered by an argument with his sister's husband, who suggested that Justin would "never amount to anything." Although he states he no longer wants to die, Justin continues to feel hopeless about his life and his ability to get through the transition process.

Discussion

This case illustrates various challenges faced by transgender individuals and the associated suicide risk factors that should be kept in mind when conducting a suicide risk assessment. These include Justin's age, which falls in the 18- to 24-year age range for highest risk in transgender individuals, previous self-injurious behaviors, recently commenced medical transition and need for support through this process, and the lack of family support for his transgendered status. In addition, diagnosing and treating psychiatric comorbidities such as depression and substance use are important. After addressing acute safety concerns, the clinician should also develop a comprehensive treatment plan that involves collaborating with the primary care physician and initiating individual and family therapy to address stressors. Finally, transgender individuals report high rates of discrimination from health care providers. Using preferred pronouns and maintaining a respectful demeanor is a part of gender affirmation.

Demographics and Race

According to the Centers for Disease Control and Prevention (CDC), in 2016, the highest rate of death from suicide (19.72 per 100,000) was among adults between 45 and 54 years of age, particularly white males. The second highest rate (18.98 per 100,000) occurred in those 85 years or older. Men die from suicide 3.5 times more commonly than women, and white males remain at consistently elevated risk (Centers for Disease Control and Prevention 2018). White males accounted for 70% of all deaths from suicides in 2016, followed by Native Americans.

Mortality due to suicide is particularly high among elderly males. Elderly females increasingly face adverse life circumstances such as limited financial resources, loss of spouse, living alone, physical illness, and functional disability (Fässberg et al. 2016). These adverse circumstances have been thought to precipitate suicidal behavior. Nevertheless, the rates of mortality from suicide among elderly women remain significantly lower than those of elderly men.

Cultural factors also may impact rates of death from suicide. Although cultural factors associated with suicidal behavior are covered elsewhere (see Chapter 6, "Cultural Humility and Structural Competence in Suicide Risk Assessment"), some protective cultural factors have been suggested. For example, although other factors contribute to high mortality rates in African American women, this population has historically had the lowest rates of suicide. Studies have highlighted various reasons for this, such as black women possessing a strong sense of heritage, history, identity, and faith, which are perceived as protective against suicide and depression (Borum 2012).

Explanations for the Gender Gap

Gender Stereotypes

Many explanations have been offered to explain the gender gap in suicide. In centuries past, Durkheim (1952) theorized that women were less prone to suicide because of their greater emotional attachments to home and family, greater religious faith, greater patience, and less developed intellectual capacity. Although this last factor cannot be credited, gender stereotypes continue to be used to explain the gap. Stereotypical beliefs such as that men are more likely to kill themselves as a result of failure and that women are more likely to die from suicide as a result of failure in romantic relationships still persist. However, evidence supports that for both men and women, mental illness, loneliness, and loss of an intimate relationship are the primary triggers for suicidal behavior (McAndrew and Garrison 2007).

Lethality of Means

Women attempt suicide more frequently than men but die from suicide less often (Värnik et al. 2008). One suspected reason for this finding is the choice of means of suicide, with men more often using firearms and women being more likely to attempt suicide by overdose. Firearm lethality far exceeds the lethality of medication overdose. Women thus are more likely to survive suicide attempts and have more opportunity to be "rescued" from a suicide attempt (Callanan and Davis 2012; Värnik et al. 2008). Methods of suicide vary by culture, age, gender, and availability (Ajdacic-Gross et al. 2008; Callanan and Davis 2012; Värnik et al. 2008). An Ohio medical examiner study comparing methods in 621 deaths from suicide found that women who died from suicide also had high rates of firearm use (38%) (Callanan and Davis 2012). This contrasts with Europe, where firearms are less available and where hanging is the most common suicide method for both men and women (Värnik et al. 2008).

Societal Stereotypes and Help-Seeking Behaviors

Möller-Leimkühler (2003) noted that women are more likely than men to seek medical and mental health services. Gender differences in help-seeking behaviors are especially pronounced in cultures that adhere to traditional social constructs emphasizing "masculine" values, such as independence, economic status, and individualism, which may prevent men from seeking help. A study of 33 countries demonstrated that individualism (defined as the self-perception as an autonomous personality not defined by or merged into collective familial or social groups) is highly correlated with death from suicide in males. In young women, however, individualism showed a negative correlation with death from suicide (Webster Rudmin et al. 2003).

Similarly, Bjerkeset et al. (2008) demonstrated that although females in the cohort had a higher incidence of depression, males in the cohort had a twofold risk of death from suicide. The researchers postulated that these differences could be attributed to the stigma associated with mental illness or the higher incidence of substance use and reduced help-seeking in males. Other researchers have noted that females are significantly overdiagnosed with major depression and other psychiatric disorders across different medical settings (Chang et al. 2009). Furthermore, the high male to female suicide ratio in the nonclinical populations could be attributed to undiagnosed psychiatric disorders among men (Liu et al. 2009).

Psychiatric Comorbidities Including Substance Use Disorders

A meta-analysis of 3,275 deaths from suicide (Arsenault-Lapierre et al. 2004) demonstrated that 87% of individuals had been diagnosed with a mental disorder prior to death. The rates of substance-related disorders, personality disorders, and childhood disorders were significantly higher in male deaths from suicide, whereas the rate of affective disorders, especially depressive disorders, was greater in female deaths from suicide. Affective and substance use disorders were the two most common diagnostic categories among all those who died from suicide (Arsenault-Lapierre et al. 2004).

Most studies have not demonstrated consistent gender differences in suicidal behavior or suicidal ideation in individuals with bipolar disorders (Diflorio and Jones 2010). Impulsivity, hostility, and aggressive personality features, present in a variety of psychiatric disorders, are much more prevalent in males and substantially heighten the risk of suicidal behavior, especially risk of death from suicide (Brezo et al. 2006; Strüber et al. 2008). Mood disorders comorbid with anxiety are associated with an increased suicide risk in males, but mood disorders alone are associated with a higher female risk of death from suicide (Arsenault-Lapierre et al. 2004; Bjerkeset et al. 2008).

Use of Hormonal Contraceptives

Skovlund et al. (2018) studied suicidal behavior and hormonal contraceptive use in women with no history of psychiatric diagnoses, antidepressant use, or contraceptive use before the age of 15 years. This Danish study used a nationwide registry to observe 475,802 women over an average of 8 years. One-half (54%) of the subjects were using hormonal contraceptives at some point during the follow-up. A total of 6,999 suicide attempts and 71 deaths from suicide were identified in this cohort. The relative risk among current and recent users of hormonal contraceptives as compared with women who had never used hormonal contraceptives was 1.97 (95% CI, 1.85–2.10) for suicide attempt and 3.08 (95% CI, 1.34–7.08) for death from suicide. The authors also found that the impact of hormonal contraceptive use on suicidal behavior was higher in adolescents, peaking 2 months after initiation of hormonal contraception. They also noted that non-oral forms of hormonal contraception conferred the highest risks. However, the study did not establish causation between suicide and contraceptive use, and further research is needed.

Special Issues in Gender and Suicide

Sexual Abuse

In a study of 8,580 British subjects, the population-attributable risk of sexual abuse to a history of suicide attempts was substantially greater among females (28%) than among males (7%). However, this may be attributed in part to underreporting in males (Bebbington et al. 2009). Martin et al. (2004) found that sexual abuse increased suicidal behaviors in women as much as threefold. Although boys tend to underreport sexual abuse, the researchers also found that substantially more sexually abused boys (55%) as compared with girls (29%) reported suicide attempts. This indicates that the response to sexual abuse may be more severe in males and merits careful history and risk assessment.

Abortion

Research on abortion often suffers from the lack of an appropriate control group. Disenfranchised females seeking an abortion should not be compared to females with a planned pregnancy but rather to those who were similarly coping with an unplanned pregnancy and were not successful in obtaining an abortion. Regardless, rates of suicidal ideation are low among females having an abortion and those denied an abortion. In one of the few studies available (Biggs et al. 2017), at 1 week post abortion, 1.9% of females reported suicidal thoughts compared with 1.3% of those who had been turned away; over the course of 5 years, rates of suicidal thinking were low in both groups.

Risk of Suicide in Pregnancy and During the Postpartum Period

Population-based studies of suicide have found a lower risk of death from suicide in pregnant and postpartum females than in the general female population (Lindahl et al. 2005; Samandari et al. 2011). Nevertheless, uncommon, violent, and dramatic methods of suicide are notable in the perinatal population in contrast to the general female population (Gold et al. 2012; Lindahl et al. 2005). Pregnant teenagers and unmarried pregnant females from cultures that particularly stigmatize unwed mothers are at elevated risk (Lindahl et al. 2005). Yet, overall, marriage is less of a protective factor against death from suicide for females than for males (Vijayakumar 2015). During pregnancy, the increased oversight of health professionals and increased social support, as well as the caring role for the fetus, are likely to decrease the risk of death from suicide overall (Lindahl et al. 2005; Samandari et al. 2011).

Despite the rarity of death from suicide in the peripartum period, thoughts of suicide are not rare in pregnancy or the postpartum period. Studies have found that at 18 weeks' gestation, approximately 10% of females endorse some thoughts of self-harm; at 32 weeks, approximately 7%; and at 6 months postpartum, 7%–15% (Lindahl et al. 2005). In an American study comparing mothers hospitalized after a nonfatal suicide attempt in the year after delivery with postpartum females who were not psychiatrically hospitalized, those who were hospitalized were more likely to be younger, of minority ethnicity, and unmarried; to have had more pregnancies and later prenatal care; and were less likely to be college graduates. Mothers with prior psychiatric hospitalizations or prior substance abuse hospitalizations were at significantly higher risk (Comtois et al. 2008). The most common means used in this population was poisoning by intentional overdose.

Using data from the U.S. National Violent Death Reporting System, researchers considered mental health, intimate partner issues, and substance use among perinatal deaths from suicide (Gold et al. 2012). When peripartum females who died from suicide were compared with other reproductive-age females who died from suicide, mental health and substance use issues were similarly prevalent in all groups. Postpartum females were more likely to have a depressed mood in the 2 weeks before death. Those who died from suicide during pregnancy or the postpartum period were more likely to have noted problems with a current or former romantic partner (Gold et al. 2012). Pregnancy is the highest risk period for intimate-partner violence victimization, and this should also be considered and assessed when evaluating pregnant females.

Suicide is the cause of approximately 20% of deaths in the postpartum period (Lindahl et al. 2005). Among those who die from suicide, stillbirth and unmarried status are overrepresented, and individuals who require psychiatric admission are also at higher risk for death from suicide (Comtois et al. 2008; Lindahl et al. 2005).

The postpartum period is the time of highest risk for the development of a mental illness in the female lifespan. Approximately one in seven mothers will develop postpartum depression (Friedman and Resnick 2009). Strides have been made in screening for perinatal depression, but great stigma associated with postpartum depression still exists, and thus many women may hide their symptoms. The lack of sleep and stress from parenting an infant may contribute to suicidal thoughts and behaviors in postpartum depression (Lindahl et al. 2005).

Postpartum psychosis, which occurs after 1–2 births per 1,000, includes symptoms of not only psychosis but also mood and cognitive symptoms (Friedman and Sorrentino 2012). Symptoms evolve rapidly, and untreated postpartum psychosis poses a risk of both suicide and infanticide (Friedman et al. 2019).

Although the risk of death from suicide is lower overall in pregnancy and postpartum, each individual patient's risk factors should be considered. Having a child at home decreases the risk of death from suicide in women. However, the risk of infanticide must be considered. One study of mothers with depression found that 41% had thoughts of harming their young child, compared to 7% of control subjects (Jennings et al. 1999). In a sample of parents who killed both their child and themselves, mothers usually committed filicide and died from suicide for altruistic reasons (Friedman et al. 2005). These may include an extended suicide, where death from suicide was the primary aim but the loving mother took the child with her in death. Alternatively, some mothers believed that they were saving the child from a fate worse than death and also killed themselves. For example, the mother of an infant with an incurable disease may believe that she is saving the child from suffering and taking him to heaven. Alternatively, a mother suffering from psychosis who kills her child and herself may have had a delusion that she was saving her child, for example, from being sold into slavery.

Menopause and Suicide

Estrogen decline during menopause may correlate with increasing mental health symptoms (Friedman et al. 2018; Usall et al. 2009). Women may experience social and developmental challenges around the menopausal transition, such as an "empty nest," as well as increased biological vulnerability to mental health issues (Friedman et al. 2018). In a sample of more than 8,000 respondents from five European nations, women in the perimenopausal period had an increased rate of suicidal ideation when compared with other groups, independent of mental disorders and sociodemographics (Usall et al. 2009). In fact, the prevalence of suicidal ideation among women in perimenopause females at 7.8% was seven times the rates for pre- and postmenopausal women.

Case Example 2: Pregnancy

Ms. Jones, age 28, was referred by her obstetrician for psychiatric consultation due to concerns about depression in pregnancy. Ms. Jones, a housewife, and her husband have recently moved to town, and she has not yet made any friends. Thus, her husband is her primary source of social support. This is Ms. Jones' second pregnancy; her first pregnancy resulted in a stillbirth, and she has significant worries about giving birth. Despite this, she has had poor attendance at prenatal care visits. She appears somewhat detached when she talks about the current pregnancy.

Ms. Jones and her husband have been having arguments that have worsened during the pregnancy. She reports no domestic violence but is feeling unsupported. Her family of origin live out of town. Upon interview, Ms. Jones reports anhedonia, depressed mood, and negative thoughts about the future. She reports poor sleep for several months, and she has not gained as much weight as her obstetrician would like. She says that she has "baby brain" and finds it difficult to concentrate or remember things well. She sometimes feels that life is not worth living, but she has not taken any steps to end her life. She is quite worried about not being a good enough mother. She reports no history of previous psychiatric treatment, suicide attempts, or substance misuse. What is Ms. Jones' risk of suicide and how could it be decreased?

Discussion

Ms. Jones presents with major depression as well as symptoms of posttraumatic stress disorder related to the loss of her previous pregnancy. At present, her overall risk of death from suicide appears to be low. However, her risk is elevated because of her depression and anxiety, her passive suicidal thoughts, her difficult relationship with her husband, and her lack of social support. She agrees that she should join some groups and meet new people. Seeking to optimize her functioning as well as minimize her risk of death from suicide, the psychiatrist discusses the benefits of psychotherapy and antidepressant medication with her. After discussing the risks of untreated mental illness (not limited to difficulty caring for oneself, risk of low birthweight, and difficulty with bonding) and potential risks from medication (Friedman and Hall 2013), Ms. Jones agrees to start a selective serotonin reuptake inhibitor and attend psychotherapy as well as prenatal groups. Interpersonal psychotherapy helps her cope with the change in her social role and her marriage. Her symptoms improve significantly, and she bonds with her healthy baby after birth.

Conclusion

Gender issues are important to consider when assessing suicide risk. Although women die from suicide less frequently than men do, they attempt suicide more frequently. Women tend to use less lethal methods in suicide attempts than do males. However, notable exceptions occur both in cultural contexts and during the reproductive years. In addition, in recent years rates of death from suicide for women have risen more rapidly, and guns remain the most common means of death from suicide in America. Social constructs and gender stereotypes may present hindrances to seeking care for men, and sexual trauma and depression may be underrecognized in men. Conversely, suicide attempts in women may be minimized as attention-seeking behaviors or be misattributed to personality disorders.

In transgender individuals, suicidal ideation is common, as are suicide attempts. Special attention should be given to risk factors in this population such as homelessness, bullying, other discriminatory behaviors, and access to health care. The individual patient, regardless of gender, requires thoughtful assessment of suicide risk. For example, the presence of children in the home is generally considered to be protective; however, the suicidal mother may plan to take her beloved children with her to heaven. New data suggest heightened risk of death from suicide with hormonal contraceptive use; however, further studies are needed.

Key Points

- Across the world (with the exception of China), men die from suicide more frequently than women do, although women have higher rates of depression and more frequent suicide attempts.

- Risk of death from suicide is increasing in recent years for both men and women but at higher rates for women.

- Transgender individuals have high rates of suicidal behavior.

- Men use firearms as a means of suicide more frequently than women, although when women use firearms, their attempts may be similarly lethal.

- Sexual abuse is a risk factor for suicidal behavior and is underreported in males.

- Although risk of death from suicide is lower overall in pregnancy and the post-partum period, individual patient risk factors need to be considered. One-fifth of postpartum deaths are due to suicide. The risk of killing the infant (infanti-cide) must also be considered in suicide risk assessments of the mother.

- Women with depression in the perimenopause should be assessed for risk of death from suicide.

References

Ajdacic-Gross V, Weiss MG, Ring M, et al: Methods of suicide: international suicide patterns derived from the WHO mortality database. Bull World Health Organ 86(9):657–736, 2008

American Psychiatric Association: Diagnostic and Statistical Manual of Mental Disorders, 5th Edition. Arlington, VA, American Psychiatric Association, 2013

Arsenault-Lapierre G, Kim C, Turecki G: Psychiatric diagnoses in 3275 suicides: a meta-analysis. BMC Psychiatry 4:37, 2004 15527502

Bebbington PE, Cooper C, Minot S, et al: Suicide attempts, gender, and sexual abuse: data from the 2000 British Psychiatric Morbidity Survey. Am J Psychiatry 166(10):1135–1140, 2009 19723788

Biggs MA, Upadhyay UD, McCulloch CE, et al: Women's mental health and well-being 5 years after receiving or being denied an abortion: a prospective, longitudinal cohort study. JAMA Psychiatry 74(2):169–178, 2017 27973641

Bjerkeset O, Romundstad P, Gunnell D: Gender differences in the association of mixed anxiety and depression with suicide. Br J Psychiatry 192(6):474–475, 2008 18515904

Borum V: African American women's perceptions of depression and suicide risk and protection: a womanist exploration. Affilia 27(3):316–327, 2012

Brezo J, Paris J, Turecki G: Personality traits as correlates of suicidal ideation, suicide attempts, and suicide completions: a systematic review. Acta Psychiatr Scand 113(3):180–206, 2006 16466403

Callanan VJ, Davis MS: Gender differences in suicide methods. Soc Psychiatry Psychiatr Epidemiol 47(6):857–869, 2012 21604180

Centers for Disease Control and Prevention: Suicide rising across the United States. Vital Signs, 2018. Available at: https://www.cdc.gov/vitalsigns/suicide/index.html. Accessed November 25, 2018.

Chang CM, Liao SC, Chiang HC, et al: Gender differences in healthcare service utilisation 1 year before suicide: national record linkage study. Br J Psychiatry 195(5):459–460, 2009 19880939

Comtois KA, Schiff MA, Grossman DC: Psychiatric risk factors associated with postpartum suicide attempt in Washington State, 1992–2001. Am J Obstet Gynecol 199(2):120.e1–120.e5, 2008 18355781

Cutler DM, Glaesen EL, Norberg KE: Explaining the rise in youth suicide, in Risky Behavior Among Youths: An Economic Analysis. Edited by Gruber J. Chicago, IL, University of Chicago Press, 2001

Diflorio A, Jones I: Is sex important? Gender differences in bipolar disorder. Int Rev Psychiatry 22(5):437–452, 2010 21047158

Durkheim E: Suicide: A Study in Sociology (1897). Translated by Spaulding JA, edited by Simpson G. London, Routledge and Kegan, 1952

Fässberg MM, Cheung G, Canetto SS, et al: A systematic review of physical illness, functional disability, and suicidal behaviour among older adults. Aging Ment Health 20(2):166–194, 2016 26381843

Friedman SH, Hall RCW: Antidepressant use during pregnancy: how to avoid clinical and legal pitfalls. Curr Psychiatr 12(2):10–17, 2013

Friedman SH, Resnick PJ: Postpartum depression: an update. Womens Health (Lond) 5(3):287–295, 2009 19392614

Friedman SH, Sorrentino R: Commentary: postpartum psychosis, infanticide, and insanity—implications for forensic psychiatry. J Am Acad Psychiatry Law 40(3):326–332, 2012 22960914

Friedman SH, Hrouda DR, Holden CE, et al: Filicide-suicide: common factors in parents who kill their children and themselves. J Am Acad Psychiatry Law 33(4):496–504, 2005 16394226

Friedman SH, Prakash C, Moller-Olsen C: Psychiatric considerations in menopause. Curr Psychiatr 17(10):11–16, 2018

Friedman SH, Prakash C, Nagle-Yang S: Postpartum psychosis: protecting mother and infant. Curr Psychiatr 18(4):12–21, 2019

Gold KJ, Singh V, Marcus SM, et al: Mental health, substance use and intimate partner problems among pregnant and postpartum suicide victims in the National Violent Death Reporting System. Gen Hosp Psychiatry 34(2):139–145, 2012 22055329

Grant JM, Mottet LA, Tanis J, et al: Injustice at Every Turn: A Report of the National Transgender Discrimination Survey. Washington, DC, National Center for Transgender Equality and National Gay and Lesbian Task Force, 2011. Available at: https://transequality.org/issues/resources/national-transgender-discrimination-survey-executive-summary. Accessed November 25, 2018.

Hedegaard H, Curtin SC, Warner M: Suicide rates in the United States continue to increase. NCHS Data Brief (309):1–8, 2018 30312151

Jennings KD, Ross S, Popper S, et al: Thoughts of harming infants in depressed and nondepressed mothers. J Affect Disord 54(1-2):21–28, 1999 10403143

Lindahl V, Pearson JL, Colpe L: Prevalence of suicidality during pregnancy and the postpartum. Arch Women Ment Health 8(2):77–87, 2005 15883651

Liu KY, Chen EY, Cheung AS, et al: Psychiatric history modifies the gender ratio of suicide: an East and West comparison. Soc Psychiatry Psychiatr Epidemiol 44(2):130–134, 2009 18661085

Martin G, Bergen HA, Richardson AS, et al: Sexual abuse and suicidality: gender differences in a large community sample of adolescents. Child Abuse Negl 28(5):491–503, 2004 15159067

McAndrew FT, Garrison AJ: Beliefs about gender differences in methods and causes of suicide. Arch Suicide Res 11(3):271–279, 2007 17558612

Möller-Leimkühler AM: The gender gap in suicide and premature death or: why are men so vulnerable? Eur Arch Psychiatry Clin Neurosci 253(1):1–8, 2003 12664306

Neeleman J, de Graaf R, Vollebergh W: The suicidal process: prospective comparison between early and later stages. J Affect Disord 82(1):43–52, 2004 15465575

Samandari G, Martin SL, Kupper LL, et al: Are pregnant and postpartum women at increased risk for violent death? Suicide and homicide findings from North Carolina. Matern Child Health J 15(5):660–669, 2011 20549551

Skovlund CW, Mørch LS, Kessing LV, et al: Association of hormonal contraception with suicide attempts and suicides. Am J Psychiatry 175(4):336–342, 2018 29145752

Strüber D, Lück M, Roth G: Sex, aggression and impulse control: an integrative account. Neurocase 14(1):93–121, 2008 18569735

Turban JL: Transgender youth: the building evidence base for early social transition. J Am Acad Child Adolesc Psychiatry 56(2):101–102, 2017 28117053

Usall J, Pinto-Meza A, Fernández A, et al: Suicide ideation across reproductive life cycle of women. Results from a European epidemiological study. J Affect Disord 116(1-2):144–147, 2009 19155069

Värnik A, Kõlves K, van der Feltz-Cornelis CM, et al: Suicide methods in Europe: a gender-specific analysis of countries participating in the "European Alliance Against Depression." J Epidemiol Community Health 62(6):545–551, 2008 18477754

Värnik P: Suicide in the world. Int J Environ Res Public Health 9(3):760–771, 2012 22690161

Vijayakumar L: Suicide in women. Indian J Psychiatry 57(2 suppl 2):S233–S238, 2015 26330640

Webster Rudmin F, Ferrada-Noli M, Skolbekken JA: Questions of culture, age and gender in the epidemiology of suicide. Scand J Psychol 44(4):373–381, 2003 12887559

CHAPTER 24

Self-Injurious Behavior

Michele Berk, Ph.D.

Claudia Avina, Ph.D.

Stephanie Clarke, Ph.D.

Self-injurious behaviors are a significant public health problem in the United States. Suicide is the tenth leading cause of death across all age groups, the second leading cause of death among 10- to 34-year-olds, and the fourth leading cause of death among 35- to 54-year-olds (Centers for Disease Control and Prevention 2018). Unlike suicide, data on the prevalence of nonsuicidal self-injury (NSSI) have not been collected on a national level, and estimates have varied across studies due to use of different samples and measurement strategies (Swannell et al. 2014). Although less is known about the epidemiology of NSSI, extant research suggests rates are high, particularly among youth. A meta-analysis of existing studies of NSSI prevalence in non-clinical samples found a lifetime prevalence of 17.2% for adolescents, 13.4% for young adults, and 5.5% for adults after controlling for methodological differences between studies (Swannell et al. 2014). Another study that used a sample of high school students from 11 U.S. states found that 18% of all students and approximately 24% of female students reported at least one NSSI act within the past 12 months (Monto et al. 2018). Both suicide attempts (SAs) and NSSI have been shown to be risk factors for future SAs (Asarnow et al. 2011; Wilkinson et al. 2011); hence, strategies for effectively reducing these behaviors are urgently needed. Given the high rates of suicide, SA, and NSSI in adolescence, the primary focus of this chapter is on this age group. However, the majority of recommendations made are also applicable to adults.

Definitions of Self-Injurious Behaviors

As shown in Table 24–1, self-injurious behaviors include both SAs and NSSI. SAs are defined as potentially self-injurious behaviors performed with some intent to die (i.e.,

TABLE 24–1.   Definitions of types of self-injurious behaviors

Suicide attempt (SA)	A potentially self-injurious behavior associated with *some evidence of intent to die*.
Nonsuicidal self-injury (NSSI)	Self-injurious behavior *not associated with intent to die* (e.g., intent may be to reduce negative emotion, to punish oneself).
Self-harm	Broader category including all intentional self-injury, with or without intent to die (i.e., SA and NSSI).

to cause one's own death) as a result of the behavior (Nock 2010). In contrast, NSSIs are defined as self-injurious behaviors performed without any intent to die (Nock 2010). NSSIs are typically associated with functions other than death, such as reducing negative emotions, punishing oneself, and reducing dissociation or feelings of numbness (Klonsky 2007). Common methods of NSSI include cutting, burning, scratching the skin, head banging, and hitting oneself (Klonsky 2007).

Inconsistent definitions of self-injurious behaviors have hindered research progress by making comparison of the findings between studies difficult. In the United States, SA and NSSI are seen as distinct behaviors differentiated based on the presence or absence of intent to die, as described earlier. In contrast, in Europe, SA and NSSI are typically grouped together into a broader category of self-harm, regardless of intent, due to the overlap between these behaviors and the difficulty of accurately determining whether intent to die was present (Ougrin et al. 2012).

Similarities and Differences Between Suicide Attempts and Nonsuicidal Self-Injury

Research has focused on elucidating the similarities and differences between SA and NSSI. Beyond the presence or absence of intent to die, SA and NSSI can also be differentiated by other factors, such as lethality or medical severity, prevalence rates, and frequency of the behavior (Glenn et al. 2017). In DSM-5 (American Psychiatric Association 2013), a new diagnostic category of "nonsuicidal self-injury disorder" has been included as a condition for further study, underscoring NSSI as distinct from SAs. Similarly, DSM-5 has also proposed a new diagnosis of "suicidal behavior disorder" as a condition for further study.

These new categories represent an important shift in the conceptualization of self-injurious behaviors. Previously, SA and NSSI were addressed diagnostically only as symptoms of other mental disorders, such as major depressive disorder and borderline personality disorder. The new proposed diagnostic categories highlight NSSI and SA as conditions worthy of treatment in their own right rather than as symptoms of other psychiatric disorders. This conceptualization is consistent with a growing consensus in the suicide literature that NSSI and SA must be targeted directly in treatment and not simply as secondary to treatment of other disorders (Meerwijk et al. 2016).

Despite the important distinctions between SA and NSSI, these behaviors are also interrelated in important ways. Research has shown that most adolescents engage in both NSSI and SA concurrently (Whitlock et al. 2013). Furthermore, the majority of adolescents who have engaged in NSSI have also attempted suicide (Nock et al. 2006).

NSSI is a robust predictor of future SAs among youth with depressive disorders (Asarnow et al. 2011; Wilkinson et al. 2011). The onset of suicidal ideation (SI) typically precedes the first onset of NSSI, and NSSI typically precedes the first SA (Glenn et al. 2017). This suggests a temporal relationship in which adolescents have already thought about suicide prior to the first onset of NSSI, but NSSI may serve as a "gateway" to SA (i.e., increase the likelihood of progression from NSSI to SA) because the individual develops the capacity to engage in increasingly dangerous self-injurious behaviors as a result of repetitive NSSIs (Whitlock et al. 2013).

In a sample of youth admitted to an adolescent inpatient unit with a prior NSSI within the past 12 months, predictors of future SAs included a greater number of years of engaging in NSSI, a greater number of different methods of NSSI used, and lack of physical pain during NSSI (Nock et al. 2006). A study of high school students found that SI, a lack of reasons for living, and more severe depressive symptoms differentiated youth with NSSI and SA from youth with NSSI alone (Muehlenkamp and Gutierrez 2007). Studies examining sex differences in rates of NSSI have found mixed results. One meta-analysis found that females were more likely to engage in NSSI than males across age groups, with this difference more pronounced in clinical versus community samples (Bresin and Schoenleber 2015). With regard to the relationship between NSSI and suicide deaths, one study found that cutting parts of the body other than the arms was associated with later suicide (Carroll et al. 2016).

These findings highlight the importance of taking NSSI seriously and targeting it aggressively in treatment as opposed to viewing NSSIs as "suicide gestures" or as merely "attention-seeking" behaviors. Minimization of the significance of NSSIs may lead to underestimation of suicide risk and inadequate safety planning. Clinicians should be aware of the likelihood that a patient reporting NSSI has likely already considered suicide, is at high risk for future SAs, and may have already made an SA. Therefore, a thorough suicide risk assessment should be performed not only for patients with current or prior SI or SA but also for any individual reporting current or past NSSI.

Clinical Approaches to Treating Suicide Attempts and Nonsuicidal Self-Injury

Given the overlap between SA and NSSI, safety-based interventions have generally targeted both types of behaviors concurrently rather than separately. In this section, we describe risk assessment and evidence-based safety interventions and highlight how each may be used to address SA and NSSI.

Risk Assessment

Every clinical contact with an individual at risk for death from suicide, including any individual with a history of NSSI, should include a detailed risk assessment. This is true even among patients who have been in long-term treatment, because suicidal and self-harm urges and behaviors often wax and wane over time. Essential components of risk assessment include but are not limited to a) current and recent SI, intent, and plan; b) current and recent urges to engage in NSSI; c) history of prior SA and NSSI; d) access to lethal means and means for NSSI; e) ability to commit to using a safety plan instead of SA or NSSI; f) enhancement of safety in the home environment (i.e., restriction of lethal means and means of NSSI, the ability of parents of adolescents to provide close monitoring); g) current status of risk and protective factors; and h) current stressors/potential triggering events.

Multiple risk factors for death from suicide have been identified; however, risk factors are neither sensitive nor specific enough for clinicians to accurately predict who will go on to attempt or ultimately die from suicide (Fowler 2012). Although research shows that risk increases with the number of risk factors present, no algorithms exist to accurately predict which combinations of risk factors are most likely to lead to suicidal behavior (Franklin et al. 2017). As a result, the determination of risk is largely dependent on clinical judgment.

Safety Interventions

Basic safety interventions should be regularly implemented when working with individuals with SA and NSSI. These interventions can be used across treatment settings and approaches and include 1) restricting access to lethal means and means of NSSI; 2) creating a written safety plan and providing emergency crisis numbers; 3) creating a hope box; 4) close parental monitoring; 5) reducing family conflict; 6) informing parents to take suicidal thoughts and behaviors seriously; and 7) reducing exposure to information that may cause contagion. Each intervention is described in more detail in Table 24–2.

Restrict Lethal Means

Means restriction—that is, removing or limiting access to potential methods of suicide—is one of the only approaches to suicide prevention that has a robust empirical basis (Mann et al. 2005). This can include firearms, medications (both prescription and over the counter), sharps (e.g., knives, scissors, razors, and pencil sharpeners, which can be broken apart to obtain blades), methods of suffocation/hanging (e.g., belts, ties), household poisons, and alcohol and other substances. Blocking access to "suicide hot spots," such as bridges, tall buildings, cliffs, and trains may also be needed if these are present in the local area (see Chapter 30, "Suicide Prevention Programs"; Public Health England 2015).

Restricting access to means of NSSI, such as razors, knives, scissors, paper clips, pins, glass, and lighters, is an important component of treatment intended to block the behavior from occurring and thus reduce the likelihood of injury. A range of unexpected items may be used for NSSI, so assessing the methods the patient has used previously is important, and clinicians should ensure those items are removed. All potentially lethal means and means of NSSI should be removed from the home if possible. Items that cannot be removed should be kept in a secured location such as a locked box or safe, although complete removal is safer.

Clinicians should repeatedly assess for access to means because patients may acquire new means between sessions or reveal possession of means that were previously kept secret. The following metaphor is useful in explaining the importance of restricting lethal means and means of NSSI to patients and families, particularly when working with parents of adolescents who feel overwhelmed and anxious about this responsibility: "Imagine that you are on a diet. Would you be more likely to break your diet if you did or did not have a chocolate cake in your kitchen?" Although patients can always acquire additional means of self-harm, removing easily available means for impulsive self-harming

TABLE 24–2.   **List of safety-based interventions**

	Specific steps to be taken
Restrict lethal means and means of NSSI	Discuss importance of removal of firearms from the home. Review removal of lethal means and means of NSSI with parent.
	Review access to lethal means and means of NSSI with teen.
	Ask teen if he/she has any lethal means or means of NSSI hidden "just in case" he/she wants to use them in the future.
Discuss parental monitoring	Review need for close monitoring and discuss amount of close monitoring currently needed.
	If 24/7 monitoring is needed, set up a plan to reassess safety within the next 1–2 days.
Create a written safety plan	Complete a written safety plan with teen.
	Review written safety plan with parent.
Create a hope box	Ask teen to place reminders of reasons to live and materials needed to implement coping skills in a box or other small container.
Provide emergency contact information	Provide parent and teen with emergency cards that list 24/7 emergency hotline numbers.
Reduce family conflict	Inform parents of the importance of reducing family conflict until teen is no longer suicidal.
Educate parents to take suicide and self-harm communications seriously	Inform parents that all communications about suicidal thoughts or urges and NSSI should be taken seriously and appropriate safety interventions implemented as needed.
Reduce contagion	Discuss plan with parent and teen for limiting access to internet content related to suicide and NSSI and discussion about suicidal thoughts and behaviors/self-harm with peers.

Note.   NSSI=nonsuicidal self-injury.

Source.   Adapted from Berk MS, Clarke S: "Safety Planning and Risk Management," in *Evidence-Based Treatment Approaches for Suicidal Adolescents: Translating Science Into Practice*. Edited by Berk MS. Washington, DC, American Psychiatric Association Publishing, 2019, p. 64. Copyright © 2019 American Psychiatric Association Publishing.

behavior may give patients time to reconsider, seek help, or be interrupted by others. To extend the metaphor to address this issue, we also say, "You can always go to the store to buy a chocolate cake, but that would take much more time and effort, and you would have more opportunities to change your mind or for somebody else to stop you."

Create a Written Safety Plan

Individuals who are in a suicidal crisis may have difficulty remembering and implementing their safe coping strategies. Therefore, developing a detailed, written safety plan in advance that individuals can follow when in crisis is an important safety intervention. The Suicide Prevention Resource Center/American Foundation for Suicide Prevention has identified a safety plan template and intervention developed by Stanley and Brown (2012) as a "best practice"; this can be adapted across settings and populations. A generic template is available online at www.sprc.org/sites/default/files/Brown_StanleySafetyPlanTemplate.pdf.

The safety plan template is organized in a stepwise manner and starts with strategies that patients can implement themselves at home. It ends with 24/7 emergency contact numbers that can be used when patients feel they are in imminent danger and need to access emergency services. Recent research conducted with a large sample of adult veterans seen in U.S. Department of Veterans Affairs (VA) emergency departments for suicidal thoughts and behaviors has shown that completing the written safety plan can reduce subsequent SAs by up to 50% (Stanley et al. 2018). Although the written safety plan was developed for suicidal individuals, we recommend that clinicians use the same template to develop a written plan for patients with NSSI only. Because a majority of individuals who have engaged in NSSI are at risk for future SA, it is important to create a safety plan addressing steps to follow if the individual experiences urges to attempt suicide in the future.

Provide Emergency Contact Numbers

All patients at risk for death from suicide, including those with a history of NSSI (and in the case of adolescents, their parents) should be given phone numbers for the local emergency departments, mobile crisis teams, and 24/7 crisis hotlines that they can keep with them at all times, such as on small business cards that fit easily in a wallet or pocket. Patient and family education should include instructions for appropriate/necessary circumstances in which to use these resources. Patients and parents should also be given clear information about the therapist's availability to respond to emergencies outside of business hours.

Create a Hope Box

Similar to the written safety plan, the "hope box" (Berk et al. 2004) is a way to prepare in advance for a suicidal crisis. It can also be used to facilitate use of coping strategies to replace NSSI. The patient is asked to create a hope box by placing reminders of reasons to live and materials needed to implement coping skills into a box or other small container. Items to place in the hope box can include photographs of favorite people and places, postcards, letters, self-soothing items such as scented candles and music, and distracting tasks such as paints and paper for painting or a funny video or list of URLs the patient can view when emotionally distressed. Copies of the written safety plan and emergency contact numbers can also be placed in the hope box. Clinicians should advise patients to keep the hope box in an easily accessed location for use when they experience urges to engage in suicidal behavior or NSSI. Patients can also be encouraged to make a travel-sized hope kit for their backpack or purse when at school or out of the home. A free "virtual hope box" app is available from the National Center for Telehealth and Technology, a U.S. Department of Defense Center of Excellence for Psychological Health and Traumatic Brain Injury (http://t2health.dcoe.mil/apps/virtual-hope-box; see Bush et al. 2017).

Discuss Parental Monitoring

Close monitoring by parents is another important safety strategy for blocking SA and NSSI in adolescents. Depending on the level of risk, parental monitoring includes a wide range of behaviors, such as frequent check-ins, not allowing adolescents to be alone in their room or in an isolated part of the home, not allowing adolescents to lock the door to their bedrooms or the bathroom, not allowing adolescents to leave the home, or not allowing adolescents to be alone at all (including sleeping in the same room or bed or parents sleeping in shifts). Parents should be directed to check in regularly with adolescents about whether they are having thoughts about suicide or urges to engage in NSSI. Clinicians should emphasize to parents that asking about suicidal thoughts does not increase the likelihood of the adolescent having suicidal thoughts or engaging in suicidal behaviors (Gould et al. 2005). Additionally, parents should be vigilant for the emergence of specific warning signs of a crisis as identified in the safety plan and of any increase of general risk factors for death from suicide.

An adolescent at high risk of death from suicide for an extended period of time should be frequently reevaluated by the clinician, given that 24/7 monitoring by parents is not sustainable over long periods of time. If the crisis persists such that parents cannot sustain the level of monitoring needed, the adolescent may need to be evaluated for an inpatient or residential level of care. The clinician's assessment of current risk should determine recommendations for the amount and duration of parental monitoring, and the degree of risk and related safety monitoring needs can vary over time.

Reduce Family Conflict

Family conflict is a key risk factor for adolescent suicidal behavior, and family cohesion has been shown to be a protective factor (Bridge et al. 2006). Parents should be provided with psychoeducation about the relationship between family conflict and adolescent suicidal behavior. The clinician should work with the family to reduce conflict and encourage parents to "choose their battles" until risk has been reduced. Parents play a critical role in maintaining youth safety by restricting access to lethal means, closely monitoring the adolescent, and seeking emergency services when needed. Creating a positive parent/teen relationship is essential in increasing the likelihood that the adolescent will reach out to the parent for help when in a suicidal crisis or experiencing urges to self-harm, regardless of suicidal intent.

Parent/teen relational difficulties have also been shown to be associated with NSSI (Martin et al. 2016). Hence, reducing family conflict is also an important safety target for youth with NSSI only.

Educate Parents to Take Suicide and Self-Harm Communications Seriously

At times, parents may minimize or misunderstand the degree of risk associated with SI, SA, and NSSI or may view these thoughts and behaviors as "attention seeking" or "manipulative." This may occur for various reasons, such as lack of knowledge or education about suicidal behavior, fear, helplessness, or the parents' desire to believe that their child is not at risk. Adolescents typically do not fake being suicidal in order to gain attention or get their way. Even if the adolescent is lying or exaggerating reports of suicidal thoughts and behaviors and self-harm for personal gain, this approach to getting needs met is highly problematic, potentially dangerous, evidence that the youth is thinking about self-harm, and a sign that mental health treatment is needed. Furthermore, clinicians should emphasize to parents that taking suicidal ideation and behaviors seriously is safer than being wrong and having something terrible happen (i.e., "better safe than sorry").

Reduce Contagion

The phrase *suicide contagion* refers to "the exposure to suicide or suicidal behaviors within one's family, one's peer group, or through media reports of suicide and can result in an increase in suicide and suicidal behaviors" (U.S. Department of Health and Human Services 2018). Teens may also be at risk for contagion of NSSI. Adolescents are particularly vulnerable to contagion of self-injurious behaviors because they are forming their identities and often rely on the behaviors of peers to guide their choices (Insel and Gould 2008). Increased use of electronic devices and social media has also increased the potential for contagion.

To reduce risk of contagion, adolescents should be encouraged to refrain from sharing information about SI, SA, and NSSI with peers. Adolescents often discuss these topics as a way to help or get help from friends. Therefore, cooperatively "brainstorming" other ways to achieve these goals may help reduce the need to share with peers and thus reduce the risk of NSSI or SA contagion. Clinicians should emphasize the importance of teens seeking assistance from an adult if they or their friends are suicidal. In addition, parents should be advised to monitor adolescents' exposure to content regarding suicide and self-harm through social network platforms and websites and to restrict access as needed.

Treatment Approaches

A surprisingly small number of empirically supported treatments are available for decreasing SA and NSSI in adolescents despite the magnitude of the problem in this age group. Only 16 randomized controlled trials of treatments for adolescents that targeted reduction in self-harm as the primary outcome variable have been published. Only eight of these trials yielded statistically significant results. Of these eight trials, success with only one treatment modality has been replicated: dialectical behavior therapy (DBT; McCauley et al. 2018; Mehlum et al. 2014). DBT also has multiple randomized controlled trials supporting its effectiveness at reducing self-harm in adults (Cristea et al. 2017). At present, no psychotherapy approaches have been designed for NSSI only.

A meta-analysis of 19 studies of therapeutic interventions for self-harm behavior in adolescents (including studies focused on brief interventions conducted in emergency department settings) found a significant advantage for therapeutic interventions versus control conditions for decreasing self-harm, with the strongest effect sizes for DBT, mentalization-based therapy, and cognitive-behavioral therapy (Ougrin et al. 2015). These treatments have also demonstrated effectiveness at reducing self-harm with adults (Cristea et al. 2017). As noted earlier, treatment studies have differed in the measurement of SA, NSSI, or a broader category of self-harm as the primary outcome variable. All of the treatments studied in randomized controlled trials have targeted either SA or self-harm (Berk 2019). None of the treatments have focused on NSSI exclusively; all include a focus on SA only or SA in addition to self-harm. Hence, treatments have focused on targeting common elements of these behaviors.

Dialectical Behavior Therapy

In the DBT model, emotion dysregulation is considered to be the primary dysfunction leading to self-injurious behaviors and other features of borderline personality disorder (Linehan 1993; Miller et al. 2007). Accordingly, DBT focuses on eliminating self-injurious behaviors by teaching more adaptive coping skills for decreasing emotion dysregulation. Standard DBT is a treatment program consisting of multiple treatment modalities. For adolescents, DBT includes a weekly individual session, a weekly multifamily skills group session, telephone coaching, a weekly consultation team meeting for therapists, and parent and family sessions as needed (Miller et al. 2007). Consistent with the safety recommendations described earlier, DBT closely monitors and targets SA and NSSI through the use of a weekly diary card. Skills such as mindfulness, emotion regulation, distress tolerance, interpersonal effectiveness, and dialectics (e.g., eliminating "either-or" thinking, helping parents/teens solve disagreements by taking into account all perspectives) are taught during the multifamily skills group and individually tailored to each client during individual psychotherapy sessions.

Hospitalization

The American Academy of Child and Adolescent Psychiatry's "Practice Parameter for the Assessment and Treatment of Children and Adolescents With Suicidal Behavior" (Shaffer and Pfeffer 2001) recommends that psychiatric hospitalization be considered if an adolescent is determined to be at high risk of imminent suicidal behavior. Potential benefits of hospitalization may include increased safety due to restricted access to lethal means, close supervision by mental health professionals, immediate access to mental health treatment, and short-term removal from problematic situations that are contributing to the current crisis (e.g., conflict with parents). Hospitalization is typically not required for NSSI unless the degree of medical severity is high. However, given the aforementioned relationship between SI, SA, and NSSI, as well as the difficulty in discerning the presence or absence of suicidal intent, hospitalization may be appropriate if the individual appears to be at imminent risk of SA or medically serious NSSI.

Potential costs of hospitalization should also be considered. At present, no research data support the effectiveness of hospitalization at reducing SA. It has been suggested that hospitalization may even increase suicide behaviors under certain circumstances (Linehan 1993). The increased risk for future SA or NSSI is a primary concern if the hospitalization reinforces these behaviors by providing positive outcomes such as removing the patient from an aversive situation or environment (e.g., not having to take an upcoming final examination) or leading to an increase in positive interpersonal responses (e.g., nurturing, caretaking, or increased attention/concern). Moreover, the removal of the patient from the natural environment limits the opportunity to practice coping effectively with suicidal and self-harm urges and behaviors in that environment, increasing the likelihood of another hospitalization in the future. Another difficulty is the potential for contagion among adolescents on the inpatient unit. Adolescents may discuss methods of SA and NSSI with each other or discuss self-harm as a normative and desirable option.

Case Example

Julia was a 16-year-old white female with a diagnosis of major depressive disorder. Her parents brought her to an intake appointment at an outpatient clinic after she had been discharged the previous day from an inpatient psychiatric unit following an SA by taking an overdose of her prescribed antidepressant medication. Julia also had a history of engaging in NSSI approximately once per month and reported using a razor to make superficial cuts on her forearms to reduce strong emotions and self-critical thoughts. These cuts had not required medical attention.

In the initial session, Julia reported experiencing passive SI ("I wish I was dead") on one occasion since hospital discharge; however, she denied active SI (e.g., thoughts about killing herself), intent, and plan. Julia also denied any current urges to engage in NSSI. Julia's parents reported they had removed all lethal means from the home while Julia was hospitalized, including a search of her bedroom and backpack for items. When the therapist asked Julia if she had any additional means hidden anywhere "just in case," Julia revealed that she had one razor blade hidden in a jewelry box in her bedroom. Her parents were informed of this and agreed to confiscate the razor.

The therapist worked with Julia to create a written safety plan to be used for both suicidal and NSSI urges. Julia reported that warning signs of increased risk were hopelessness ("when I start to feel nothing will ever change and I will feel this way forever"), strong feelings of shame, and perceived rejection by friends. She identified several coping strategies she could use to reduce self-harm urges when warning signs occurred, including drawing, listening to music, watching shows on Netflix, and texting with friends. The therapist questioned Julia about the pros and cons of texting with friends as a coping strategy and discussed the risk of contagion or being triggered by negative peer interactions. Julia agreed to only text a particular friend with whom she has had a consistently good relationship, to not discuss self-harm with this friend, and to notify her parents rather than friends if she feels she is in imminent danger of self-harm. As part of the written safety plan, Julia listed people she could contact in a crisis and identified a reason for living ("because I love my family and would not want to hurt them"). The safety plan also included how to reach the therapist in a crisis, local 24/7 emergency crisis hotline numbers, and a reminder to call 911 or to go to the nearest emergency department if she believed she could no longer stay safe. The safety plan was shared with Julia's parents. Both Julia and her parents were also given wallet-sized cards with the emergency numbers.

The therapist asked Julia to create a hope box and to bring it in to review together. Julia and the therapist spent some time making a list of items Julia could place in the hope box, including paper and pencils for drawing, a list of songs that make her feel happy, a picture of her family, and a copy of her written safety plan. Julia stated she believed she would be able to notify her parents and use the safety plan and hope box as steps to keep herself safe if she experienced urges to attempt suicide or engage in NSSI prior to the next session. The therapist also spoke with Julia's parents about close monitoring. Although Julia denied SI, intent, and plan as well as urges to engage in NSSI during the session, because of her recent hospital discharge for an SA, the therapist recommended that the parents remain with Julia at all times (including having a parent sleep in her room or check on her during the night) until safety could be reassessed. A follow-up session was scheduled for 2 days later in order for the therapist to closely monitor Julia's safety during this high-risk time of transition from inpatient to outpatient care. Julia's parents agreed to closely monitor her, stated they felt they could keep her safe in the home, and agreed to call 911 or take Julia to the emergency department if they believed she was no longer safe. Based on this assessment, the therapist determined that Julia was safe to return home with her parents.

Julia's parents were also informed of the association between family conflict and increased risk of death from suicide in teens and were encouraged to "pick their battles" and prioritize safety. Julia's parents expressed concern about her many absences from school and missed school assignments. The therapist validated these concerns and agreed that they should be addressed in treatment in the future but, for now, recommended the parents avoid arguments and avoid making critical statements about this topic until safety was established. Finally, the therapist recommended that Julia enroll in a comprehensive DBT program, given that it presently has the most empirical evidence for decreasing suicidal and self-harm behaviors in adolescents.

Conclusion

SAs and NSSI are significant public health problems, particularly among teens. Although both are forms of self-injurious behaviors, they can be distinguished based on the intent to die associated with the behavior, with SA being associated with at least some intent to die (Nock 2010) and NSSI not being associated with any intent to die. The focus of recent research has been on identifying the similarities and differences between SA and NSSI in ways that best inform risk assessment and treatment approaches. Of particular importance is recent research showing that NSSI increases the likelihood of future SA and that SI often precedes the first onset of NSSI (Glenn et al. 2017).

These findings underscore the need to take NSSI seriously, to assume that patients engaging in NSSI are at high risk for future SAs, and to engage in risk assessment and safety planning accordingly. DBT has been shown to decrease self-injurious behaviors across multiple clinical trials with adolescents and adults and is considered to be the gold standard treatment for self-harm (Miller 2015). DBT targets both SA and NSSI by identifying the function of the behavior (e.g., reducing emotional distress) for the given individual and finding ways to obtain that function safely using DBT-based coping skills.

Key Points

- Suicide attempts (SAs) and nonsuicidal self-injury (NSSI) are two closely related but distinct forms of self-injurious behavior.

- Youth who engage in NSSI are at high risk for future SA and may have considered suicide prior to their first engagement in NSSI.

- Given its association with suicide ideation and SA, all NSSI should be taken seriously and not dismissed as "suicide gestures" or "attention-seeking" behaviors.

- The clinician should conduct basic safety planning interventions with all youth with histories of SA or NSSI and their parents/caretakers.

- At present, dialectical behavior therapy is the only treatment showing decreases in self-harm behaviors in adolescents that has been replicated.

References

American Psychiatric Association: Diagnostic and Statistical Manual of Mental Disorders, 5th Edition. Arlington, VA, American Psychiatric Association, 2013

Asarnow JR, Porta G, Spirito A, et al: Suicide attempts and nonsuicidal self-injury in the treatment of resistant depression in adolescents: findings from the TORDIA study. J Am Acad Child Adolesc Psychiatry 50(8):772–781, 2011 21784297

Berk MS: Introduction, in Evidence-Based Treatment Approaches for Suicidal Adolescents: Translating Science Into Practice. Edited by Berk MS. Washington, DC, American Psychiatric Association Publishing, 2019, pp 1–18

Berk MS, Clarke S: Safety planning and risk management, in Evidence-Based Treatment Approaches for Suicidal Adolescents: Translating Science Into Practice. Edited by Berk MS. Washington, DC, American Psychiatric Association Publishing, 2019, pp 63–84

Berk MS, Henriques GR, Warman DM, et al: Cognitive therapy for suicide attempters: overview of the treatment and case examples. Cogn Behav Pract 11(3):265–277, 2004

Bresin K, Schoenleber M: Gender differences in the prevalence of nonsuicidal self-injury: a meta-analysis. Clin Psychol Rev 38:55–64, 2015 25795294

Bridge JA, Goldstein TR, Brent DA: Adolescent suicide and suicidal behavior. J Child Psychol Psychiatry 47(3–4):372–394, 2006 16492264

Bush NE, Smolenski DJ, Denneson LM, et al: A virtual hope box: randomized controlled trial of a smartphone app for emotional regulation and coping with distress. Psychiatr Serv 68(4):330–336, 2017 27842473

Carroll R, Thomas KH, Bramley K, et al: Self-cutting and risk of subsequent suicide. J Affect Disord 192:8–10, 2016 26707346

Centers for Disease Control and Prevention: 10 Leading Causes of Death by Age Group—United States 2016. Atlanta, GA, Center for Disease Control and Prevention, 2018. Available at: https://www.cdc.gov/injury/wisqars/pdf/leading_causes_of_death_by_age_group_2016-508.pdf. Accessed November 26, 2018.

Cristea IA, Gentili C, Cotet CD, et al: Efficacy of psychotherapies for borderline personality disorder: a systematic review and meta-analysis. JAMA Psychiatry 74(4):319–328, 2017 28249086

Fowler JC: Suicide risk assessment in clinical practice: pragmatic guidelines for imperfect assessments. Psychotherapy (Chic) 49(1):81–90, 2012 22369082

Franklin JC, Ribeiro JD, Fox KR, et al: Risk factors for suicidal thoughts and behaviors: a meta-analysis of 50 years of research. Psychol Bull 143(2):187–232, 2017 27841450

Glenn CR, Lanzillo EC, Esposito EC, et al: Examining the course of suicidal and nonsuicidal self-injurious thoughts and behaviors in outpatient and inpatient adolescents. J Abnorm Child Psychol 45(5):971–983, 2017 27761783

Gould MS, Marrocco FA, Kleinman M, et al: Evaluating iatrogenic risk of youth suicide screening programs: a randomized controlled trial. JAMA 293(13):1635–1643, 2005 15811983

Insel BJ, Gould MS: Impact of modeling on adolescent suicidal behavior. Psychiatr Clin North Am 31(2):293–316, 2008 18439450

Klonsky ED: The functions of deliberate self-injury: a review of the evidence. Clin Psychol Rev 27(2):226–239, 2007 17014942

Linehan MM: Cognitive-Behavioral Treatment of Borderline Personality Disorder. New York, Guilford, 1993

Mann JJ, Apter A, Bertolote J, et al: Suicide prevention strategies: a systematic review. JAMA 294(16):2064–2074, 2005 16249421

Martin J, Bureau JF, Yurkowski K, et al: Family-based risk factors for non-suicidal self-injury: considering influences of maltreatment, adverse family-life experiences, and parent-child relational risk. J Adolesc 49:170–180, 2016 27086083

McCauley E, Berk MS, Asarnow JR, et al: Efficacy of dialectical behavior therapy for adolescents at high risk for suicide: a randomized clinical trial. JAMA Psychiatry 75(8):777–785, 2018 29926087

Meerwijk EL, Parekh A, Oquendo MA, et al: Direct versus indirect psychosocial and behavioural interventions to prevent suicide and suicide attempts: a systematic review and meta-analysis. Lancet Psychiatry 3(6):544–554, 2016 27017086

Mehlum L, Tørmoen AJ, Ramberg M, et al: Dialectical behavior therapy for adolescents with repeated suicidal and self-harming behavior: a randomized trial. J Am Acad Child Adolesc Psychiatry 53(10):1082–1091, 2014 25245352

Miller AL: Introduction to a special issue dialectical behavior therapy: evolution and adaptations in the 21(st) century. Am J Psychother 69(2):91–95, 2015 26160616

Miller AL, Rathus JH, Linehan MM: Dialectical Behavior Therapy With Suicidal Adolescents. New York, Guilford, 2007

Monto MA, McRee N, Deryck FS: Nonsuicidal self-injury among a representative sample of US adolescents, 2015. Am J Public Health 108(8):1042–1048, 2018 29927642

Muehlenkamp JJ, Gutierrez PM: Risk for suicide attempts among adolescents who engage in non-suicidal self-injury. Arch Suicide Res 11(1):69–82, 2007 17178643

Nock MK: Self-injury. Annu Rev Clin Psychol 6:339–363, 2010 20192787

Nock MK, Joiner TE Jr, Gordon KH, et al: Non-suicidal self-injury among adolescents: diagnostic correlates and relation to suicide attempts. Psychiatry Res 144(1):65–72, 2006 16887199

Ougrin D, Tranah T, Leigh E, et al: Practitioner review: self-harm in adolescents. J Child Psychol Psychiatry 53(4):337–350, 2012 22329807

Ougrin D, Tranah T, Stahl D, et al: Therapeutic interventions for suicide attempts and self-harm in adolescents: systematic review and meta-analysis. J Am Acad Child Adolesc Psychiatry 54(2):97–107, 2015 25617250

Public Health England: Preventing Suicides in Public Places: A Practice Resource. London, Public Health England, 2015. Available at: https://assets.publishing.service.gov.uk/government/uploads/system/uploads/attachment_data/file/481224/Preventing_suicides_in_public_places.pdf. Accessed November 26, 2018.

Shaffer D, Pfeffer CR: Practice parameter for the assessment and treatment of children and adolescents with suicidal behavior. J Am Acad Child Adolesc Psychiatry 40(7 suppl):24S–51S, 2001 11434483

Stanley B, Brown K: Safety planning intervention: a brief intervention to mitigate suicide risk. Cogn Behav Pract 19:256–264, 2012

Stanley B, Brown GK, Brenner LA, et al: Comparison of the safety planning intervention with follow-up vs usual care of suicidal patients treated in the emergency department. JAMA Psychiatry 75(9):894–900, 2018 29998307

Swannell SV, Martin GE, Page A, et al: Prevalence of nonsuicidal self-injury in nonclinical samples: systematic review, meta-analysis and meta-regression. Suicide Life Threat Behav 44(3):273–303, 2014 24422986

U.S. Department of Health and Human Services: What Does "Suicide Contagion" Mean, and What Can Be Done to Prevent It? (website). Washington, DC, U.S. Department of Health and Human Services, 2018. Available at: https://www.hhs.gov/answers/mental-health-and-substance-abuse/what-does-suicide-contagion-mean/index.html. Accessed August 1, 2019.

Whitlock J, Muehlenkamp J, Eckenrode J, et al: Nonsuicidal self-injury as a gateway to suicide in young adults. J Adolesc Health 52(4):486–492, 2013 23298982

Wilkinson P, Kelvin R, Roberts C, et al: Clinical and psychosocial predictors of suicide attempts and nonsuicidal self-injury in the Adolescent Depression Antidepressants and Psychotherapy Trial (ADAPT). Am J Psychiatry 168(5):495–501, 2011 21285141

PART V

Special Topics

CHAPTER 25

Social Media and the Internet

Patricia R. Recupero, J.D., M.D.

In recent years, much has changed with respect to the role of the internet and social media in suicide and its prevention. The research literature on the topic has expanded dramatically. Data from social media and from information and communications technology have taken an increasingly critical role in death investigations, and patients' digital activities are often an important focus for psychiatric case formulation and treatment planning. This chapter presents an update on what is known about the relationship between suicide and social media and the internet, with suggestions for clinicians who are treating patients at risk for death from suicide. The chapter is organized into three sections to offer starting points for further reading and treatment planning: 1) "Social Networking and Behavior," 2) "Information Access," and 3) "Growing Role of Artificial Intelligence and Software."

Social Networking and Behavior

Although the topic remains controversial and additional research is needed, some evidence suggests that specific types of internet and social media activities may increase suicide risk, particularly among youth and young adults. Some scholars argue that the proliferation of social media may be a contributing factor to the concurrent rise in suicide rates (Aboujaoude 2016; Luxton et al. 2012). The research literature in this area vastly exceeds what can be covered in this brief overview, but clinicians should be familiar with some of the major trends, including harassment and humiliation; baiting, incitement, and suicide voyeurism; problematic internet use and media-related risk factors; disclosure of suicidal ideation via social media; and peer support and protective factors.

Harassment and Humiliation

Digital victimization, such as cyberbullying, is linked to a number of important suicide risk factors, including various psychiatric symptoms, emotional difficulties, thwarted belongingness, and perceived burdensomeness. Cyberbullying victimization has been correlated with suicidal ideation, seeking suicide-related content online, problematic internet use, and suicide attempts (Mitchell et al. 2018). In 2017, 14.9% of high-school youth in the United States were victims of cyberbullying, and victimization rates were greater among sexual minority youth (27.1% of lesbian, gay, or bisexual youth and 22% of those unsure of their sexual identity), who experience higher rates of death from suicide (Division of Adolescent and School Health 2018; see also Chapter 23, "Suicide and Gender").

Cyberharassment may include public humiliation or extortion, such as the real or threatened exposure of sensitive personal information. This may include sexts (sexually explicit personal photographs) sent to former romantic partners; bullies masquerading as prospective partners (catfishing); or online publishing of private information (a practice known as "doxing") such as one's home address, family members' contact information, and social security numbers. Public shaming via social media tends to go viral quickly, frequently resulting in targets being harassed and insulted by strangers and, often, losing their jobs. Depression and suicidal ideation are correlated with these types of harassment, and they may contribute to other suicide risk factors, such as the feeling of entrapment. Researchers have also described a self-sabotaging form of social networking in vulnerable individuals, wherein one posts or directs damaging content toward oneself. Patchin and Hinduja (2017) called this behavior "digital self-harm" and defined it as "the anonymous online posting, sending, or otherwise sharing of hurtful content about oneself" (Patchin and Hinduja 2017, p. 761).

Baiting, Incitement, and Suicide Voyeurism

Although little academic research has explored these phenomena, cases of suicide baiting or incitement and voyeurism garner a considerable amount of coverage in the popular press. In today's hyperconnected world, these behaviors often involve social networking applications. Livestreamed suicides appear to be growing more frequent, and baiting comments are commonplace in social media. Trolls (internet users who post inflammatory content to provoke arguments or upset other users) seek out vulnerable individuals for abusive vitriol, and baiting statements such as "the world would be better off without you" are, unfortunately, omnipresent in the comment feeds of popular social networking sites such as YouTube, Reddit, and Twitter. Phillips and Mann (2019) explored a small sample ($N=26$) of cases in which a suicidal person disclosed an intention to die from suicide via webcam; in 11 of those cases (44%), suicide baiting was observed. Viewers offered helpful assistance (e.g., efforts to dissuade the suicide attempt) in 88% of cases, but the suicidal person followed through with the attempt in 92% of cases. Depression-support chat rooms are also plagued by trolls who engage in jeering, verbal abuse, and suicide baiting.

Young persons may engage in high-risk behavior to solicit more "likes" and subscribers on social media, and participation in viral challenges and games may increase the risk of self-harm and suicidal behavior (Nesi and Prinstein 2018). These challenges may involve potentially fatal behavior (e.g., the "choking game"), and some challenge-based electronic games reportedly feature suicide baiting in the final task. Cases of suicide incitement linked to the internet and social media, such as the 2014 Massachusetts case of a teenage girl who, via text messages, encouraged her boyfriend to kill himself, present significant challenges with respect to prosecution and deterrence (Binder and Chiesa 2018). However, many jurisdictions have criminalized actions of aiding, advising, or encouraging someone to attempt suicide (e.g., California Penal Code 2019).

Problematic Internet Use and Media-Related Risk Factors

Empirical research supports a connection between problematic internet use and suicide risk. Although the interactions are complex and require further research, problematic use of technology and social media has been correlated with suicidal ideation, suicide attempts, social isolation, and other risk factors (Cheng et al. 2018), with increasing screen time predicting decreasing psychological well-being in youth (Twenge et al. 2018). The inclusion of internet gaming disorder as a condition for further study in DSM-5 (American Psychiatric Association 2013) reflects a growing consensus in the psychiatric community that problematic use of electronic media is a significant clinical concern that treatment providers should expect to encounter in their regular practice, perhaps with increasing frequency. During the clinical interview, just as one asks patients about their consumption of alcohol and use of drugs, inquiries about the patient's media habits should be routine. Table 25–1 presents some suggested assessment questions and discussion prompts to help psychiatrists elicit more detailed information about a patient's internet and social media use and whether current use may be cause for concern.

Internet use may also affect suicide risk when the behavior is not considered excessive or abnormal. For example, the term "phubbing" was coined to describe the practice of snubbing one's conversation partner(s) in favor of scrolling through social feeds on one's smartphone, and this behavior is fairly common. Uncivil commentary in social media is also prevalent. These aspects of the technology may increase feelings of social disconnection and thwarted belongingness. Preliminary research supports a relationship between normative social media use and suicide risk factors such as depression, self-harm, and social isolation, although this relationship is a complex interaction between multiple individual risk and protective factors (Luxton et al. 2012). To determine the likely effect of social media and internet use on an individual patient's suicide risk, the clinician must gain an understanding of the patient's unique strengths and vulnerabilities, situational risk and protective factors, and the ways in which they use information and communications technology.

Disclosure of Suicidal Ideation via Social Media

The disclosure of suicidal ideation via social networking sites and other social media is now fairly common. Such posts range from vague hints (e.g., "wish I weren't here," "can't take this anymore") to explicit announcements of an intent to die from suicide and "goodbye" messages that are, in some ways, analogous to written suicide notes. The disclosure of suicidal ideation via social media has led to successful rescues of individuals in imminent risk and, frequently, an outpouring of social support and encouragement for the suicidal person.

Unfortunately, vulnerable individuals face the risk that their posts will be met with derision and suicide baiting, although such malicious behavior does not appear to be the normative response. There is also a risk that suicidal persons will use the internet

TABLE 25–1.   Suggested clinical interview questions and discussion prompts

Harassment and humiliation

Is there anyone that you interact with online who isn't respectful toward you?

Has anyone ever posted something online about you without your permission?

Baiting, incitement, and suicide voyeurism

Has anyone you interact with on [Twitter/Reddit/4chan/YouTube] ever told you that you should kill yourself or that the world would be a better place without you?

Online, have you seen people posting comments like "If you were really suicidal you would do it tomorrow" or "You're just looking for attention. Pathetic."?

Have you ever watched a video of someone's suicide or suicide attempt (or self-harm) online?

Problematic internet use and media-related risk factors

How many hours do you spend online in a typical day, including using your smartphone?

Have you ever had difficulty tearing yourself away from your phone?

Do you scroll through your news feed when you are with your friends or family? Do your friends or family members ever do this when you are together?

Have any of your friends or family said you should cut down on your internet or phone use?

Have you tried to cut down on your time on social media or done a "digital detox" (or thought about it)?

Have you ever felt guilty about how you use your smartphone?

Disclosure of suicidal ideation via social media

Are you open with your [friends online/followers] about what you're going through?

Has anyone ever said that something you posted on [Facebook/Twitter/Instagram] made them feel worried or concerned about you? Or prompted them to ask you if you were okay?

Peer support and protective factors

Are your followers supportive, for the most part?

Do you belong to any Facebook groups?

Are there any things that you find easier to talk about online than face-to-face?

Information access

Have you used your phone or the internet to visit sites or forums related to death or dying?

When you have felt suicidal in the past, have you ever looked up different ways to kill yourself online? (If yes: What did you find?)

Have you ever come across materials online that present suicide as a good idea when someone is suffering greatly from emotional pain or other circumstances? (If yes: Explore whether the patient has interacted with others in the forum.)

What suicide methods have you considered? (Pay attention to the patient's answer; a plan involving nitrogen or helium asphyxiation, charcoal burning, or any unusual method may be a clue that the patient has been researching methods online, and this may be a critical point from a risk-management perspective.)

to arrange suicide pacts with others (Luxton et al. 2012). Although their sample size was small and consistent with the statistical rarity of suicide, Phillips and Mann (2019) found a troubling rate of high-lethality means when plans for suicides were announced online. Furthermore, the permanency of internet content and the stigma attached to suicide may present additional problems, such as future discrimination against the person or their loved ones.

From a clinical risk-management perspective, there may be good reason to review patients' recent social media activity in cases of undetermined suicidal intent or unknown toxicology in a suicide attempt in acute situations. Waters et al. (2018) described an illustrative case example in which a suicide victim had posted her suicide plan on social media, but the post was not discovered in time; had it been found, she would have received different emergency medical treatment that may have saved her life. In cases of murder-suicide and mass violence, the perpetrator's violent fantasies, threats, and suicidal intent often are posted online before the incident, sometimes in the form of manifestos or statements made through video-sharing applications. Although "patient-targeted Googling" and reviewing patients' social media activity remain controversial in the psychiatric literature, these practices could be lifesaving in certain clinical situations. Mental health professionals who do such searches, however, should consider factors such as the reliability of the information, boundary concerns, mandated reporting laws, and confidentiality and privacy issues. The frequency of suicidal ideation disclosures on social media, coupled with the reluctance of many suicidal patients to be forthcoming with clinicians, raises a number of ethical concerns for health care professionals.

Peer Support and Protective Factors

Peer support via social media is playing an increasingly prominent role in mental health and suicide prevention. Scholars and patient advocates have called for better integration of evidence-based practices into existing peer-support networks as dialogues regarding mental health and suicide already take place on social networking channels with or without the participation of mental health professionals and public-health agencies. High-risk suicidal youth often go online for social support, and these connections and exchanges can be positive or negative.

Fortunately, organizations and individuals involved in mental health advocacy work have developed a variety of different social media–based suicide-prevention initiatives and tools. Most of the prominent social networking services now provide a feature whereby someone who is concerned about a friend can quickly activate interactive suicide-prevention resources for the person. As discussed later, technology is evolving toward automated recognition of acute suicide risk through electronic tools such as content-flagging algorithms. With these algorithms, posting a comment such as "I want to kill myself" may trigger an automated chatbot to message the person with resources such as phone numbers for crisis hotlines and links to crisis-intervention websites.

Social media and the internet play important roles in bereavement support and suicide postvention (i.e., risk reduction and promotion of healing following a death from suicide), possibly shaping the sociological factors involved in suicide. For example, media coverage of the suicides of LGBTQ teens who were bullied due to their sexual orientation or gender identity, and subsequent sharing through social media, helped to increase public awareness of the health disparities and minority stress experienced by many LGBTQ youth. This prompted increased support for vulnerable youth and for organizations such as the Trevor Project that are engaged in suicide-prevention advocacy. The internet and social media have also enabled the formation of larger networks of social support for marginalized groups, including robust peer-support resources for persons with mental illness and substance use disorders, which may help to reduce their suicide risk. From a clinical perspective, understanding the ways in which a patient seeks support from peers online can provide a better picture of their overall risk and may identify important protective factors to draw upon in treatment planning.

Information Access

The ease and speed of information access through the internet has had a considerable impact on trends and risk factors for death from suicide throughout the world. Internet-based information access is an important factor to consider when performing risk assessments and developing treatment plans for patients at risk for death from suicide. In the more than 10 years since I published a study investigating the phenomenon of "Googling suicide" (Recupero et al. 2008), the literature on this topic has expanded dramatically. For example, recent research has demonstrated that

- Persons who seek out suicide-related information online tend to have higher levels of suicidal ideation and intent as well as numerous suicide risk factors compared with those who do not use the internet for suicide-related reasons (Padmanathan et al. 2018).
- Suicide-related internet use is more prevalent among children and adolescents than among middle-aged and older adults (Padmanathan et al. 2018).
- The motivation for suicide-related internet use varies; sometimes a person is searching for information about methods, but sometimes he or she is seeking social support. In either case, however, what the person finds may be harmful or beneficial.

Pro-suicide forums and pro-suicide content are still easily accessible on the web, just as they were 10 years ago (Mörch et al. 2018). Patients may also encounter misinformation online, such as antipsychiatry messaging and active discouragement of treatment for mental illness. Psychiatrists may find it helpful to ask patients what they have read about mental health and its treatment; much of such reading these days is performed online, through smartphones. Embracing a collaborative approach and directing patients to helpful psychoeducation with empirically supported information online may help to support treatment engagement and a strong therapeutic alliance.

Suicide Methods

Information access was historically understood to be a factor in the higher rates of death from suicide among medical professionals via specialized knowledge about methods with greater lethality (e.g., calculating lethal dose of prescription medication). The internet and social media have impacted the accessibility of this type of information, increasing the likelihood that suicidal patients will be aware of different high-lethality methods such as inert-gas asphyxiation, formerly a rare choice of method. Detailed descriptions of various suicide methods and step-by-step directions for carrying them out are very easily and quickly accessible online by suicidal persons. Rising rates of suffocation-based suicides, particularly among children and adolescents, are cause for concern given the ease with which youth may learn such methods through social media; these types of methods are not amenable to means-restriction interventions such as suicide barriers on bridges and firearm purchase restrictions (Skinner and McFaull 2012). The internet also provides easy access to lethal means, particularly through darknet channels (Mörch et al. 2018). The purchase of firearms or their components, chemicals, plant toxins, synthetic opioids, and various novel psychoactive substances may be facilitated through social media, even when their sale is illegal.

Contagion Effects

Suicide contagion is a potential concern with respect to information access in the social networking age. Celebrity deaths from suicide often prompt subsequent upticks in suicide-related internet searches and commentary on social networking sites such as Twitter, but the significance of these trends varies, particularly on the individual patient level. In 2017, Netflix released an adaptation of a novel about a teenage girl's suicide, *13 Reasons Why*, amid a flurry of controversy and interest. Some experts in suicide prevention advocacy expressed concerns about the show's content. In the days after the series premiered, Ayers et al. (2017) found a 19% increase in suicide-related internet search queries across both potentially harmful (e.g., "how to kill yourself") and helpful ("suicide hotline") searches. Two widely-reported studies (Bridge et al. 2019; Niederkrotenthaler et al. 2019) also found significant increases in rates of youth suicide overall after the show was released.

Epidemiology and Public Health

Currently, epidemiological research literature findings are inconsistent as to whether changes in the rate of internet searches for suicide information can predict increases in suicide attempts or death rates for the general population or specific subsets of the population. Some studies have found such a correlation whereas others have not (Bruckner et al. 2014). Predictive analytics tools such as Google Trends are not yet precise enough to reliably predict suicide clusters, but this may change in the near future given the pace of research in this area.

Although advocates have promulgated media reporting guidelines to help mitigate contagion-related risks of irresponsible reporting, private individuals who have considerable reach through social media are not bound by equivalent ethical standards. Furthermore, some social media "influencers" have been accused of monetizing their appeal to vulnerable followers through endorsements of marginal business entities that market unregulated services and products to persons struggling with mental health difficulties. For this reason, clinicians may find it helpful to inquire whether the patient follows any content creators on sites such as YouTube, Twitter, and Instagram and whether their channels or feeds contain any content related to mental health, suicide, or psychiatric treatment.

The internet and social media have also enabled new forms of suicide prevention and media messaging campaigns designed to increase awareness and decrease stigma (Luxton et al. 2012; Till et al. 2017; Torous et al. 2018). After a death from suicide is widely covered in the popular press, the subsequent dialogue on social media about the death is now punctuated by comments sharing crisis-information resources, such as the phone number for the National Suicide-Prevention Lifeline or the Crisis Text Line. Additionally, some gatekeeper training programs, intended to help laypersons identify individuals at risk for death from suicide or otherwise in need of psychiatric treatment and to facilitate treatment entry, have been adapted for internet-based deployment.

Clinical Implications of Internet-Based Information Access

Evidence that adaptive, help-seeking internet use results in reduced suicidal ideation or intent over time is limited. This suggests that changes in suicide-related internet activity may be important markers for a patient's level of risk acuity, particularly in patients with fluctuating levels of suicidal ideation and intent over time. As Padmanathan et al. (2018) argued, "Internet use may be a proxy for [suicidal] intent" (p. 469). Table 25–1 suggests several questions to help guide clinical discussions about a patient's internet and social media use when the patient is at risk for death from suicide.

Growing Role of Artificial Intelligence and Software

Perhaps the most significant technological change for suicide assessment and management since the previous edition of this textbook has been the pace of advances in artificial intelligence and software applications, many of which involve the internet and social media. In 2019, academic journals published a seemingly endless stream of studies evaluating the use and potential of machine learning and algorithms for suicide prevention. The following discussion offers clinicians a brief overview of some key trends in this rapidly developing field, focusing specifically on their use in social media and the internet.

Predictive Analytics

One of the most promising recent developments has been the creation of predictive analytics to forecast the likelihood that an individual will attempt suicide based on their language patterns and features of their social media activity. These algorithms can enable automated detection of persons at high suicide risk for targeted intervention. For example, researchers have found that

- The language someone uses on Facebook (Eichstaedt et al. 2018) or the photos one shares and likes on Instagram (Torous et al. 2018) can predict the likelihood of depression.
- Clinically significant suicide risk can be accurately identified in social media communications by machine-learning algorithms, enabling automated intervention even before a troubling social post is flagged by other users for suicidal content.

Torous et al. (2018) provided a helpful and comprehensive overview of the current status of research on machine learning and smartphones for suicide prevention, predicting that clinically useful tools with strong empirical support will be available by 2023.

Proliferation of Mental Health Software ("Apps") and Internet Interventions

In the 2010s, smartphones began to replace other forms of communication for many individuals. Like other resources formerly based in brick-and-mortar facilities, crisis intervention services have been shifting toward electronic, internet-based options. Text messaging and chat functions are in increasing demand for crisis intervention, particularly among younger persons, many of whom prefer these media (e.g., Crisis

TABLE 25–2. **Factors to consider in evaluating mental health applications**

American Psychiatric Association Application Evaluation Model	Chan et al. 2015
1. Gather background information	**Usefulness**
2. Risk/Privacy and security	Validity and accuracy
3. Evidence	Reliability
4. Ease of use	Effectiveness
5. Interoperability	Time and number of sessions
	Usability
	Satisfaction and reward
	Usability
	Disability accessibility
	Cultural accessibility
	Socioeconomic and generational accessibility
	Integration and infrastructure
	Security
	Workflow integration
	Data integration
	Safety
	Privacy

Text Line) over telephone-based services. Similarly, demand for internet-based mental health treatment options remains high, and content developers have responded accordingly with an overwhelming variety of mental health applications ("apps") for smartphones. Clinicians should recognize that a significant portion of their cases today will involve patients who are using social media and smartphone apps for adjunctive mental health support, and it would be prudent to help patients make informed decisions about which apps to use.

Several apps and app-facilitated interventions have been designed specifically for suicide prevention. Among those under development, As Safe as Possible (ASAP; Kennard et al. 2018) and MYPLAN (Buus et al. 2018) have some initial positive results from clinical trials. ASAP is specifically designed for patients just discharged from inpatient hospitalization, which is a time of especially high suicide risk. Not all apps are well suited for all patients, however, and study results for other apps are mixed. Clinicians are encouraged to consult the American Psychiatric Association's (APA; 2018) App Evaluation Model or similar tools for guidance before discussing mental health apps with patients. Table 25–2 compares the APA's evaluation model and another excellent option (Chan et al. 2015) that clinicians may wish to consider when evaluating the risks and benefits of a particular application or program. In addition to patient- or client-facing software, there are applications designed to assist health care providers with suicide risk assessment and management, such as the Substance Abuse and Mental Health Services Administration's Suicide Safe app.

High demand for mental health services and limited access among those who need treatment have helped to spur the development and adoption of internet-based self-help approaches. Results from empirical research studies of these treatment modalities thus far have been inconsistent. Furthermore, app-facilitated services, analogous to ride-sharing apps such as Uber, are now available, marketing unlicensed private individuals as "trained specialists" to help individuals with mental health difficulties. Whether such business models will be pursued for the unlicensed practice of psychotherapy remains to be seen, but vulnerable individuals may engage these services due to their lower cost than traditional psychotherapy and medical treatment. From the clinical perspective, high-quality evidence is insufficient to recommend the use of adjunctive self-help programs online. However, because these programs may be marketed to suicidal persons via social media, it is advisable to ask the patient about all strategies they are using or considering to manage their symptoms, including digital tools and self-help approaches.

The development of ecological momentary assessment has been a boon to mental health researchers, and its use seems poised to expand significantly in suicidology and clinical risk management over the next several years (Kleiman et al. 2018). *Ecological momentary assessment* refers to the assessment of variables in real time, typically via smartphone. For example, patients may download and install an app that prompts them at specific time intervals to respond to questions from validated measures of suicide risk assessment, such as those discussed in Chapter 1 ("Suicide Risk Assessment"), that have been adapted for mobile electronic use. This real-time monitoring of dynamic risk factors enables earlier intervention for patients approaching crisis points, improved understanding of how suicide risk variables interact to increase the likelihood of decompensation or recovery, and strategies to focus on specific risk and protective factors for maximum treatment efficiency (Torous et al. 2018).

Wearables and sensor technology can provide even more detailed information about a patient's condition (Torous et al. 2018): digital pills recently approved by the U.S. Food and Drug Administration can now provide evidence of medication compliance; smartwatches can track a patient's movements; smartphones can detect the pace and volume of the user's speech; and data analysis tools can help to detect changes in these patterns over time. In the near future, clinicians are likely to see valid, empirically based tools that can, for example, reliably predict the onset of a manic or depressive episode in bipolar disorder.

Several empirically supported treatment methods and screening tools have been adapted for internet-based use. Internet-based cognitive-behavioral therapy (iCBT), for example, has been shown to reduce several suicide risk factors, including suicidal ideation, substance abuse, and symptoms of depression and anxiety. Among medical interns, a population at statistically greater risk for death from suicide, the use of brief, web-based iCBT was associated with a reduced likelihood of suicidal ideation (Guille et al. 2015). Electronic screening for depression and suicidal ideation may improve suicide risk detection and engagement in high-risk populations, such as men, who may be reluctant to endorse suicidal ideation or planning in face-to-face clinical interviews. Like smartphone apps and iCBT, some text-messaging interventions have also been found helpful for lessening suicide risk, although data are insufficient to recommend their adoption at this time.

Important risk management issues should be considered for the use of internet-based treatment methods, such as telepsychiatry, in patients at high risk for death from suicide. These complex issues are beyond the scope of this chapter, but the research literature on general clinical telepsychiatry and telemental health often covers suicide-related risks. Clinicians who are new to videoconferencing and other types of electronic treatment (such as iCBT) should first consult the existing clinical practice guidelines for their use, of which there are many. A partial listing of professional organizations that have published such guidance includes the APA, the American Telemedicine Association, the American Academy of Child and Adolescent Psychiatry, the Federation of State Medical Boards, the American Medical Association, and the American Psychological Association.

Conclusion

Due to the increasingly central role that technology plays in our day-to-day lives, the importance of understanding a suicidal patient's internet and social media use cannot be overstated. Electronic social networking has transformed the ways in which we connect with one another, for better and for worse. The internet has dramatically changed the landscape of information access for persons at risk of death from suicide and their loved ones, directly impacting the formation of suicide plans and suicide postvention. Finally, mental health professionals should pay close attention to emerging developments in the clinical applications of artificial intelligence and software, because these technologies are poised to take on a central, potentially lifesaving role in the practice of evidence-based suicide risk management.

Key Points

- Specific types of social networking may affect dynamic risk factors for death from suicide, such as suicidal ideation, depressive symptoms, and social support.

- Cyberharassment, incitement through social media, and similar behaviors may increase a patient's suicide risk.

- The disclosure of suicidal ideation is common in social media, and such posts are often met with supportive responses from peers, potentially facilitating treatment entry.

- The internet may directly affect a patient's decision to attempt suicide and may also influence the chosen method. Information about suicide methods with high lethality, some of which are not amenable to means restriction, is readily accessible online.

- Patients with higher levels of suicide risk are more likely to search for information about suicide online.

- Predictive analytics and smartphone apps are actively shaping the field of suicide research, and clinical use of these tools in the assessment and management of suicidal patients is likely to increase significantly in the near future.

References

Aboujaoude E: Rising suicide rates: an under-recognized role for the internet? World Psychiatry 15(3):225–227, 2016 27717270

American Psychiatric Association: Diagnostic and Statistical Manual of Mental Disorders, 5th Edition. Arlington, VA, American Psychiatric Association, 2013

American Psychiatric Association: App Evaluation Model (website). Washington, DC, American Psychiatric Association, 2018. Available at: https://www.psychiatry.org/psychiatrists/practice/mental-health-apps/app-evaluation-model. Accessed November 1, 2018.

Ayers JW, Althouse BM, Leas EC, et al: Internet searches for suicide following the release of 13 Reasons Why. JAMA Intern Med 177(10):1527–1529, 2017 28759671

Binder G, Chiesa L: The puzzle of inciting suicide. American Criminal Law Review 56(1):65–133, 2018

Bridge JA, Greenhouse JB, Ruch D, et al: Association between the release of Netflix's 13 Reasons Why and suicide rates in the United States: an interrupted time series analysis. J Am Acad Child Adolesc Psychiatry 2019 Epub ahead of print

Bruckner TA, McClure C, Kim Y: Google searches for suicide and risk of suicide. Psychiatr Serv 65(2):271–272, 2014 24492910

Buus N, Erlangsen A, River J, et al: Stakeholder perspectives on using and developing the MY-PLAN suicide prevention mobile phone application: a focus group study. Arch Suicide Res 2018 Epub ahead of print

California Penal Code Section 401. (2019) Available at: https://leginfo.legislature.ca.gov/faces/codes_displaySection.xhtml?lawCode=PENandsectionNum=401.andhighlight=trueandkeyword=suicide. Accessed January 8, 2019.

Chan S, Torous J, Hinton L, et al: Towards a framework for evaluating mobile mental health apps. Telemed J E Health 21(12):1038–1041, 2015 26171663

Cheng YS, Tseng PT, Lin PY, et al: Internet addiction and its relationship with suicidal behaviors: a meta-analysis of multinational observational studies. J Clin Psychiatry 79(4):e1–e15, 2018 29877640

Division of Adolescent and School Health: Youth Risk Behavior Survey Data Summary and Trends Report, 2007–2017. Atlanta, GA, Centers for Disease Control and Prevention, 2018

Eichstaedt JC, Smith RJ, Merchant RM, et al: Facebook language predicts depression in medical records. Proc Natl Acad Sci USA 115(44):11203–11208, 2018

Guille C, Zhao Z, Krystal J, et al: Web-based cognitive behavioral therapy intervention for the prevention of suicidal ideation in medical interns: a randomized controlled trial. JAMA Psychiatry 72(12):1192–1198, 2015 26535958

Kennard BD, Goldstein T, Foxwell AA, et al: As Safe As Possible (ASAP): a brief app-supported inpatient intervention to prevent postdischarge suicidal behavior in hospitalized, suicidal adolescents. Am J Psychiatry 175(9):864–872, 2018 30021457

Kleiman EM, Turner BJ, Fedor S, et al: Digital phenotyping of suicidal thoughts. Depress Anxiety 35(7):601–608, 2018 29637663

Luxton DD, June JD, Fairall JM: Social media and suicide: a public health perspective. Am J Public Health 102(suppl 2):S195–S200, 2012 22401525

Mitchell SM, Seegan PL, Roush JF, et al: Retrospective cyberbullying and suicidal ideation: the mediating roles of depressive symptoms, perceived burdensomeness, and thwarted belongingness. J Interpers Violence 33(16):2602–2620, 2018 26862162

Mörch CM, Côté LP, Corthésy-Blondin L, et al: The darknet and suicide. J Affect Disord 241:127–132, 2018 30118946

Nesi J, Prinstein MJ: In search of likes: longitudinal associations between adolescents' digital status seeking and health-risk behaviors. J Clin Child Adolesc Psychol 2018 Epub ahead of print

Niederkrotenthaler T, Stack S, Till B, et al: Association of increased youth suicides in the United States with the release of 13 Reasons Why. JAMA Psychiatry 2019 Epub ahead of print

Padmanathan P, Biddle L, Carroll R, et al: Suicide and self-harm related internet use: a cross-sectional study and clinician focus groups. Crisis 39(6):469–478, 2018

Patchin JW, Hinduja S: Digital self-harm among adolescents. J Adolesc Health 61(6):761–766, 2017 28935385

Phillips JG, Mann L: Suicide baiting in the internet era. Computers in Human Behavior 92:29–36, 2019

Recupero PR, Harms SE, Noble JM: Googling suicide: surfing for suicide information on the internet. J Clin Psychiatry 69(6):878–888, 2008 18494533

Skinner R, McFaull S: Suicide among children and adolescents in Canada: trends and sex differences, 1980–2008. CMAJ 184(9):1029–1034, 2012 22470172

Till B, Tran US, Voracek M, et al: Beneficial and harmful effects of educative suicide prevention websites: randomised controlled trial exploring Papageno v. Werther effects. Br J Psychiatry 211(2):109–115, 2017 28522433

Torous J, Larsen ME, Depp C, et al: Smartphones, sensors, and machine learning to advance real-time prediction and interventions for suicide prevention: a review of current progress and next steps. Curr Psychiatry Rep 20(7):51, 2018 29956120

Twenge JM, Martin GN, Campbell WK: Decreases in psychological well-being among American adolescents after 2012 and links to screen time during the rise of smartphone technology. Emotion 18(6):765–780, 2018 29355336

Waters B, Hara K, Ikematsu N, et al: An unusual case of suicide by methanol ingestion. Forensic Sci Int 289:e9–e14, 2018 29908646

CHAPTER 26

Physician-Assisted Dying

Nathan Fairman, M.D., M.P.H.

Clinicians who take care of patients near the very end of their lives might be surprised to find a chapter on physician-assisted dying (PAD) in a book, aimed at psychiatrists, about suicide risk assessment and management. In the United States, the practice of PAD, often positioned as a "palliative option of last resort," is an intervention in which terminally ill adults with intact decisional capacity, having met certain qualification steps, may be prescribed a lethal dose of a drug, which they can choose to self-administer, in order to bring about a peaceful death.

Whether aid in dying should be considered a form of suicide in the "traditional" sense is still a subject of debate. Using a narrow definition of suicide as any "death caused by self-directed injurious behavior with intent to die as a result of the behavior" (Centers for Disease Control and Prevention 2018), PAD should perhaps be considered a form of suicide. However, in a "traditional" suicide, for example, a young man with schizophrenia who shoots himself under the influence of command hallucinations, a broad range of obligations falls to the psychiatrist to protect individuals made vulnerable by a state of diminished autonomy. There is broad agreement that efforts to prevent this outcome—involving mental health professionals, law enforcement agents, mental health institutions, and public health agencies—are warranted on ethical, professional, and legal grounds. By contrast, a typical case of PAD might involve a woman in the final stages of an advanced cancer who works with her doctor to qualify for an aid-in-dying drug and then uses it with the hope of minimizing her suffering as she dies. The professional and legal obligations that arise in such a case remain unclear; PAD stands apart in important ways from the kind of suicide that has been the focus of other chapters in this book.

Including PAD in a discussion about suicide risk assessment and management points to the importance of being able to draw distinctions between different acts that may influence the timing of death. This challenge has emerged in recent decades, in particular in the setting of caring for individuals with terminal diseases, because advances in medical therapeutics have increasingly left seriously ill patients with choices that offer stark tradeoffs between quality and quantity of life. The American philosopher John Hardwig (2009) captured this as an historical shift in which individuals have moved from working to avoid a death that was likely to come too soon to trying to avoid a death that has come too late:

> The differences between this new death and the death of former times are profound. When the sensible fear is that death will come too soon, the reasonable course is to flee it—try to postpone it or put it off…. However, many of us now worry that death will come too late—long after life has lost its usefulness and its savor, long after we have ceased to have a "life," perhaps long after we even are ourselves. When the more sensible fear is that death will come too late, the reasonable course is to make death come sooner—to seek it out. Learning how to go to meet death is, I believe, one of the basic tasks of our time. (p. 38)

Psychiatrists do not generally play a central role in the care of the dying, although some advocate that they should (Fairman et al. 2016). However, the practice of PAD and the implementation of aid-in-dying laws raise questions that often call for the expertise of psychiatrists. For example, in the specific setting of caring for individuals nearing the end of life, can a space exist within which patients can be allowed, under certain conditions, to deliberately bring about their own deaths—without triggering the standard psychiatric assumptions about mental illness, incapacity, and the pursuant professional duties to intervene? Perhaps more critically, do psychiatrists have a role to play in identifying that space or in providing care to patients struggling with this end-of-life issue?

A review of suicide risk assessment and management benefits from a discussion of PAD for two reasons. First, although most of the practice of PAD falls outside the scope of psychiatric care, some individuals who pursue aid in dying will have significant psychiatric symptoms or comorbid mental illness, and there may be a critical need for psychiatric diagnostic assessment and treatment recommendations as well as a need for assistance with clarifying decisional capacity. Second, the geographic footprint of legal aid in dying in the United States has expanded substantially in the past decade, a trend that appears likely to continue. Hence, in the future, more and more psychiatrists can expect to be practicing in states where dying patients may request and obtain a lethal dose of medication to end their lives. For these reasons, it has become increasingly important for psychiatrists to be knowledgeable about the practice of aid in dying, its legal status, how it is positioned among the range of options in end-of-life care, how it is viewed by professional organizations, and the roles that psychiatrists might play in the implementation of laws where the practice is legal.

Nomenclature

Opinions about the legitimacy of PAD are deeply divided, and proponents and opponents frequently spar over language used to describe this practice. In public discourse, chosen labels seem to primarily serve a rhetorical purpose, often advancing a particular advocacy position. One might envision these efforts on a continuum (see Figure 26–1): at one end, "death with dignity" conveys the peaceful, autonomous ending that many would like to have, while at the other end, "assisted suicide" links the practice to a wide range of morally objectionable acts (Macauley 2018). Those terms often appear to serve a signaling function (i.e., to indicate which camp the speaker is in) rather than a clarifying one (i.e., to assist patients and families with thinking clearly about interventions in the setting of end-of-life care).

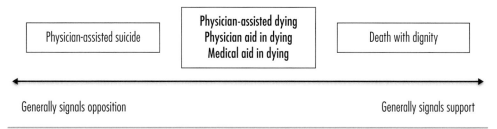

FIGURE 26–1. Continuum of nomenclature for physician-assisted dying.

From a legal standpoint, in all states where the practice is regulated, PAD is defined in explicit statutory language as "*not* suicide." In California, for example, where the End of Life Option Act went into effect in 2016, the law states "death resulting from the self-administration of an aid-in-dying drug is not suicide" (California End of Life Option Act 2016). The fact that ethics and philosophy literature still commonly refer to PAD as suicide, and sometimes categorize it as a form of "voluntary active euthanasia," may contribute to some confusion on this point (Dworkin 2007). Generally, philosophical discussions about PAD accept the notion that suicide can be either rational or irrational and that some suicides warrant particular kinds of intervention (e.g., involuntary detainment or public health investments in prevention) while others do not. These efforts essentially seek to retain the use of the word *suicide* while uncoupling the narrow definition from its broader moral, religious, social, and political attachments (Dworkin 2007; Hardwig 2009).

Finally, older references in the medical literature often use the term "physician-assisted suicide." Advocacy groups opposed to the practice of PAD retain this nomenclature; conversely, advocacy organizations that promote PAD laws often use the phrase "death with dignity." In general, more recent discourse in the medical literature has moved away from the language of suicide. In light of ethically relevant differences between the practice of aid in dying and so-called traditional suicide, and reflecting the importance of maintaining a "patient-centered" orientation to medical care, most current work in the clinical context uses one of the following terms: *physician-assisted dying, physician aid in dying,* or *medical aid in dying.* The American Academy of Hospice and Palliative Medicine (2016), which maintains a position of "studied neutrality" on PAD, uses the term *physician-assisted dying.* That nomenclature is followed here.

Status of Physician-Assisted Dying

Although this chapter's focus is limited to the practice of PAD in the United States, assisted dying is also available in several jurisdictions internationally, including Switzerland, Belgium, the Netherlands, Luxembourg, Colombia, and Canada (Emanuel et al. 2016; Orentlicher 2016). Of note, the eligibility criteria for PAD in other countries tend to be less restrictive than in the United States in ways that can raise particular challenges for psychiatrists. For example, laws in several countries do not stipulate explicitly that patients have a terminal disease (e.g., with a prognosis of less than 6 months as in all U.S. jurisdictions). As a result, in some places individuals with serious mental illness who can demonstrate significant suffering and intact decisional capacity may qualify for PAD. Indeed, recent studies have shed light on the use of PAD by individuals with psychiatric disorders in the Netherlands (Kim et al. 2016), raising concerns for many about the adequacy of regulatory safeguards in that setting.

Another important difference is that several countries permit voluntary active euthanasia. The physician's active role in administering the lethal drug rather than the patient self-administering the drug distinguishes voluntary active euthanasia from PAD. To be clear, mental illness cannot be the qualifying diagnosis for PAD in any U.S. jurisdiction. To the contrary, statutory and regulatory safeguards in the United States are generally intended, among other things, to ensure that terminally ill individuals with significant mental illness are *not* eligible for PAD, although their effectiveness in achieving that goal is subject to debate. Similarly, the practice of euthanasia is not legal anywhere in the United States.

Landscape of Physician-Assisted Dying in the United States

Legal, regulated aid in dying became part of the landscape of end-of-life care in the United States in 1997, when the Oregon Death With Dignity Act went into effect. Since then, the practice has expanded substantially: as of August 2019, PAD was legal in Oregon, Washington, Vermont, Montana, California, Colorado, Hawaii, and New Jersey, encompassing approximately 18% of the U.S. population. PAD legislation has also passed in the District of Columbia, but its status is indeterminate due to federal government restrictions. Because further expansion in the states may continue, increasing numbers of psychiatrists may find themselves practicing in jurisdictions where PAD is legal and regulated.

Regulation and Safeguards

With the exception of Montana, where a state Supreme Court ruling permits PAD and no statutory structure for the practice exists, all other U.S. jurisdictions follow a general set of guidelines and safeguards (Table 26–1). In all states, qualifying individuals must be adult residents of the state, must have a terminal disease (prognosis less than 6 months), and must possess intact decisional capacity as determined independently by two physicians. Statutory language defines the elements of informed consent that, along with other safeguards, must be met in order for individuals to qualify.

Applicants must make requests both verbally and in writing, and in all states the qualification process involves a waiting period of at least 2 weeks (except Hawaii, which mandates a 20-day interval). Participation in the practice of PAD is explicitly voluntary for patients, providers, and institutions, and state laws stipulate penalties for activity found to be coercive. Finally, state agencies must collect data and provide publicly available annual reports summarizing assisted-dying activity. Of note, in all states reporting is triggered when an individual has successfully completed the qualification process and has been prescribed an aid-in-dying drug. As a result, no state-level data characterizing the population that pursues aid-in-dying unsuccessfully are available, and judgments about the effectiveness of the safeguards can only be made on the basis of data about qualified individuals.

TABLE 26–1.   **General process/safeguards for physician-assisted dying in the United States[1]**

Participants include

> Patient: Adult, resident of the state, terminally ill, able to provide informed consent, able to self-administer medication

> Attending physician: Determines patient is terminally ill, capable of providing informed consent, able to self-administer medication, and acting voluntarily; counsels patient; prescribes if patient qualifies

> Consulting physician: Provides independent assessment to determine that patient is terminally ill and capable of providing informed consent

> Mental health specialist (when required): Consulted if either attending or consulting physician is concerned that patient lacks decisional capacity or has impaired judgment due to mental illness[2]

The process involves

> Two verbal requests by the patient to the attending physician

> A "waiting period" between the two verbal requests of at least 15 days[3]

> One written request from the patient to the "attending physician"—signed by two witnesses

Participation is voluntary—for patients, physicians, and institutions.

Statutes define *terminal illness* as a medical condition likely to result in death within 6 months.

Statutes define elements of informed consent.

Statutes stipulate mandated documentation requirements for attending physician, consulting physician, and mental health specialist.

Statutes require reporting (to state health department) by attending physician when an aid-in-dying drug is prescribed and when a qualified patient dies.

Death resulting from ingestion of an aid-in-dying drug by a qualified individual is not considered suicide.

Note.   [1]These features are generally shared, with small differences, among the states with legislatively regulated aid in dying. As noted, the practice is legal in Montana but not regulated by statute.
[2]Specific criteria that trigger mental health specialist assessment vary slightly between states (see Table 26–2). In Hawaii, *all* applicants are required to have a mental health assessment.
[3]In Hawaii, the cooling off period is at least 20 days.

As noted earlier, state laws provide several ways in which PAD is treated differently than death from suicide from a legal standpoint. All statutes explicitly distinguish PAD from death from suicide for the purposes of completing a death certificate, with respect to benefits from insurance policies, with respect to legal vulnerability for participating health care providers, and with respect to state-level public health efforts to monitor and prevent "traditional" suicide.

Most states have a conditional requirement for an assessment by a mental health specialist if the attending or consulting physician has concerns about the presence of a mental illness or impaired judgment. Such assessments are aimed at ensuring that all qualified applicants, even those with signs of depression or another mental illness, are able to exercise autonomy without significant impairments in judgment. By contrast, the law in Hawaii is the first in the United States to stipulate a mandatory psychiatric review. All applicants there, even those without signs of mental illness or evidence of impaired decisional capacity, are required to have a mental health evaluation as part of the qualification process. Small but potentially meaningful differences in the statutes define the trigger and purpose of a mental health specialist assessment in each state (Table 26–2).

Public and Professional Responses to Physician-Assisted Dying

Attitudes toward assisted-dying practices have been difficult to reliably capture. Among other factors, significant framing effects exist with questions about aid in dying; as Emanuel et al. (2016) noted:

> Support varies substantially depending on the wording of survey questions; the provision of details about the patients, their prognosis, their medical diagnosis, and symptoms; how the interventions are characterized; and whether the questions are focused on ethical acceptability, legalization, or some other endorsement. (p. 81)

Nonetheless, opinion polls have generally found high levels of public support for different forms of assisted dying when limited to the setting of end-of-life care in individuals with significant suffering. Since 2000, for example, public support for euthanasia has hovered around 70% in the United States, and in a recent Gallup poll, 65% of Americans indicated support for "assisted suicide" (Brenan 2018).

Perhaps unsurprisingly, physician attitudes toward assisted-dying practices appear to be highly variable and dynamic, and few current, methodologically sound data to characterize the diversity of views are available. In an annual Medscape survey, 58% of physician participants in 2018 responded favorably to the query "should physician-assisted suicide or physician-assisted dying be made legal for terminally ill patients?"—an increase from 46% in 2010 (Martin 2018). A number of smaller, older, but methodologically more rigorous studies have found generally lower levels of support among physicians as compared to the public, but with high variability over time, geographic location, and specialty (Emanuel et al. 2016).

Few surveys of psychiatrists' attitudes toward PAD exist. After passage of the Oregon Death with Dignity Act, Ganzini et al. (1996) surveyed Oregon psychiatrists regarding their views as to the permissibility of PAD. Regarding the care of terminally ill patients with intact decisional capacity, 68% of psychiatrists endorsed the view that physicians should be permitted "to write a prescription for medication whose sole purpose would be to allow the patient to end his or her life." Of note, respondents reported low levels of confidence that they could reliably determine, in a single assessment, whether or not a psychiatric disorder was impairing judgment in a patient seeking aid in dying: 51% were not at all confident and 43% were only somewhat confident. A subsequent survey of forensic psychiatrists found similar levels of general support for PAD (66%) in at least some circumstances, along with high levels of support for more stringent evaluation criteria including mandatory psychiatric assessment, judicial review, and an automatic finding of incompetence in patients with major depressive disorder (Ganzini et al. 2000).

As with physician attitudes, professional organizations have taken a range of positions on the practice of PAD. For more than two decades, the American Medical Association (2019) has maintained a position that "physician-assisted suicide is fundamentally incompatible with the physician's role as healer, would be difficult or impossible to control, and would pose serious societal risks," although its position has

TABLE 26–2. Mental health specialist assessments in U.S. PAD jurisdictions

State	Trigger	Clinician	Purpose	Definitions*
Oregon Death with Dignity Act (1997)	Required if the physician believes the individual "may be suffering from a psychiatric or psychological disorder or depression causing impaired judgment."	Licensed psychiatrist or psychologist	To determine whether "the patient is capable and not suffering from a psychiatric or psychological disorder or depression causing impaired judgment."	*Capable* means that the patient "has the ability to make and communicate health care decisions"; *impaired judgment* is not defined.
Washington Death with Dignity Act (2008)	Identical to Oregon statute	Licensed psychiatrist or psychologist	To determine whether "the patient is competent and not suffering from a psychiatric or psychological disorder or depression causing impaired judgment."	*Competent* means that the patient "has the ability to make and communicate an informed decision"; *impaired judgment* is not defined.
Vermont Patient Choice and Control at End of Life Act (2013)	Does not have a specific trigger. "The physician either verified that the patient did not have impaired judgment or referred the patient for an evaluation by a psychiatrist, psychologist, or clinical social worker licensed in Vermont for confirmation that the patient was capable and did not have impaired judgment."	Licensed psychiatrist, psychologist, or clinical social worker	To provide "confirmation that the patient was capable and did not have impaired judgment."	*Capable* means that the patient "has the ability to make and communicate health care decisions"; *impaired judgment* means "that a person does not sufficiently understand or appreciate the relevant facts necessary to make an informed decision."

TABLE 26–2.   Mental health specialist assessments in U.S. PAD jurisdictions *(continued)*

State	Trigger	Clinician	Purpose	Definitions*
California End of Life Option Act (2016)	Required if there are "indications of a mental disorder."	Psychiatrist or licensed psychologist	To determine whether "the individual has the capacity to make medical decisions and is not suffering from impaired judgment due to a mental disorder."	*Capacity to make medical decisions* means that the patient "has the ability to understand the nature and consequences of a health care decision, the ability to understand its significant benefits, risks, and alternatives, and the ability to make and communicate an informed decision"; *impaired judgment* is not defined.
Colorado End-of-Life Options Act 2016	Required if the physician believes that the individual "may not be mentally capable of making an informed decision."	Licensed psychiatrist or psychologist	To determine "whether the individual is mentally capable and making informed decisions."	*Mental capacity* and *mentally capable* mean that the individual "has the ability to make and communicate an informed decision."

TABLE 26–2. **Mental health specialist assessments in U.S. PAD jurisdictions** *(continued)*

State	Trigger	Clinician	Purpose	Definitions[*]
Hawaii "Our Care, Our Choice" Act (2019)	Required in all cases	Licensed psychiatrist, psychologist, or clinical social worker	To determine whether "the patient is capable, and that the patient does not appear to be suffering from undertreatment or nontreatment of depression or other conditions which may interfere with the patient's ability to make an informed decision."	*Capable* means that the individual "has the ability to understand the patient's choices for care, including risks and benefits, and make and communicate health care decisions"; *impaired judgment* is not defined.
New Jersey Aid in Dying for the Terminally Ill Act (2019)	Required if the physician believes that the individual "may not be capable because the patient may have a psychiatric or psychological disorder or depression that causes impaired judgment."	Licensed psychiatrist, psychologist, or clinical social worker	To determine whether "the patient is capable and not suffering from a psychiatric or psychological disorder or depression causing impaired judgment."	*Capable* means that the individual "has the capacity to make health care decisions and communicate them to a health care provider"; *impaired judgment* is not defined.

Note. [*]*Informed decision* is defined in detail in every state.
PAD=physician-assisted dying.

recently been under review by the Council on Ethical and Judicial Affairs. The American Academy of Family Physicians (2018), on the other hand, removed its opposition to PAD in 2018, favoring instead a position of "engaged neutrality" similar to the position of the American Academy of Hospice and Palliative Medicine. By contrast, the American College of Physicians reaffirmed its opposition to PAD in 2017, stating that the practice is "problematic given the nature of the physician–patient relationship, affects trust in the relationship and in the profession, and fundamentally alters the medical profession's role in society" (Snyder Sulmasy and Mueller 2017). The American Psychiatric Association has a position on "medical euthanasia" in "non–terminally ill adults," a practice illegal everywhere in the United States, but it does not maintain an independent position or policy on the practice of PAD. The impact of professional organization positions on efforts to legalize aid in dying is unknown, although the California Medical Association's adoption of a neutral position on PAD was widely felt to remove a significant political obstacle to passage of the End of Life Option Act.

Individuals Who Pursue Physician-Assisted Death

Demographics

Demographic data about users of aid in dying come primarily from state surveillance programs. In Oregon, which now has more than 20 years of experience with PAD, participants have been 72 years old on average (range, 25–102 years), male (52%), predominantly white (96%), and highly educated (72% with at least some college). For nearly 80% of participants, cancer was the underlying terminal disease, with amyotrophic lateral sclerosis (at 8%) the second most common (Hedberg and New 2017). Monitoring data from Washington have generally revealed a similar population: older adults with cancer who are disproportionately white and well educated (Washington State Department of Health 2018). Even in California, which has a substantially more diverse population than Oregon and Washington, a similar picture has emerged: PAD recipients in California in 2017 averaged 74 years of age, were 88.9% white, and were highly educated—72.9% had at least some college education (California Department of Public Health 2018). In all three states, more than 80% of participants had been enrolled in hospice care.

Reasons for Pursuing Physician-Assisted Dying

Statutes in Oregon and Washington ask prescribing physicians to report patients' reasons for pursuing PAD. In Oregon, the most common motivations have been concerns about loss of autonomy (91%), decreased ability to engage in enjoyable activities (89%), and loss of dignity (68%) (Hedberg and New 2017). Surveillance in Washington has produced a strikingly similar pattern of motivations: loss of autonomy (90%), decreased ability to engage in enjoyable activities (87%), and loss of dignity (73%) (Washington State Department of Health 2018).

Several small studies have sampled patients themselves to characterize their reasons for pursuing PAD. Ganzini et al. (2009) surveyed 56 Oregonians who requested PAD. The chief motivating factors were the desire to control the circumstances of death, the desire to die at home, concerns about the loss of independence, and concerns about future pain or poor quality of life. Although respondents expressed moderate concern about future physical symptoms, they were generally not concerned with physical symptoms at the time of making an aid-in-dying request.

Smith et al. (2015), using patient self-report, examined differences in attachment style among individuals pursuing PAD compared with a matched set of individuals with advanced disease who did not seek PAD. Those seeking aid in dying were significantly more likely to have a dismissive attachment style and a pattern of interpersonal connection marked by high levels of independence and self-reliance. Additionally, those seeking PAD also exhibited higher levels of hopelessness, lower levels of spirituality, and higher levels of symptoms of depression.

Depression in Individuals Pursuing Physician-Assisted Dying

The prevalence of depression among individuals who seek PAD has been difficult to characterize, as has its potential impact in motivating the pursuit of PAD. A larger body of work, more broadly pertaining to individuals with advanced disease, has examined rates of depression, desire for hastened death, and other related phenomena. Findings have shown that symptoms of depression are common, that depression and feelings of hopelessness appear strongly linked to preferences for hastening death (Breitbart et al. 2000), and that effective treatment of depression can reduce the desire to die (Breitbart et al. 2010). However, how reliably those data generalize to the population of patients interested in PAD, or to the smaller population of individuals who qualify for assisted dying, is unknown.

Data focused on the small set of individuals pursuing PAD are limited. In Oregon, patients and their family members often report that depression is not an important factor in seeking aid in dying (Bharucha et al. 2003). However, as noted earlier, Smith et al. (2015), using standardized measures of depression, found that individuals seeking to qualify for aid in dying exhibited significantly higher levels of depression compared with a matched set of individuals with advanced disease who were not pursuing PAD. The best available study in the United States is a small cross-sectional survey of 58 individuals pursuing a lethal prescription in Oregon. Using a validated depression screening instrument and structured clinical interview, Ganzini et al. (2008) reported that among those who sought an aid-in-dying drug, 26% met criteria for depression. Of note, none of the depressed individuals who received an aid-in-dying drug was assessed by a mental health specialist as part of the qualification process, and each was determined to have decisional capacity.

Despite the evidence suggesting that some individuals seeking to qualify for PAD may experience depression, state-level surveillance data show that mental health specialist assessments are rarely requested. In more than 20 years of practice in Oregon, only 5% of qualified patients were referred for a mental health assessment (Hedberg and New 2017). In Washington, only 2% of qualified patients in 2017 were referred for a mental health specialist assessment (Washington State Department of Health 2018). As noted, state-level data do not permit conclusions about patients who are unsuccessful in attempting to qualify for PAD, so the possibility that mental health assessments might be effective in screening individuals inappropriate for PAD cannot be assessed.

Finally, substantial variation is found in institutional processes that implement procedures for PAD qualification. In describing the implementation of PAD at a comprehensive cancer center, Loggers et al. (2013) reported that no patients with current or previous depression elected to move forward with seeking PAD. This suggests that elements related to the process of qualification at that institution (e.g., the role of a clinical navigator) may serve a safeguarding or gatekeeping function. By contrast, some institutions may require a mental health assessment for all applicants, but few data are available to evaluate whether those processes provide an important safeguard, add a burdensome or unnecessary barrier, or have some other impact on the implementation of PAD (Bourgeois et al. 2018).

Psychiatric Practice and Aid in Dying

Mental Health Specialist Assessments in Physician-Assisted Dying Jurisdictions

Requests for assistance in dying are not uncommon in the setting of caring for individuals near the end of life, and a number of guidelines exist to help clinicians respond to such requests. These guidelines share several general elements, including cultivating self-awareness about personal attitudes and emotional responses; conducting a thorough, nonjudgmental exploration of the meaning beneath the patient's request; facilitating collaboration with other clinical experts and stakeholders; maintaining familiarity with "last resort" options in palliative care; ensuring expert assessments of decisional capacity and depression (if appropriate); and seeking to relieve suffering and avoid abandonment while maintaining professional integrity (Bascom and Tolle 2002).

Less guidance exists for psychiatrists involved in providing mental health assessments in PAD programs. Table 26–3 provides a framework for conducting a PAD mental health assessment, synthesized from existing guidelines.

PAD psychiatric evaluations are generally focused on assessing decisional capacity and determining whether patients experience impaired judgment from a mental disorder. Although such assessments may be generally familiar to psychiatrists, several unique features of working with dying patients warrant mention. First, physician participants should be aware of their own attitudes and judgments about the practice of aid in dying, because some evidence suggests that moral judgments may masquerade as clinical opinion when ethically controversial interventions such as PAD are being considered (Ganzini et al. 2000). Clinicians with strongly polar views about the morality of PAD might consider recusing themselves from participation or at least disclosing their attitudes to patients and referring providers. Second, depression is often difficult to diagnose in the setting of advanced disease, so mental health specialists need to be adept at distinguishing depression from its lookalikes, including normal sadness, grief, demoralization, and other related conditions (Fairman et al. 2016).

In addition, in the context of PAD, the anticipated outcomes, risks, and benefits of ingesting an aid-in-dying drug are fairly straightforward (and thus may not require a high level of decisional capacity). However, patients often have difficulty understanding and appreciating the potential outcomes, risks, and benefits of routine strategies, such as hospice and palliative care, used to manage end-of-life care. In fact, in many cases, helping the patient understand the effectiveness of routine end-of-life care strategies will reduce the patient's interest in pursuing aid in dying. Finally, be-

---

TABLE 26–3. **General approach to mental health assessment in PAD programs**

In most jurisdictions, the evaluation encompasses

    1) An assessment of decisional capacity: Does the patient

        Understand relevant information about the medical situation and the risks, benefits, expected outcomes of PAD and reasonable alternatives

        Appreciate the implications of the various interventions to the situation

        Reason about options in a logical way

        Communicate a stable choice

    2) A diagnostic assessment of mental illness, if present

General process:

    Review records

    Assess patient (generally alone)

    Obtain collateral from family/caregivers (if permitted)

    Communicate findings to attending physician

    Complete required documentation

Other considerations:

    Standardized screening instruments/rating scales may be helpful (e.g., Patient Health Questionnaire–9, Generalized Anxiety Disorder–7, Montreal Cognitive Assessment).

    Participants should maintain familiarity with law and institutional policy, which may vary.

    Participants should be cognizant of personal attitudes/moral judgments about PAD; consider recusal if there is a potential for bias or disclose potential for bias to attending physician.

    The presence of a mental disorder should not, in and of itself, disqualify an individual from PAD.

    If reversible conditions impair decisional capacity, brief intervention and reassessment may be appropriate.

    Participants may provide recommendations for treatment or other resources to address psychological/emotional distress when appropriate and consistent with goals of care.

Note. PAD=physician-assisted dying.

Source. Adapted from Appelbaum (2007), Bourgeois et al. (2018), Oregon Death with Dignity Act (1997), Stewart et al. (2011), and Yager et al. (2018).

cause the particular requirements for a PAD mental health assessment (i.e., the trigger for assessment, the purpose of assessment, details about documentation and reporting) may vary between jurisdictions (see Table 26–2) and across institutions, psychiatrists involved in PAD evaluations will need to be certain that their practice is in compliance with local laws and policies.

Beyond Assessments of Decisional Capacity

Interest in aid in dying may be linked to a variety of factors, including many uniquely within the scope of psychiatric practice, such as affective, cognitive, intrapersonal, dynamic, and social factors. As a result, many experts recommend an enlargement of the psychiatrist's role beyond merely assessing for decisional capacity. Muskin (1998), for example, argued for attention to intrapersonal conflict and dynamic processes that may underlie and give meaning to a patient's request to die. Similarly, Block and Billings (1995) laid out a series of domains in which the psychiatrist's expertise may be advantageous when a patient desires hastened death. These domains include providing an expert diagnostic assessment; clarifying conflict between the patient and loved ones (or the patient and clinicians); attending to suffering in physical, psychological, social, and spiritual domains; and creating a setting that allows colleagues and patients to work productively and to share in the moral and emotional responsibilities that surround difficult cases.

Conclusion

Robust debates and deep disagreements continue in public, political, and professional spheres as to the ethical permissibility of aid in dying and the participation of medical professionals in practices that influence the timing of death. The expansion of aid-in-dying laws reflects a social and political acknowledgment that some forms of self-determined death can be tolerated, in narrow and tightly regulated circumstances. Support for regulated PAD challenges the field of psychiatry to become more adept at identifying ethically and clinically relevant distinctions among different forms of life-ending acts. Psychiatrists have a role to play in helping to define (and perhaps delimit) those circumstances. Perhaps more importantly, *all* patients nearing the end of life, not just the very small set of individuals who might pursue assisted dying, are vulnerable to significant psychological, emotional, interpersonal, and existential distress. Psychiatrists are uniquely suited to play an important role in improving the care of the dying, including caring for patients who wish to control the manner and timing of their death.

Key Points

- Physician-assisted dying (PAD) is considered a "palliative option of last resort," in which terminally ill adults with intact decisional capacity are prescribed a lethal dose of medication that they may choose to use to bring about a peaceful, self-determined death.

- PAD is legal in eight U.S. states, encompassing nearly one-fifth of the U.S. population.

- In states where PAD is regulated by statute, a fairly uniform set of safeguards exists to structure the practice. In these states, death resulting from ingestion of an aid-in-dying drug by a qualified individual is not considered suicide.

- In general, discussions about suicide concern individuals who are mentally ill but, for the most part, not dying; conversely, discussions about PAD in the United States concern individuals who are dying but, for the most part, are not mentally ill.

- A mental health specialist assessment may be required in some or all cases to provide an evaluation of decisional capacity and determine whether a patient experiences impaired judgment due to a mental disorder. In states where the mental health assessment is not compulsory, few patients receive such an assessment.

- Psychiatric involvement is significantly valuable in the care of the dying, including in the context of PAD requests.

References

American Academy of Family Physicians: COD addresses medical aid-in-dying, institutional racism. 2018 Congress of Delegates, October 18, 2018. Available at: https://www.aafp.org/news/2018-congress-fmx/20181010cod-hops.html. Accessed January 31, 2018.

American Academy of Hospice and Palliative Medicine: Statement on Physician-Assisted Dying. Chicago, IL, AAHPM, June 24, 2016. Available at: http://aahpm.org/positions/pad. Accessed January 31, 2019.

American Medical Association: Code of Medical Ethics Opinion 5.7: Physician-Assisted Suicide. Chicago, IL, American Medical Association, 2019. Available at https://www.ama-assn.org/delivering-care/ethics/physician-assisted-suicide. Accessed January 31, 2019.

Appelbaum PS: Clinical practice: assessment of patients' competence to consent to treatment. N Engl J Med 357(18):1834–1840, 2007 17978292

Bascom PB, Tolle SW: Responding to requests for physician-assisted suicide: "These are uncharted waters for both of us...." JAMA 288(1):91–98, 2002 12090867

Bharucha AJ, Pearlman RA, Back AL, et al: The pursuit of physician-assisted suicide: role of psychiatric factors. J Palliat Med 6(6):873–883, 2003 14733679

Block SD, Billings JA: Patient requests for euthanasia and assisted suicide in terminal illness: the role of the psychiatrist. Psychosomatics 36(5):445–457, 1995 7568652

Bourgeois JA, Mariano MT, Wilkins JM, et al: Physician-assisted death psychiatric assessment: a standardized protocol to conform to the California End of Life Option Act. Psychosomatics 59(5):441–451, 2018 29653821

Breitbart W, Rosenfeld B, Pessin H, et al: Depression, hopelessness, and desire for hastened death in terminally ill patients with cancer. JAMA 284(22):2907–2911, 2000 11147988

Breitbart W, Rosenfeld B, Gibson C, et al: Impact of treatment for depression on desire for hastened death in patients with advanced AIDS. Psychosomatics 51(2):98–105, 2010 20332284

Brenan M: Americans' strong support of euthanasia persists. Gallup Politics, May 31, 2018. Available at: https://news.gallup.com/poll/235145/americans-strong-support-euthanasia-persists.aspx. Accessed January 31, 2019.

California Department of Public Health: California End of Life Option Act 2017 Data Report. June 2018. Available at https://www.cdph.ca.gov/Programs/CHSI/CDPH%20Document%20Library/2017EOLADataReport.pdf. Accessed January 31, 2019.

California End of Life Option Act (AB-15) (2016). Available at https://leginfo.legislature.ca.gov/faces/billNavClient.xhtml?bill_id=201520162AB15. Accessed January 31, 2019.

Centers for Disease Control and Prevention: Self-Directed Violence Surveillance: Uniform Definitions and Recommended Data Elements. Atlanta, GA, National Center for Injury Prevention and Control, 2018. Available at https://www.cdc.gov/violenceprevention/pdf/self-directed-violence-a.pdf. Accessed January 31, 2019.

Colorado End-of-Life Options Act, Article 48, Title 25, Colorado Revised Statutes (C.R.S.) (2016)

Dworkin G: Physician-assisted death: the state of the debate, in The Oxford Handbook of Bioethics. Edited by Steinbock B. New York, 2007, pp 375–392

Emanuel EJ, Onwuteaka-Philipsen BD, Urwin JW, et al: Attitudes and practices of euthanasia and physician-assisted suicide in the United States, Canada, and Europe. JAMA 316(1):79–90, 2016 27380345

Fairman N, Hirst JM, Irwin SA: Clinical Manual of Palliative Care Psychiatry. Washington, DC, American Psychiatric Publishing, 2016

Ganzini L, Fenn DS, Lee MA, et al: Attitudes of Oregon psychiatrists toward physician-assisted suicide. Am J Psychiatry 153(11):1469–1475, 1996 8890683

Ganzini L, Leong GB, Fenn DS, et al: Evaluation of competence to consent to assisted suicide: views of forensic psychiatrists. Am J Psychiatry 157(4):595–600, 2000 10739419

Ganzini L, Goy ER, Dobscha SK: Prevalence of depression and anxiety in patients requesting physicians' aid in dying: cross sectional survey. BMJ 337:a1682, 2008 18842645

Ganzini L, Goy ER, Dobscha SK: Oregonians' reasons for requesting physician aid in dying. Arch Intern Med 169(5):489–492, 2009 19273779

Hardwig J: Going to meet death: the art of dying in the early part of the twenty-first century. Hastings Cent Rep 39(4):37–45, 2009 19711633

Hawaii "Our Care, Our Choice Act" (H.B. 2739) (2019)

Hedberg K, New C: Oregon's Death with Dignity Act: 20 years of experience to inform the debate. Ann Intern Med 167(8):579–583, 2017 28975232

Kim SY, De Vries RG, Peteet JR: Euthanasia and assisted suicide of patients with psychiatric disorders in the Netherlands 2011 to 2014. JAMA Psychiatry 73(4):362–368, 2016 26864709

Loggers ET, Starks H, Shannon-Dudley M, et al: Implementing a death with dignity program at a comprehensive cancer center. N Engl J Med 368(15):1417–1424, 2013 23574120

Macauley RC: Ethics in Palliative Care. New York, Oxford University Press, 2018

Martin K: Medscape Ethics Report: Life, Death, and Pain (website). New York, Medscape LLC, 2018. Available at: https://www.medscape.com/slideshow/2018-ethics-report-life-death-6011014. Accessed January 21, 2019.

Muskin PR: The request to die: role for a psychodynamic perspective on physician-assisted suicide. JAMA 279(4):323–328, 1998 9450720

New Jersey Aid in Dying for the Terminally Ill Act. (A1504) (2019). Available at: https://www.njleg.state.nj.us/bills/BillView.asp?BillNumber=S1072. Accessed July 29, 2019.

Oregon Death With Dignity Act (ORS 127.800–995) (1997)

Orentlicher D: International perspectives on physician assistance in dying. Hastings Cent Rep 46(6):6–7, 2016 27875642

Smith KA, Harvath TA, Goy ER, et al: Predictors of pursuit of physician-assisted death. J Pain Symptom Manage 49(3):555–561, 2015 25116913

Snyder Sulmasy L, Mueller PS: Ethics and the legalization of physician-assisted suicide: an American College of Physicians position paper. Ann Intern Med 167(8):576–578, 2017 28975242

Stewart C, Peisah C, Draper B: A test for mental capacity to request assisted suicide. J Med Ethics 37(1):34–39, 2011 21097939

Vermont Patient Choice and Control at End of Life Act (VT Stat Annot Sec 1, 18 V.S.A. Ch 113) (2013)

Washington Death With Dignity Act (RCW 70.245) (2008)

Washington State Department of Health: Washington State 2017 Death With Dignity Act Report. March 2018. Available at https://www.doh.wa.gov/Portals/1/Documents/Pubs/422-109-DeathWithDignityAct2017.pdf. Accessed January 31, 2019.

Yager J, Ganzini L, Nguyen DH, et al: Working with decisionally capable patients who are determined to end their own lives. J Clin Psychiatry 79(4):17r11767, 2018 29873952

CHAPTER 27

Suicide Risk Management

Mitigating Professional Liability

Donna Vanderpool, M.B.A., J.D.

Although psychiatry is one of the least-often sued medical specialties (Studdert et al. 2016), patient death from suicide or suicide attempt is one of the two most frequent identifiable causes of loss in lawsuits and claims (demands for money outside of litigation) filed against psychiatrists. Psychopharmacology errors, the other most frequent cause of loss, only recently surpassed suicide as the most identifiable cause. The most frequent allegation in lawsuits and claims against psychiatrists is "incorrect treatment"; attorneys will use this broad allegation in initial pleadings and then develop more specific allegations of wrongdoing by the psychiatrist as the malpractice case develops (Table 27–1). Therefore, cases involving both suicide and psychopharmacology can also be found in the "incorrect treatment" category.

Most lawsuits against psychiatrists are allegations of medical malpractice, but other causes of action, such as wrongful death, can also be brought. In addition to lawsuits, psychiatrists may also face administrative actions related to a patient's death from suicide, such as licensing board investigations and medical staff privilege suspensions. All of these actions are reportable to the U.S. Department of Health and Human Services' National Practitioner Data Bank (NPDB; 2018), and information reported to the NPDB can follow physicians throughout their career.

Legal Basics

Elements of Medical Malpractice

The statutory requirements to file a medical malpractice action vary by state, but all states require the plaintiff (the patient, the patient's representative, or the patient's estate) to prove four key elements in order to prevail in a medical malpractice lawsuit.

351

TABLE 27–1.   **Cause of loss: claims and lawsuits, The Psychiatrists' Program, 2009–2018**

Primary allegation[1]	Percentage of claims and lawsuits
Incorrect treatment[2]	34%
Medication issues	19%
Suicide/Attempted suicide	13%
Other	8%
Incorrect diagnosis	6%
Unnecessary commitment	5%
Breach of confidentiality	5%
Improper supervision[3]	2%
Vicarious liability	2%
Improper discharge	2%
Forensic (e.g., expert testimony, independent medical examiner)	1%
Duty to warn/protect	1%
Abandonment	1%
Boundary violation	1%

Note.   [1]"Primary allegation" is the main allegation by plaintiffs' attorneys of what the psychiatrist did wrong.
[2]"Incorrect treatment" will represent a high percentage of cases because plaintiffs' attorneys often use a broad, general allegation initially; this category includes all types of cases, including suicide and psychopharmacology.
[3]The category labeled "improper supervision" refers to supervision of patients as well as of other providers.
Source.   Professional Risk Management Services, Inc. (PRMS). Copyright © 2019 Professional Risk Management Services, Inc. (PRMS); used with permission.

These four elements of a medical malpractice case have been referred to as the "four Ds": duty, dereliction, damages, and direct causation.

- Duty: The plaintiff has to prove that the physician had a duty to the patient to meet the standard of care. Typically, a duty is created once a doctor–patient treatment relationship is established.
- Dereliction (negligence): The plaintiff has to prove that the care delivered did not meet an acceptable standard of care or that the physician breached the duty.
- Damages (injury): The plaintiff has to prove that the patient experienced damage, which can be physical, financial, or emotional.
- Direct causation: The plaintiff has to prove that the defendant physician's negligence directly caused the patient's injuries. Plaintiffs generally have to show that "but for" the defendant's actions, the plaintiff's suicide would not have occurred. Often plaintiffs' experts fail to establish the required connection between the defendant's actions and the suicide.

Medical malpractice is defined as the act or continuing conduct of a physician that does not meet the standard of care and results in harm to the patient. Note that a plaintiff must prove all four elements; therefore, a suicide is not necessarily evidence of negligence in and of itself. An adverse outcome can happen even in light of prudent professional judgment and adequate treatment. Without negligence, there can be no malpractice. However, negligence alone is not enough without direct causation. For example, in *Providence Health Center v. Dowell* (2008), the Texas Supreme Court agreed with the plaintiff that the defendants were negligent but then said that the negligence did not cause the suicide:

> In IHS Cedars, we said: "the conduct of the defendant may be too attenuated from the resulting injuries to the plaintiff to be a substantial factor in bringing about the harm." In this case, the defendants' negligent conduct was their failure to comprehensively assess his risk for suicide. Because there is no evidence that Lance could have been hospitalized involuntarily, that he would have consented to hospitalization, that a short-term hospitalization would have made his suicide unlikely, that he exhibited any unusual conduct following his discharge, or that any of his family or friends believed further treatment was required, the defendants' negligence was too attenuated from the suicide to have been a substantial factor in bringing it about. (pp. 329–330)

Allegations of Negligence in Suicide Cases

A review of suicide lawsuits handled by The Psychiatrists' Program ("the Program"), a large malpractice insurer for psychiatrists in the United States, identified the many possible allegations in suicide cases, which can be found in Table 27–2.

Standard of Care

Medical malpractice litigation turns on whether the psychiatrist met the standard of care. There is no one-size-fits-all standard of care. Reasonable clinicians might differ in opinion about what they would do in a given clinical situation. However, factors can be used to evidence the applicable standard of care in any clinical care situation, including

- Federal and state statutes (enacted by legislatures)
- Federal and state regulations (promulgated by government agencies)
- Federal and state case law (legal opinions previously decided by state and federal courts)
- Other materials from regulatory bodies (e.g., guidelines and policy statements from state and federal regulatory agencies, including state licensing boards)
- Authoritative clinical guidelines from reputable organizations (but not health plans' utilization review guidelines)
- Policies and guidelines from professional organizations (e.g., ethics statements and resource documents from the American Medical Association and the American Psychiatric Association)
- Professional literature (e.g., treatises, clinical textbooks, and journal articles)
- Accreditation and institutional standards, policies, and procedures

Clinical guidelines by themselves do not set the standard of care. Rather, guidelines are just one piece of evidence that the judge and jury will use to determine the applicable standard of care in a given case. Physicians who provide treatment that deviates from widely accepted guidelines may not have been negligent in their treatment, but the reasoning behind such deviations should be adequately documented and should be supported by current practice or the professional literature.

TABLE 27–2.	Allegations of negligence in suicide cases, from The Psychiatrists' Program

Failure to obtain an adequate history

Failure to contact the prior treating physician

Failure to obtain history from the family, including past suicidal behaviors

Failure to determine which treatments had previously failed

Failure to review prior medical records

Failure to perform a full mental status examination

Failure to properly evaluate and record the patient's risk for death from suicide

Failure to reach a rational diagnosis based on careful examination and patient history

Failure to weigh psychodynamic factors

Failure to diagnose medication intoxication and dependency

Failure to diagnose suicidal thoughts and behaviors

Failure to take reasonable steps to ensure patient safety

Failure to take protective measures (e.g., placing the patient on constant observation)

Failure to remove dangerous items (e.g., shoelaces, sharps, weapons)

Failure to develop a comprehensive treatment plan

Failure to hospitalize

Failure to communicate with other treating providers

Failure to communicate with patient's family or significant others

Improper reliance on "no-harm" contracts

Failure to weigh the benefits of electroconvulsive therapy in a timely manner

Negligent psychopharmacological management

Failure to provide adequate postdischarge care

Failure to maintain hospital records showing the diagnosis, full diagnostic evaluation, and adequate clinical notes

Failure to record a full mental status examination

Failure to document adequate suicide assessment

Some lawyers and lay persons believe that to avoid liability related to patients with suicidal behaviors, treating psychiatrists are expected to predict whether a particular patient will attempt suicide and prevent all suicide attempts, however unforeseeable. Fortunately, however, courts recognize that psychiatrists do not have superhuman powers of prediction. In *Tuten v. Farizborzian* (2012) the appellate court held:

> The science of psychiatry represents the penultimate grey area. Numerous cases underscore the inability of psychiatric experts to predict, with any degree of precision, an individual's propensity to do violence. Indeed, "[p]sychiatrists themselves would be the first to admit that however desirable an infallible crystal ball might be, it is not among the tools of their profession." (p. 1067)

The review of the Program's suicide claims and lawsuits brought against psychiatrists indicates the following standard of care expectations:

- Whether suicide risk indicators and protective factors for the patient with suicidal behaviors were adequately identified and evaluated

- Whether a reasonable treatment plan was developed based on the assessment of the patient's clinical needs
- Whether the treatment plan was appropriately (i.e., not negligently) implemented and modified based on an ongoing assessment of the patient's clinical status
- Whether the provider was professionally current regarding the assessment and treatment of patients with suicidal behaviors (e.g., knew suicide risk indicators and protective factors, knew current treatment options/interventions including medications, therapy, hospitalization)
- Whether documentation in the patient record was adequate to support that appropriate care was provided in terms of the assessment, treatment, and ongoing monitoring of the patient

What is expected, as in any other psychiatrist–patient interaction, is that the psychiatrist will meet the standard of care. A patient's death from suicide cannot be predicted; however, the risk of death from suicide may be foreseeable. For example, when discharging a patient who had been hospitalized due to suicidal ideation, a psychiatrist cannot predict that a suicide will or will not occur after discharge, because there is no crystal ball. However, it is foreseeable that the failure to assess the patient for suicidal thoughts and behaviors prior to discharge may lead to a substantial risk of injury. A review of trial verdicts involving psychiatrists sued for a patient's suicide reported in VerdictSearch between 1997 and 2017 showed that 27% of the outpatient deaths from suicide occurred within 4 days of hospital discharge (VerdictSearch.com 2018). *Foreseeability*, a legal term, does *not* mean predicting the future. Foreseeability in a suicide case is related to the clinical reasonableness of the suicide risk assessment. In other words, based on the information available, did the psychiatrist know—or should the psychiatrist have known—that the patient was at risk of death from suicide, and if such foreseeability existed, did the psychiatrist take the appropriate steps to address suicide risk factors.

Damages

Three types of monetary damages can be sought by plaintiffs in medical malpractice cases:

1. *Special damages*, or economic damages, are damages that can be calculated and are quantifiable. These can include, but are not limited to, lost earnings and lost earning capacity, medical bills, and other financial losses allegedly incurred from the injury resulting from the psychiatrist's negligence.
2. *General damages*, or noneconomic damages, include damages without a quantifiable dollar amount. For example, some states allow a plaintiff to recover for pain and suffering and mental anguish. Noneconomic damages can also include *loss of consortium*, a term used to refer to the deprivation of the benefits of a family relationship due to injuries caused by the malpractice. These damages are often difficult to ascertain and may require expert testimony to support them as well as to dispute them. General damages can also include a financial element of lack of future earning capacity. Because future earnings are speculative, they fit under general damages rather than quantifiable special damages.
3. *Punitive damages*, or compensatory damages, are usually only recovered when the physician should have known he or she was behaving in a harmful manner. Puni-

tive damages are not based on actual injuries sustained; rather, they are a way to punish the physician for intentional or grossly negligent conduct. Although it is not uncommon to see punitive damages sought in medical malpractice cases, particularly if the plaintiff wants to settle the case but the defendant physician does not, it is uncommon to see punitive damages actually awarded in a medical malpractice case. Malpractice insurance policies typically exclude coverage for punitive damages.

Some states have passed laws that place limitations on, or cap, the amount of money that can be awarded in a medical malpractice lawsuit. Juries are often not instructed about the damages cap because judges and attorneys do not want juries using the cap as a starting point when awarding damages. Instead, juries are encouraged to award the amount they find fair, and the damages are modified by the court as necessary. Most states have no damage cap at all, which could be because none has been enacted or because the caps they enacted were ruled unconstitutional by a state court.

Malpractice Insurance Issues

Professional malpractice insurance is a contract between an insurer and an insured individual or group that provides coverage for professional liability claims. The two main types of medical malpractice insurance policies are referred to as "occurrence" and "claims-made."

With an *occurrence policy*, coverage is provided for an incident giving rise to a claim or lawsuit that occurs while the policy is in effect, regardless of when the claim is reported to the insurance company and even if the claim is reported after the policy has expired. Policyholders are given a new set of policy limits each year that an occurrence policy is renewed. Previous years' limits remain available for claims that may arise from incidents occurring during those previous years.

In *claims-made policies*, coverage is provided only for claims that both occur and are reported while the policy is in effect. If the incident giving rise to the claim occurred while the insured had coverage but is reported after the policy has expired, the insurer does not provide coverage, unless extended reporting coverage ("tail" coverage) has been purchased. When this type of policy is renewed, policyholders are given a new set of policy limits but do not keep the prior years' limits. Tail coverage does not extend the policy period but rather extends the time during which coverage will be provided for claims that may be reported.

Statute of Limitations

Statutes of limitations are laws passed by legislative bodies that set the maximum time after an event within which legal proceedings may be initiated. A statute of limitations is an affirmative defense, meaning it does not preclude a case from being filed, but it is one of the defenses a defendant psychiatrist may specifically raise and plead. A mere denial in an answer (filed by the defendant responding to the allegations in the plaintiff's complaint) will not raise the defense; a defendant must specifically plead a statute of limitations defense.

Statutes of limitations for medical malpractice vary by state and can be complex because most states have a variety of time deadlines and extensions of the deadlines. There are different limitations for different causes of actions. For example, in New York, for a medical malpractice action, the plaintiff has 2.5 years to file suit from the conclusion of the treatment that allegedly caused harm to the patient, but the New York statute of limitations for wrongful death actions is 2 years after the death. Special rules apply to minors and persons with a mental disability that allow the statute to be "tolled" or extended and give the plaintiff an additional number of years to file a lawsuit.

Professional Judgment Rule

Under the *professional judgment rule*, a rule of evidence, courts will give great deference to treating physicians as long as they have some basis for the treatment decisions. That reasonable basis has already been created by the physician—years prior to the lawsuit and at the time care was provided—by contemporaneously documenting the basis for the clinical decision making. One court (*Park v. Kovachevick* 2014) noted the following:

> It is well settled that "a doctor is not liable in negligence merely because a treatment, which the doctor as a matter of professional judgment elected to pursue, proves ineffective".... Liability is imposed "only if the doctor's treatment decisions do not reflect his or her own best judgment or fall short of the generally accepted standard of care" [*Nestorowich v. Ricotta* 2002]. Although a plaintiff's expert may have chosen a different course of treatment, "this, without more, 'represents, at most, a difference of opinion among [medical providers], which is not sufficient to sustain a prima facie case of malpractice'" [*Ibguy v. State of New York* 1999 quoting *Darren v. Safier* 1994]. "When a psychiatrist chooses a course of treatment, within a range of medically accepted choices, for a patient after proper examination and evaluation, the doctrine of professional medical judgment will insulate such psychiatrist from liability" [*Durney v. Terk* 2007]. (p. 190)

Suicide Case Resolutions

A review of cases reported to VerdictSearch (a nationwide database of verdicts and settlements) between 1997 and 2017 that involved psychiatrists sued for a patient's suicide showed that in 76% of the cases a verdict was returned for the defendant psychiatrist. In 15% of the cases, a verdict was returned for the plaintiff. Verdict amounts against the defendant psychiatrists in these cases ranged from $19,000 to $4,200,000. As discussed in the next section, a jury verdict is different from a court judgment. The remaining 9% of cases in VerdictSearch settled, with reported settlements ranging from $0 (the psychiatrist was part of a global settlement in which the other defendants paid) to $1,700,000 (unassigned between the multiple defendants, so it is unknown what the psychiatrist actually paid, if anything).

Verdict Versus Judgment

The distinction between a jury verdict and a court's judgment can be significant. The court can reduce the jury's verdict amount for any number of reasons, including caps on damages or a finding that the evidence failed to support the jury's verdict amount. The court can even reject the jury's finding for the plaintiff and any associated verdict amount. One way this can occur is by the court entering a "judgment notwithstanding the verdict." The court can also decide to keep the jury's verdict for the plaintiff but amend the jury's verdict amount.

Risk Management: The Three Cs

The best risk management strategy is to provide good clinical care. One framework of risk management strategies to deliver good clinical care consists of the three Cs: collecting information, communicating, and carefully documenting.

Collecting Information

Collecting information, specifically identifying risk factors (including those that can be modified), identifying protective factors, and inquiring as to suicidal ideation, intent, and plan composes three critical components of a suicide risk assessment. The remaining two components are using the collected information to determine the risk level and treatment plan and then documenting the assessment and treatment plan. The complete elements of a comprehensive suicide risk assessment are covered in Chapter 1 of this text ("Suicide Risk Assessment").

Psychiatrists should not rely on another clinician's suicide risk assessment. Psychiatrists are responsible for conducting their own assessment, even if it has been done by another member of the treatment team. Psychiatrists may also be held liable for the negligence of other clinicians under their supervision under the legal concept of *respondeat superior* ("let the superior make answer"). Under this doctrine, an employer or principal may be held liable for an employee's or agent's wrongful acts committed within the scope of employment. This concept also applies to attending physicians who supervise residents in training. In malpractice actions against residents, the attending is typically the party held liable.

Communicating

Many clinicians have had patients agree to a "no-harm" or suicide prevention contract as a guarantee of patient safety. These "contracts" have no legal force and cannot take the place of an adequate suicide risk assessment, but it may be appropriate for such a contract to be one part of a comprehensive treatment plan as a measure of the therapeutic alliance. They may be useful in letting the patient know that the clinician is there for them, and it may be clinically significant if the patient cannot agree to the contract. However, it is the psychiatrist's responsibility to evaluate the patient's overall suicide risk and ability to participate in the treatment plan. Overreliance on such contracts may lessen a clinician's awareness or observations of a patient's suicide risk.

With the patient's permission, the involvement and education of the patient's family and significant others about the patient's condition and treatment may be helpful in ensuring patient safety and preventing a lawsuit in the event of a bad outcome. The patient, other health care providers, and the patient's family should be appropriately warned about the potential for suicide and significant risk factors. The family may be particularly helpful in keeping the patient safe, such as by removing firearms. If the patient will not consent to communicating with family or others, remember that some exceptions to patient confidentiality exist, such as when a patient is in danger of harming him- or herself or others (American Psychiatric Association 2013, section 4, annotation 8). Accordingly, even without patient consent, consider alerting family members and significant others to the risk of outpatient suicide when the risk is significant, the family does not seem aware of the risk, and the family might contribute to the patient's safety.

Some clinicians, wishing to zealously protect a patient's confidentiality, erroneously believe they cannot listen to what family members have to tell them about a patient. Listening to others—without confirming the person is a patient or any treatment details—does not constitute a breach of confidentiality and may provide invaluable information and insight into the patient's suicide risk.

In addition to communicating with family, communication with other health care professionals involved in the patient's care, especially when the patient is being treated in a split treatment situation, is important (see Chapter 5, "Split Treatment"). In order for the care given by an individual clinician to be as effective as possible, the patient's overall care should be coordinated. It is also prudent to alert covering psychiatrists about high-risk patients.

Carefully Documenting

Clinicians should document their decision-making process, including not only what they did and why but also what they considered but rejected and why. Documentation allows for the treatment plan to be understood by others, such as subsequent treating clinicians or by an expert witness in subsequent litigation. Documenting the decision-making process underlying treatment decisions is key to building a supportive record, primarily for the purpose of continuity of care but also for legal defense. The major aspects of care should be documented. The American Psychiatric Association's *Practice Guidelines for the Assessment and Treatment of Patients With Suicidal Behaviors* (Jacobs et al. 2003) described what should be documented in the record as follows:

- Risk assessments
- Decision-making processes
- Descriptions of changes in treatment
- Communications with other clinicians
- Telephone calls from patients or family members
- Prescription log or copies of actual prescriptions
- Medical records of previous treatment, if available, particularly those related to past suicide attempts

Additionally, some state legislatures and licensing boards require certain minimum information to be made part of the treatment record. Psychiatrists should be familiar with the requirements in their states.

Documentation should include more than just a form with boxes checked; the clinical judgment needs to be documented. Not only should the initial suicide risk assessment be documented but also subsequent assessments and modifications to the treatment plan. A well-documented decision-making process in the record greatly limits plaintiff attorneys and their experts from making up their own story about what happened in treatment. The written treatment record stands as a testament of treatment provided and the reasoning behind it. The record composes a significant and substantial part of the defense against any claim of malpractice against the psychiatrist. Highly defensible cases in which the psychiatrist delivered seemingly flawless treatment have been lost or settled because of poor documentation by the psychiatrist. A chart with careful documentation of the psychiatrist's reasoning process and suicide assessments is a powerful defense tool in that it 1) allows the psychiatrist and his or her expert to testify as to specifics; 2) makes the psychiatrist's testimony more believable; and 3) places the psychiatrist's attorney in a better position to convince the jury that the patient's expert is engaging in secondhand guessing after the fact (Professional Risk Management Services 2015a).

Plaintiff attorneys who sue psychiatrists in suicide cases describe the importance of documentation of the suicide risk assessment as follows (Simpson and Stacy 2004):

> Documentation is a cornerstone of the defense of a potential suicide case…. Good care combined with good documentation is the surest way to avoid being a defendant in a malpractice case…[n]othing will stop a malpractice lawyer dead in his or her tracks quicker than a well-documented chart reflecting careful and thoughtful suicide assessment…. What needs to be documented? The short answer is that the medical record must reflect a *proper* suicide assessment. In most cases, simply asking a few rote questions such as "Are you suicidal," "Do you have a plan" and/or "Do you have the means" is grossly inadequate for defending against allegations of negligence…. A chart reflecting an understanding and appreciation for a patient's particular risk factors and reflecting that the physician elicited critical information regarding specific suicidal thoughts and methods, and the extent of planning and action taken with regard to these methods, will go a long way toward dissuading a good plaintiff's lawyer from taking the case. We also search the record for pertinent *negative* findings concerning the patient's suicidal ideation, planning, and intent. Notes indicating that the clinician ruled out certain risk factors support the conclusion that the clinician performed a proper assessment…. If one documents a reasonable and fairly complete thought process and clinical considerations—in addition to the final decision—it is difficult for a plaintiff's expert to criticize that final decision. (pp. 1–4)

A patient's treatment record should never be altered, especially after a death from suicide or suicide attempt. The strength of the treatment record as evidence in a malpractice case is based upon the idea that a contemporaneous record of actions and observations can reasonably be relied upon to be true and unbiased. Altering the record undermines this assumption and can result in an otherwise defensible case being rendered totally indefensible. Correcting mistakes in the record after a death from suicide or other event should only be done with the advice of defense counsel or risk management.

After a Patient Suicide

In the event of a patient's death from suicide, psychiatrists can take steps to mitigate their risk of being successfully sued (Professional Risk Management Services 2015b). A clinician should contact their medical malpractice insurance company to report the event. They should not discuss the case with others and should seek guidance from their malpractice insurance company or defense attorney on communicating with others about the patient and the patient's treatment.

Psychiatrists should be prepared to deal with their emotions following patient death from suicide (see Chapter 32, "Psychiatrist Reactions to Patient Suicide and the

Clinician's Role"). This hopefully would include remembering that not all adverse events are the result of medical errors and that not all medical errors result in a claim or lawsuit. After a patient death from suicide, psychiatrists should ensure proper medical record management. This includes keeping the record secure and keeping correspondence with a malpractice insurance company or defense attorney separate from the clinical record. Clinicians should seek guidance prior to releasing copies of the record.

Because confidentiality survives the patient's death, guidance should be obtained from the malpractice carrier or risk manager prior to processing requests for information such as from law enforcement, family members, medical examiners, health insurance companies, or facilities, including requests to participate in peer reviews, incident reviews, quality assurance reviews, and so on.

Interactions with a decedent's family should be driven by the family and will depend on the amount of interaction between the psychiatrist and the family during the patient's treatment. Family members, including spouses, may not always have the right to access confidential treatment information (unless appointed to represent the estate, under most states' laws). However, an appreciation of confidentiality obligations need not prevent a psychiatrist from offering support and expressing care and concern for the patient's family, including recommending appropriate resources for counseling or treatment. A clinician should only consider attending the patient's funeral if invited by the family.

Conclusion

Treating patients with suicidal behaviors is one of a psychiatrist's greatest professional liability risk exposures. However, the best strategy to keep patients safe, and thereby minimize risk, is to provide good clinical care. Focusing on collecting information, communicating, and carefully documenting the care can minimize professional liability risk. After a patient death from suicide, a variety of requests might be made for information about the patient. Psychiatrists should seek guidance from their medical malpractice insurer or risk manager on how to respond properly. Not all patient deaths from suicide result in a claim or lawsuit; in fact, most do not, likely due (at least in part) to good documentation. However, if sued, keep in mind that defendant physicians prevail in the overwhelming majority of malpractice suits filed against them.

Key Points

- To prevail in a medical malpractice lawsuit, a plaintiff must prove all four elements—duty, dereliction of duty, damages, and direct causation.

- Psychiatrists are not required to predict a patient's death from suicide; however, the risk of death from suicide may be foreseeable. The psychiatrist is responsible for developing a reasonable treatment plan based on a thorough suicide risk assessment and implementing it appropriately.

- A suicide risk assessment consists of identifying risk and protective factors; inquiring about suicidal ideation, intent, and plan; determining the risk level and treatment plan; and documenting the assessment and treatment plan.

- Suicide risk is assessed at the beginning of and throughout treatment. These assessments should be adequately documented in the treatment record.

- "No-harm contracts" or patient rating scales are not substitutes for a comprehensive suicide risk assessment. They may be relevant, but only as one part of a psychiatrist's comprehensive risk assessment.

- Patient safety and the safety of others are exceptions to patient confidentiality.

- Documentation allows others to understand what happened in your treatment and provides support for a subsequent court to defer to professional judgment.

- Confidentiality survives a patient's death. Clinicians should contact a malpractice insurance company or risk manager before releasing a copy of a deceased patient's record.

References

American Psychiatric Association: Principles of Medical Ethics With Annotations Especially Applicable To Psychiatry, 2013 Edition. Arlington, VA, American Psychiatric Association, 2013. Available at: https://www.psychiatry.org/psychiatrists/practice/ethics. Accessed November 30, 2018.

Darren v Safier, 207 A.D.2d 473, 474 (2d Dept 1994)

Durney v Terk, 42 A.D.3d 335 (1st Dept 2007)

Ibguy v State of New York, 261 A.D.2d 510 (2d Dept 1999)

Jacobs D, Baldessarinin R, Conwell Y, et al: Practice Guideline for the Assessment and Treatment of Patients With Suicidal Behaviors. Arlington, VA, American Psychiatric Association, 2003. Available at: https://psychiatryonline.org/pb/assets/raw/sitewide/practice_guidelines/guidelines/suicide.pdf. Accessed August 12, 2019.

National Practitioner Data Bank: Reportable Actions (website). Fairfax, VA, National Practitioner Data Bank, 2018. Available at: https://www.npdb.hrsa.gov/hcorg/WhatYouMustReportToTheDataBank.jsp#reportableActions. Accessed December 9, 2018.

Nestorowich v Ricotta, 97 N.Y.2d 393, 398, 740 N.Y.S.2d 668, 767 N.E.2d 125 (2002)

Park v Kovachevick, 116 A.D.3d 183 (NY Sup. Ct. 2014)

Professional Risk Management Services: Lessons to be learned: a review of post-suicide malpractice lawsuits. Rx for Risk 23(1), 2015a

Professional Risk Management Services: Treatment of the suicidal patient: part II. Rx for Risk 23(3), 2015b

Providence Health Center v Dowell, 262 S.W.3d 324, 329–330 (Tex. Sup. Ct. 2008)

Simpson S, Stacy M: Avoiding the malpractice snare: documenting suicide risk assessment. J Psychiatr Pract 10(3):185–189, 2004 15330226

Studdert DM, Bismark MM, Mello MM, et al: Prevalence and characteristics of physicians prone to malpractice claims. N Engl J Med 374(4):354–362, 2016

Tuten v Farizborzian, 84 So.3d 1063, 1067 (Fla. App. 1st Dist. 2012)

VerdictSearch.com: Trial Verdicts Involving Psychiatrists Sued for a Patient's Suicide, 1997–2017 (report). New York, ALM Intelligence, 2018

CHAPTER 28

The Psychological Autopsy and Retrospective Evaluation of Suicidal Intent

Charles L. Scott, M.D.

Phillip Resnick, M.D.

A retrospective evaluation of suicidal intent plays a pivotal role in various types of litigation surrounding an individual's death. Whereas the actual *cause* of death may be clear (e.g., gunshot wound to the head or crush injury from a car accident), the *mode* of death examines the person's intent (or lack thereof) to die. When assessing the mode of death, the examiner determines whether the death was from natural causes, an accident, a suicide, or a homicide. In approximately 5%–20% of deaths the mode of death is unclear; these are referred to as "equivocal deaths" (Botello et al. 2013). Common situations in which the cause of death is clear but the mode of death is not include autoerotic asphyxia, a fatal motor vehicle accident, and death resulting from playing Russian roulette.

Any one of these scenarios could result from either suicidal intentions or from a tragic accident. When the circumstances surrounding a death are unclear, litigation may follow to answer such unresolved questions, especially if financial or legal consequences ensue. Multiple areas of potential litigation may follow a death from unclear reasons, and some of these are noted in Table 28–1. This chapter provides an overview of how a psychological autopsy may assist in solving forensic mysteries surrounding potential suicides in both civil and criminal litigation.

TABLE 28–1.   **Areas of potential litigation following death from unclear reasons**

Life, health, or disability benefits from insurance policies that allow financial recovery for accidents but not suicides

Homeowner's policies that exclude coverage for intentionally violent acts

Legal actions related to workers' compensation benefits

Malpractice actions alleging suicide

Product liability claims

Motor vehicle insurance claims

Contested wills

Awarding of military benefits to surviving family members

Criminal prosecution when homicide by a third party rather than suicide of the decedent is alleged

Determination of whether death from police intervention was "suicide by cop"

Source.   Simon 1990.

Psychological Autopsy Overview

A *psychological autopsy* represents a structured approach to help evaluate individuals' intent related to actions or circumstances that resulted in their death. Robins et al. (1959) conducted the first retrospective psychological study of suicides through a detailed analysis of 134 consecutive deaths from suicide that occurred during a 1-year period. This retrospective investigation of a deceased's mental state was further developed during the 1950s by the Suicide Prevention Center in Los Angeles, California, to assist coroners' accuracy in the determination of death (Botello et al. 2013).

Schneidman (1981) coined the term *psychological autopsy* to describe the method by which an evaluator conducts a retrospective review in equivocal deaths to determine whether the death involved suicidal *intent*. Three important legal components of intent are that it 1) is a state of mind, 2) is about consequences of an act (or omission) and not about the act itself, and 3) extends not only to having in mind a purpose (or desire) to bring about given consequences but also to having in mind a belief (or knowledge) that given consequences are substantially certain to result from the act (Keeton et al. 1984).

More simply stated, suicidal intent involves a person's understanding that an action he or she takes will result in his or her own death. Whereas suicidal intent involves an appreciation of the permanent consequences of the suicidal act, *motive* refers to the reasons that the person wants to die. Such reasons may include a desire to have insurance money cover a family debt in the face of overwhelming financial stress or the hope that suicide will provide escape from personal problems or emotional pain.

In many types of litigation after a death from suicide, the evaluator will need to consider both intent and motive to determine if the deceased's suicide was "sane" or "insane." One often-cited definition of an "insane" suicide was described more than 100 years ago in the U.S. Supreme Court case *Mutual Life Insurance Company v. Terry* (1873). The Supreme Court wrote:

> If the death is caused by the voluntary act of the assured, he knowing and intending that his death shall be the result of his act, but when his reasoning faculties are so far

---

TABLE 28–2.   **Factors suggesting cognitive ability to understand suicidal actions and consequences**

Leaving a suicide note stating intent to die

Writing (e.g., in journals, posts) about desires or plans to die

Telling others of suicidal thoughts

Researching successful ways to die from suicide

Prepping the location to minimize collateral blood or tissue splatter

Having a prior near-lethal suicide attempt

Giving away belongings in advance of suicide

Recently creating, updating, or altering a will

TABLE 28–3.   **Factors suggesting ability to resist suicidal impulses**

Delaying suicide attempt until alone and cannot be stopped by others

Stopping suicidal actions if interrupted

Choosing a particular location to die from suicide and taking time to get to that location

Waiting until selected means to kill oneself is available

Taking steps prior to the suicide that require time and delay an immediate suicide

Taking time to write a suicide note

Telling others of suicidal thoughts and behaviors prior to attempt

No evidence of intoxication that could increase impulsivity

---

impaired that he is not able to understand the moral character, the general nature, consequences and effect of the act he is about to commit, or when he is impelled thereto by an insane impulse, which he has not the power to resist, such death is not within the contemplation of the parties to the contract and the insurer is liable. (p. 242).

This definition highlights three important factors used (alone or in combination) to assess suicidal intent and motive when distinguishing "insane" versus "sane" suicides in various jurisdictions. First, did the deceased have an underlying mental disorder? The evaluator will use the psychological autopsy approach outlined later to establish likely psychiatric symptoms and potential diagnoses present at the time of the suicide. However, the presence of a mental disorder alone is generally insufficient to demonstrate that the individual died from an "insane" suicide. Second, was the mental disorder of such severity that the person did not know or understand that these actions could actually result in his or her own death? This analysis examines individuals' cognitive awareness that they could die as a result of their action. Table 28–2 highlights factors to consider when evaluating whether or not the person consciously intended to die from suicide. Third, was the person so mentally ill that he or she could not resist the impulse to attempt suicide? This analysis reviews the person's ability to control suicidal impulses. Table 28–3 summarizes factors that may indicate the person's suicide was volitional and not an irresistible impulse.

Of note, many factors relevant to evaluating if a suicide was impulsive may also overlap with factors indicating that the person knew that he or she was going to die from suicide. For example, taking time to write a suicide note telling people goodbye

TABLE 28–4.	Areas to review for psychological autopsy

Basic identifying information (e.g., age, sex, marital status, occupation)

Specific details of the death

Outline of the decedent's history to include previous suicide attempts

Family psychiatric history (e.g., suicides and mood disorders)

Decedent's personality and lifestyle characteristics

Decedent's historical pattern of reaction to stress and emotional lability

Recent stressors or anticipated conflicts

Relation of alcohol and drugs to the decedent's lifestyle and death

Quality of the decedent's interpersonal relationships

Changes in the decedent's routine, schedule, and habits before death

Information relating to the "lifeside" of the decedent (i.e., successes and plans)

Rating of lethality

Reaction of informants to the decedent's death

Assessment of suicidal intention

Source.   Jacobs and Klein-Benheim 1995; Schneidman 1981.

indicates that the person knew that he or she could die from these actions (e.g., had the cognitive awareness) and had the behavioral control to take the time to write a farewell letter (e.g., had volitional control to temporarily delay their suicide).

Definitions of an "insane" suicide vary among jurisdictions, and the evaluator may not need to substantiate that the deceased had both a cognitive and volitional impairment in reasoning. Examiners must be familiar with the relevant statute and case law used to determine sane from insane suicides in their jurisdiction and how such distinctions apply in various types of suicide-related litigation.

Components of the Psychological Autopsy

Schneidman (1981) recommended that forensic evaluators review 14 areas when conducting the psychological autopsy (Jacobs and Klein-Benheim 1995). Table 28–4 outlines important areas to review when conducting a psychological autopsy.

To accomplish such an analysis, the evaluator examines two sources of information when conducting the psychological autopsy (Isometsä 2001). The first source involves extensive interviews of family members, friends, and other individuals close to the deceased. The second source is a thorough review of collateral records. Collateral documents that should be considered for review include the deceased's psychiatric records, medical records, suicide notes, personal journals, computer hard drive, social media postings and interactions, employment records, and academic records (when indicated). Evaluators should also review relevant legal documents such as the person's will or new insurance policies, police reports, witness statements, accident reports, and autopsy reports.

Although often admitted into evidence in a courtroom proceeding, psychological autopsies have been criticized for lacking basic psychometric test qualities such as reliability and validity. Other limitations include inconsistent retrospective assessments of psychiatric illness, potential recall bias by surviving informants, and medical ex-

---

TABLE 28–5.   **Suicide and mental state checklist**

---

1. Pathological evidence (autopsy) indicates self-inflicted death.
2. Toxicological evidence indicates self-inflicted harm.
3. Statements by witnesses indicate self-inflicted death.
4. Investigatory evidence (e.g., police reports, photographs from scene) indicates self-inflicted death.
5. Psychological evidence (observed behavior, lifestyle, personality) indicates self-inflicted death.
6. Statements of the deceased indicate self-inflicted death.
7. Evidence indicates that decedent recognized high potential lethality of means of death.
8. Decedent had suicidal thoughts.
9. Decedent had recent and sudden change in affect (emotions).
10. Decedent had experienced serious depression or mental disorder.
11. Decedent had made an expression of farewell, indicated desire to die, or acknowledged impending death.
12. Decedent had made an expression of hopelessness.
13. Decedent had experienced stressful events or significant losses (actual or threatened).
14. Decedent had experienced general instability in immediate family.
15. Decedent had recent interpersonal conflicts.
16. Decedent had history of generally poor physical health.

Source.   Jobes et al. 1986; Simon 1998.

aminers who may be prone to return a finding of suicide in individuals with a known psychiatric illness (Hjelmeland et al. 2012).

To address these concerns, the Centers for Disease Control and Prevention developed the Empirical Criteria for Determination of Suicide (ECDS). This instrument has 16 items that review a person's mental state at the time of his or her death and has been shown to be 92% accurate in differentiating between a suicide and an accident. The 16 items included on this instrument are listed in Table 28–5 (Jobes et al. 1986; Simon 1998).

The ECDS serves to supplement the evaluator's clinical judgment and may provide useful data to support opinions reached in the psychological autopsy.

Conducting the Psychological Autopsy

Surviving family members, friends, and colleagues of the decedent may be reluctant to speak with an examiner after the decedent's death. Because the evaluator may have only one opportunity to interview a key informant, reviewing the collateral documents carefully in advance when formulating interview questions is helpful. The evaluator should be sensitive to a variety of feelings that the person interviewed may experience. Such feelings range from extreme grief accompanied by guilt, sadness, or anger to suspicion and mistrust regarding the examiner's role. In some circumstances, if the examiner determines that the cause of death was an intentional suicide, the individual being interviewed may endure a financial loss and therefore may have substantial reluctance to participate in the postmortem analysis. Such individuals also may have significant motivation to misrepresent information. Asking interviewees what they think the outcome of the litigation should be may assist in evaluating their potential bias.

Although some family members may be reluctant to discuss suicidal communications, a sudden death from suicide may be genuinely surprising to most family members. Research indicates that only one-third to one-half of all victims examined in a psychological autopsy had communicated explicit statements of suicidal thoughts and behaviors to their family members or health care professionals during the months before their death (Isometsä et al. 1994; Robins et al. 1959). Likewise, a clinician may not know that his or her patient was contemplating taking his or her own life. In a Finnish review of 100 suicides of persons who had met with a health care professional on the day of their suicide, only 21% had communicated their suicidal intent to their clinician (Isometsä 2001; Isometsä et al. 1995).

When are the best times to conduct these interviews? Postmortem researchers of suicide have conducted interviews of informants a few weeks to 6 months after the victim's death. Brent et al. (1988) reported that when interviews were performed between 2 and 6 months after the suicide, no significant relation was found between the timing of the interview and the reporting of important diagnostic history and familial variables. However, studies also have found that survivors are more satisfied when interviews are conducted less than 10 weeks following the death rather than later (Runeson and Beskow 1991).

Various approaches have been proposed for contacting informants to arrange the interview. Researchers have found that contacting informants by letter, followed by a telephone call 1 week later, resulted in a high acceptance rate, with 77% of the approached families agreeing to be interviewed (Brent et al. 1988). In contrast, other researchers have achieved a low rejection rate by first contacting the survivors by telephone before sending a letter. By speaking directly with the informant during the initial contact, the evaluator is able to assess the reaction of the survivor (Beskow et al. 1990). When a letter is used to contact a close survivor, improved outcomes may be achieved through attempts to personalize the letter by referring to the deceased as "your son," "wife," "partner," or other appropriate phrase (Cooper 1999). Procedures that require the informant to complete a personality inventory of the deceased in advance of the interview have generated negative reactions from interviewees and are not recommended (Beskow 1979).

The evaluator must use caution when setting up the interview to avoid potentially sensitive dates such as the decedent's birthday or the anniversary of his or her death. The examiner needs to be flexible and sensitive to the emotional needs of the interviewee. In a pilot study that examined factors increasing the acceptability of the interview, Cooper (1999) determined that asking questions surrounding the death during an early stage of the interview was recommended to alleviate anxiety as soon as possible. In addition, the use of the phrase "sudden death" instead of "suicide" was generally preferred, especially in those cases in which the informant did not believe the death was a result of suicide.

The evaluator needs to anticipate the potential grief, guilt, or distress that an informant may experience during the interview. A refusal to participate during the first contact should be respected. Examiners may invite potential interviewees to contact them when and if they are ready to do so. Although the investigator may discuss the factual circumstances of the death, information that has been concealed from relatives or close friends generally should not be disclosed (Beskow et al. 1990). In summary, the psychological autopsy is a delicate examination that balances the need to obtain sufficient relevant information with the requirement to treat both the survivors and the deceased person with dignity and respect.

Psychological Autopsy and Litigation

Inheritance Litigation

Many life insurance policies differentiate the extent of death benefits according to whether the death was due to natural or accidental causes rather than a suicide, as in the following example:

> Mrs. and Mr. Barnes are enjoying their routine Sunday morning coffee and newspaper. Mr. Barnes leaves the room to take his shower while Mrs. Barnes begins tackling the weekly crossword puzzle. After 5 minutes, Mrs. Barnes hears a loud shot from their bedroom and rushes to the room, where she discovers her husband lying dead on the floor. His .45-caliber revolver is in his right hand, and he has a gunshot wound to his head. Mr. Barnes never communicated any suicidal thoughts to her, and she reports that he was not depressed. Mr. and Mrs. Barnes each took out a life insurance policy 18 months prior that included an exclusion clause for any suicide that occurred within the first 2 years of the policy. The insurance company refuses to pay benefits to Mrs. Barnes, stating that she is not entitled to benefits because her husband's death was a suicide. Mrs. Barnes' attorney contacts a psychiatrist seeking his assistance in conducting a psychological autopsy to help determine and offer an opinion about whether the decedent died from suicide.

When conducting an assessment of a deceased person's suicidal intent, the evaluator should seek the relevant insurance policy language. In particular, the psychiatrist should examine whether the policy governed by the relevant jurisdictional statute and case law distinguishes "sane" from "insane" suicides as discussed earlier. The jurisdictional definition of "insane" suicide must be determined when conducting the psychological autopsy. The referring attorney should provide the relevant standard. In some jurisdictions, a person who dies from suicide but is assessed as insane is determined not to have intentionally died from suicide; therefore, the beneficiaries have a right to the policy proceeds.

The following example illustrates a situation in which life insurance benefits may be granted if insane suicides are not specifically excluded from policy coverage:

> Mr. Cole, a psychotic man with the delusional belief that he is immortal and cannot be killed, shoots himself in the head with a revolver. Although Mr. Cole may have understood that he was pulling the trigger of a loaded weapon, if his delusional beliefs prevented him from understanding that he would die as a result of this gunshot wound, his death could be determined an insane suicide.

Some insurance companies have revised their policies specifically to exclude the recovery of benefits for death from suicide, whether sane or insane. In *Bigelow v. Berkshire Life Insurance Company* (1876), the U.S. Supreme Court upheld the exclusion of insane suicides from coverage under a particular life insurance policy, thereby preventing the distribution of life insurance benefits following a death from suicide re-gardless of the mental state of the deceased.

In general, perpetrators who take a person's life cannot inherit or profit from their crime. This concept is often referred to as the "slayer rule." For example, if a son shoots his father because his father was about to alter his will to exclude the son, that son could not profit from his father's death. In *Mutual Life Insurance Company of New York v. Armstrong* (1886), the U.S. Supreme Court specifically held that murderers should not financially profit as a beneficiary of their victim's estate. In this case, Benjamin Hunter obtained a life insurance policy for $10,000 on John Armstrong in which Mr. Hunter had himself named as beneficiary. Mr. Hunter subsequently killed Mr. Armstrong, attacking him at night and killing him by lethal blows to the head. Mr. Hunter was eventually arrested, convicted, and hanged for this murder. In regard to whether or not New York Life Insurance Company was required to pay Mr. Hunter prior to his execution, the U.S. Supreme Court held that "it would be a reproach to the jurisprudence of the country, if one could recover insurance money payable on the death of a party whose life he had feloniously taken" (*Mutual Life Insurance Company of New York v. Armstrong* 1886, p. 600).

Does this same principle apply if a person commits a homicide and then dies from suicide? In other words, would the homicide victim's assets be included in the deceased perpetrator's estate if the perpetrator had been included in the victim's will? Addressing this question requires consideration of two important factors. First, in some jurisdictions, negligent homicides are not included under the slayer rule because the person committing the homicide did not intend to kill the victim and profit from the victim's death. Consider the situation in which a husband accidentally runs over and kills his wife when exiting their garage in his car. He becomes so grief stricken that he dies from suicide 2 weeks later. Some states would allow the husband to inherit his wife's assets if named in her will, despite having caused her death, because he had no actual intent to kill her and profit from her death.

Second, many jurisdictions allow consideration as to whether a homicide perpetrator is "sane" or "insane" in the homicide-suicide context. Consider the following scenario:

> John, a divorced man with three children from a prior marriage, marries Barbara, a self-made billionaire owner of her own startup company. Barbara decides to leave all of her financial assets to John and not one penny to her own children.
>
> Over the next decade, John becomes increasingly demented and develops the delusional belief that Barbara is dying from cancer. When he asks Barbara about her health, she adamantly denies having cancer. He becomes convinced that she is "being brave" to keep him from worrying. He begins hearing her voice begging him to kill her and mercifully end her pain. He has no insight that he is psychotic and actually experiencing auditory hallucinations. In his delusional state, John does not believe that ending Barbara's life is wrong. In fact, due to his mental disorder, he believes he is morally compelled to aid his dying wife to relieve her suffering.
>
> John feels tormented by his dilemma and decides to honor his "wife's wishes" and join her in heaven by immediately killing himself after killing her. One night, he smothers Barbara with a pillow, takes a revolver, lays next to her dead body, places the revolver in his mouth, and pulls the trigger with the intent to die. Investigators rule that the two deaths resulted from a homicide-suicide based on extensive psychotic writings and notes left by John. Barbara's children legally challenge their mother's fortune going to her murderer's estate, regardless of whether or not he died from suicide. In this situa-

tion, courts may allow evidence to be presented in regard to John's sanity at the time he murdered his wife and then took his own life. In essence, John's ghost is on trial, and the evaluator will apply the relevant statutory definition of criminal insanity to render an expert opinion on John's mental state at the time he killed Barbara.

Workers' Compensation

Workers' compensation awards monetary benefits for individuals who sustain work-related injuries. The Longshore and Harbor Workers' Compensation Act (LHWCA; 1927) is a federal law that provides medical and other benefits to certain maritime employees such as longshoremen and harbor workers. A common requirement for all workers' compensation programs is that the workplace injury must "arise out of and in the course of employment." In other words, an injury that occurred outside and unrelated to the work environment does not qualify for workers' compensation. For example, an employee who sustains a knee injury when skiing on vacation will not be able to claim workers' compensation. In addition, employees who purposely injure themselves are not usually eligible for workers' compensation (Gold et al. 2017).

For many years, only physical injury claims were compensated under workers' compensation programs. However, mental health claims related to a workplace injury are now allowed in all states depending on the context of how the mental injury developed. Mental injury claims related to workplace injury have been broadly classified into the following three categories (Gold et al. 2017):

1. Physical-mental injury claims: In this category, a person's physical injury at work can conceivably lead to a mental injury. Imagine a firefighter who sustains third-degree burns while trying to save the life a young infant from a burning building, with resulting scarring and severe pain. This firefighter's significant and painful injury could lead to depression or another related mental disorder, all mental claims resulting from his original workplace injury.
2. Mental-physical injury claims: Claims in this category involve a causal relationship to workplace emotional distress and a resulting physical condition. To illustrate, an overworked employee with severe work-related stress and anxiety may experience a heart attack, stomach ulcers, or severe headaches.
3. Mental-mental injury claims: In this category, a worker claims that some emotional trauma has resulted in a mental disorder. For example, an employee who works as a first responder and observes severe trauma in others might allege that he or she experienced posttraumatic stress disorder as a result. Not all states allow compensation for mental-mental claims, and they are often difficult to substantiate.

When an employee dies from suicide, can compensation boards award surviving family members workers' compensation death benefits? In general, examiners may use two approaches when examining whether to award compensation benefits under this circumstance as summarized in the following discussion.

Irresistible Impulse Approach

The "irresistible impulse approach" analyzes whether the deceased employee had a mental disorder that made him or her unable to resist the impulse to die from suicide. *In re Sponatski* (1915) is the key case cited for establishing this approach in evaluating workers' compensation suicide cases. Mr. Sponatski was working when hot molten lead splashed into his eyes. He was taken emergently to the hospital, and while experiencing agonizing pain from his burn injury, he jumped from a hospital window to his death. The court upheld the decision of the Industrial Commission to award his family death benefits and established the following irresistible impulse rule often used in subsequent cases to determine workers' compensation benefits:

> Where there follows as the direct result of a physical injury an insanity of such violence as to cause the victim to take his own life through an uncontrollable impulse or in a delirium of frenzy, without conscious volition to produce death, having knowledge of the physical consequences of the act, then there is a direct and unbroken causal connection between the physical injury and the death. But where the resulting insanity is such as to cause suicide through a voluntary willful choice determined by a moderately intelligent mental power, which knows the purpose and physical effect of the suicide act even though the choice is dominated and ruled by a disordered mind, then there is a new and independent agency which breaks the chain of causation arising from the injury. (*In re Sponatski* 1915, p. 468)

Evaluators applying the irresistible impulse test must carefully consider the degree of the employee's suicide planning as well as any impairments in impulse control.

Chain of Causation Approach

An increasing number of jurisdictions no longer require proof that employees were unable to resist suicidal impulses when determining workers' compensation benefits in suicide cases. Instead, if the survivors can show that a workplace injury started a "chain of causation" between the qualifying workplace injury and the resulting death from suicide, then benefits may be awarded. The case of *Kealoha v. Director, Office of Workers Compensation Programs* (2013) provides an excellent example of this alternate approach. William Kealoha worked as a ship laborer. While at work, he fell from a barge and landed on a steel floor. He experienced blunt trauma to the head, chest, and abdomen; fractured a rib and his scapula; and developed chronic knee and back pain as a result of his fall. He filed for compensation through the LHWCA, and protracted litigation over his claim followed.

In 2003, Mr. Kealoha attempted suicide by shooting himself in the head. Although he survived, he sustained significant permanent injuries. He sought additional workers' compensation benefits related to the litigation over his claim and the injuries resulting from his suicide attempt. A psychiatrist evaluated Mr. Kealoha and diagnosed him with major depressive disorder due to multiple traumas and chronic pain, posttraumatic stress disorder, and a cognitive disorder. This psychiatrist also testified that Mr. Kealoha's 2001 fall aggravated his preexisting problems with impulse control and resulted in his becoming increasingly depressed, angry, and anxious. According to this expert, the 2001 fall set into a motion of chain of events that ultimately resulted in his suicide attempt.

At Mr. Kealoha's initial hearing, the administrative law judge applied the irresistible impulse test and found that because evidence indicated Mr. Kealoha had planned his suicide, he was not eligible for compensation. On appeal, the Ninth Circuit Court of Appeals held the following:

> a suicide or injuries from a suicide attempt are compensable under the Longshore Act when there is a direct and unbroken chain of causation between the compensable work-

related injury and the suicide attempt. The claimant need not demonstrate that the suicide or attempt stemmed from an irresistible suicidal impulse. (*Kealoha v. Director, Office of Workers Compensation Programs* 2013, pp. 524–525)

The chain of causation standard is easier to prove than the irresistible impulse approach. This standard allows consideration of awarding benefits in suicide cases even when the individual may have preexisting mental disorders that made the employee more vulnerable to becoming suicidal. If the psychological autopsy shows that the work-related injury played a significant role in the employee's mental state culminating in death from suicide, then compensation benefits will likely be awarded.

Criminal Cases

The psychological autopsy may also provide useful information in the evaluation of defendants involved in the criminal justice system. Most commonly, a psychological autopsy is requested by defendants charged with homicide to support their defense that the death with which they are charged was actually a result of the decedent's or victim's suicide. In the case of *United States v. St. Jean* (1995), a husband charged with the premeditated murder of his wife argued that his wife's death was as likely a result of a suicide as a homicide, and therefore reasonable doubt existed as to his guilt. To rebut this assertion, the prosecutor called an expert who had conducted a psychological autopsy of the decedent and was prepared to testify that none of the factors normally associated with suicide was present. The defense challenged the admissibility of the psychological autopsy results, alleging that they were unreliable and that the evaluator was not an expert in suicidology. The court allowed the expert's testimony, and the results of the psychological autopsy were deemed admissible on appeal (Biffl 1996; *United States v. St. Jean* 1995).

Results from psychological autopsies also may be allowed in cases involving criminal child abuse. *Jackson v. State* (1989) is a frequently cited case in which a psychological autopsy examined the relationship between a mother's alleged abusive behavior and her daughter's subsequent death from suicide. In this case, a mother altered her 17-year-old daughter's birth certificate so that she could work as a nude dancer in a nightclub. The teenager subsequently shot herself, and a psychiatrist was prepared to testify that the mother's behavior was a substantial factor in the daughter's death from suicide.

Although the defense argued that psychological autopsies were not reliable and therefore not admissible, the court reasoned that the jury could determine the reliability of this testimony and allowed the psychological autopsy results into evidence. A psychiatrist specializing in suicidology testified that the abusive relationship with the mother was a substantial contributing cause of the teenager's death from suicide. The mother was found guilty of child abuse, and this verdict was challenged. A Florida appellate court held that the state had presented sufficient evidence to establish that psychological autopsies examining deaths from suicide had gained acceptance in the field of psychiatry and that the trial judge did not err in allowing the psychiatrist's testimony (*Jackson v. State* 1989).

In a subsequent Ohio case, a father was alleged to have repeatedly sexually abused his daughter. After she died from suicide, he was charged with nine counts of sexual battery and involuntary manslaughter. A psychological autopsy was conducted to determine if the father's alleged sexual abuse was connected with his daughter's death from suicide. The father filed a motion to exclude the results of the psychological autopsy. Although the courts ultimately determined that the father could not be charged with involuntary manslaughter for his daughter's death from suicide, they commented that the results of the psychological autopsy could be relevant to the charges of sexual abuse. The court also emphasized that the possible relation of the father's sexual abuse to his daughter's death from suicide could be considered as evidence during his sentencing phase (*State v. Huber* 1992).

Conclusion

The psychological autopsy retrospectively assesses a deceased's mental state and intent. The evaluator conducting the psychological autopsy must be familiar with jurisdictional definitions of "insane" vs. "sane" suicides, consider collateral information, and make appropriate approaches to interviewing surviving friends and family. The psychological autopsy is an important assessment tool in both civil and criminal litigation and can identify hidden aspects of a person's life that explain any lingering mystery that shrouds his or her death.

Key Points

- The *cause* of death explains how a person died; the *mode* of death explains why the person died.

- A psychological autopsy can help evaluate whether a person died from natural causes, an accident, a homicide, or a suicide.

- Evaluators should be familiar with how "insane" versus "sane" suicides are defined in their jurisdiction.

- The psychological autopsy involves a combination of in-depth interviews with surviving family members and friends and an extensive review of collateral records.

- Workers' compensation benefits in employee suicide cases may be awarded to beneficiaries based on either an assessment of an irresistible impulse to die from suicide or a proven chain of causation between the workplace injury and the death from suicide.

References

Beskow J: Suicide in mental disorder in Swedish men. Acta Psychiatr Scand Suppl (277):1–138, 1979 286500

Beskow J, Runeson B, Asgård U: Psychological autopsies: methods and ethics. Suicide Life Threat Behav 20(4):307–323, 1990 2087767

Biffl E: Psychological autopsies: do they belong in the courtroom? Am J Crim Law 24:123–145, 1996

Bigelow v Berkshire Life Insurance Company, 93 U.S. 284 (1876)

Botello T, Noguchi T, Sathyavagiswaran L, et al: Evolution of the psychological autopsy: fifty years of experience at the Los Angeles County Chief Medical Examiner-Coroner's Office. J Forensic Sci 58(4):924–926, 2013 23551031

Brent DA, Perper JA, Kolko DJ, et al: The psychological autopsy: methodological considerations for the study of adolescent suicide. J Am Acad Child Adolesc Psychiatry 27(3):362–366, 1988 3379020

Cooper J: Ethical issues and their practical application in a psychological autopsy study of suicide. J Clin Nurs 8(4):467–475, 1999 10624264

Gold LH, Metzner JL, Buck JB: Psychiatric disability evaluations, workers' compensation, fitness-for-duty evaluations, and personal injury litigation, in Principles and Practice of Forensic Psychiatry. Edited by Rosner R, Scott CL. New York, Taylor and Francis, 2017, pp 307–318

Hjelmeland H, Dieserud G, Dyregrov K, et al: Psychological autopsy studies as diagnostic tools: are they methodologically flawed? Death Stud 36(7):605–626, 2012 24563941

In re Sponatski, 108 N.E. 466, 468 (Mass 1915)

Isometsä ET: Psychological autopsy studies—a review. Eur Psychiatry 16(7):379–385, 2001 11728849

Isometsä ET, Henriksson MM, Aro HM, et al: Suicide in major depression. Am J Psychiatry 151(4):530–536, 1994 8147450

Isometsä ET, Heikkinen ME, Marttunen MJ, et al: The last appointment before suicide: is suicide intent communicated? Am J Psychiatry 152(6):919–922, 1995 7755124

Jackson v State, 553 So.2d 719, 720 (Fla Dist Ct App 1989)

Jacobs D, Klein-Benheim M: The psychological autopsy: a useful tool for determining proximate causation in suicide cases. Bull Am Acad Psychiatry Law 23(2):165–182, 1995 8605401

Jobes DA, Berman AL, Josselson AR: The impact of psychological autopsies on medical examiners' determination of manner of death. J Forensic Sci 31(1):177–189, 1986 3944561

Kealoha v. Director, Office of Workers Compensation Programs, 713 F.3d 521, 524–25 (9th Cir. 2013)

Keeton W, Dobbs D, Keeton R, et al: Prosser and Keeton on Torts, 5th Edition. St. Paul, MN, West Publishing, 1984, pp 33–66

Longshore and Harbor Workers' Compensation Act, 33 U.S.C. §§ 901–950, 1927

Mutual Life Insurance Company of New York v Armstrong, 117 U.S. 591 (1886)

Mutual Life Insurance Company v Terry, 15 Wall 21 L.Ed 236, 242 (1873)

Robins E, Gassner S, Kayes J, et al: The communication of suicidal intent: a study of 134 consecutive cases of successful (completed) suicide. Am J Psychiatry 115(8):724–733, 1959 13617503

Runeson B, Beskow J: Reactions of survivors of suicide victims to interviews. Acta Psychiatr Scand 83(3):169–173, 1991 2031460

Schneidman ES: The psychological autopsy. Suicide Life Threat Behav 11(4):325–340, 1981

Simon RI: You only die once—but did you intend it? Psychiatric assessment of suicide intent in insurance litigation. Tort Insur Law J 25:650–662, 1990

Simon RI: Murder masquerading as suicide: postmortem assessment of suicide risk factors at the time of death. J Forensic Sci 43(6):1119–1123, 1998 9846387

State v Huber, 597 N.E.2d 570 (Ohio C.P. 1992)

United States v St. Jean, WL 106960, at 1 (A.F. Ct Crim App 1995)

PART VI

Prevention

CHAPTER 29

Suicide and Firearms

Liza H. Gold, M.D.

Firearms are the most common means of suicide in the United States; suicide is also the most common category of death associated with firearms. For the past decade, firearms have consistently been associated with more suicide deaths than all other means of suicide combined. In 2017, 23,854 people died from firearm suicide. This number represents 60% of all deaths due to firearm injury, 50% of all deaths from suicide, and 44.6% of teen deaths from suicide (Centers for Disease Control and Prevention 2019).

Lethal means restriction has been empirically demonstrated to decrease rates of suicide deaths (Mann and Michel 2016). When access to commonly used and highly lethal means of suicide such as firearms is restricted, suicide mortality decreases. In 2017, the Small Arms Survey estimated that U.S. civilians owned 393.3 million legal and illegal firearms, a rate of 120.5 firearms per 100 persons (Karp 2018), far higher than any other comparable country in the world. The profound connection between suicide, mental illness, and firearms underscores the need for clinicians to inquire about patients' access to firearms, particularly when patients are in crisis. In addition, to reduce risk of suicide before a crisis arises, clinicians should routinely and systematically discuss lethal means restriction and firearm risk management with patients and their families.

Lethality and Means of Suicide

Lethality is defined as the potential for death associated with an act intended to cause one's own death (Berman et al. 2003). Suicidal intent and lethality are independent dimensions of any suicide attempt. Factors that influence the lethality of a given method include inherent deadliness, ease of use, accessibility, ability to abort midattempt, and acceptability as a method of suicide to the individual (Miller et al. 2012). Firearms are inherently deadly, relatively easy to use, and highly accessible in the United States. Their use leaves relatively little time to change one's mind and abort a suicide attempt, and use of firearms is culturally syntonic in wide sectors of American society.

The case fatality rate for firearm suicide is far higher than that of suffocation (hanging) and poisoning (overdose), the next most common means of suicide (Table 29–1). Thus,

TABLE 29–1.   **Lethality of suicide means**

Means	Case fatality ratio, %	Suicide deaths 2017, %	Suicide deaths 2007, %
Firearms	85–90	50.6	50.2
Drowning	66–84	1.0	1.0
Suffocation/Hanging	61–83	27.7	23.6
Falling/Jumping	31–79	2.4	2.1
Cutting/Piercing	1–3	1.8	1.8
Poisoning/Overdose	<0.5–2	13.9	18.4

Source.   Centers for Disease Control and Prevention 2019; Consortium for Risk-Based Firearm Policy 2017.

even though less than 5% of all suicide attempts in the United States involve firearms, firearms are the means of half of all deaths from suicide (Anestis et al. 2017; Miller et al. 2012). Individuals who die from firearm suicide are more likely to die on their first attempt than individuals who use other means (Anestis et al. 2017). Moreover, the lethality of firearm use in suicide is more significant than demographic protective factors: suicide mortality is higher among males than females, independent of age, and higher among adults than among minors except when firearms are used (Shenassa et al. 2003).

How Means Restrictions Works

Restriction of a particular lethal means does not always prevent death from suicide. Nevertheless, in other countries and in the United States where restriction of commonly used and highly lethal means have been implemented, the decline in the rate of suicide by the restricted method has been associated with decreased method-specific suicide rates and typically with decrease of overall suicide rates (Barber and Miller 2014; Mann and Michel 2016).

In addition, many suicide attempts are impulsive, and the risk of death from suicide is often transitory (Barber and Miller 2014; Liu et al. 2017). When steps are taken to restrict access to highly lethal methods such as firearms, individuals intent on a suicidal act may temporarily or permanently delay an attempt. This can provide time for a suicidal crisis to pass, for the individuals to change their minds or abort attempts, or for the individuals or concerned others to find opportunities for intervention.

Gun owners are no more likely than non–gun owners to experience suicidal ideation (Anestis et al. 2017). However, gun owners endorsing suicidal ideation are seven times likelier to develop a suicide plan involving a gun than are non–gun owners endorsing suicidal ideation (Betz et al. 2011). The impulsive and unplanned nature of many suicides implies that individuals tend to use the method most readily accessible to them. Three in ten Americans report owning a gun and four in ten adults report living in a household with a gun (Pew Research Center 2017). Most firearm suicide deaths occur in the home (Anglemyer et al. 2014).

Substance use, particularly the use of alcohol, has long been recognized as one of the strongest risk factors for death from suicide (see Chapter 1, "Suicide Risk Assessment," and Chapter 9, "Substance-Related Disorders"). Notably, researchers have found individuals who died from firearm suicide to have the highest mean levels of blood alcohol concentration compared with those who died from hanging or poisoning (Conner et al. 2014). Another study found that individuals who had any level of acute alcohol consumption were 5.9 times as likely to die from firearm suicide as those who had no acute alcohol consumption and, in cases of excessive acute alcohol consumption, were 77.1 times more likely to die from firearm suicide (Branas et al. 2011).

Although individuals may attempt to substitute another method when highly lethal means are restricted, other methods are less lethal and fewer attempts prove fatal. Evidence indicates that restriction of one method of suicide does not inevitably lead to a compensating rise in the use of other methods (Mann and Michel 2016; Yip et al. 2012). In addition, a nonfatal attempt combined with waning impulses or crisis resolution may also result in accessing assistance. Despite the fact that a history of a suicide attempt is one of the most significant risk factors in assessments of risk of death from suicide, 85%–95% of individuals who have survived a suicide attempt do not ultimately die from suicide (Barber and Miller 2014).

Finally, unlike other methods of suicide, means restriction in regard to firearms neutralizes a significant and independent suicide risk factor. More than a dozen case-control studies in the United States have consistently found that having a gun in the home is a major risk factor for death from suicide for all household members, not just the gun owner (Anestis and Houtsma 2018; Anglemyer et al. 2014; Miller et al. 2013). This large relative risk of suicide varies from two- to tenfold depending on the age group and the manner in which firearms are stored, with less-safely stored guns conferring greater risk (Miller et al. 2016). The increased risk of death from suicide for all members of the household in which guns are available is independent of serious psychiatric disorders and rates of suicidal ideation or attempts (Betz et al. 2011; Miller et al. 2013).

Strategies for Restriction of Firearms to Reduce Suicide Mortality

Strategies for suicide prevention based on lethal means restriction fall into two categories. *Population-based strategies* typically require multidisciplinary and systemwide institutional design and implementation and general community support. *Individual-level strategies* involve improving the ability to recognize suicide risk on a case-by-case basis and intervene appropriately. These interventions are not limited to professionals and institutions; they are also available to acquaintances, family, and friends of high-risk individuals, who often are the first to recognize a crisis (Simon and Gold 2016).

Population-Based Strategies

General restriction of access to common means of suicide, which is not dependent on individual assessment or professional skills, is a population-based suicide prevention strategy. This has been demonstrated to be an effective strategy to reduce suicide when the restricted method is both highly lethal and common and when the restriction is supported by the community. Following legislation and policy changes reducing access to firearms in other countries, overall rates of suicide and rates of suicide by firearm decreased, particularly among youth (Barber and Miller 2014; Mann and Michel 2016; Yip et al. 2012).

Restricting access to firearms has also been found effective in decreasing rates of suicide in the United States. Among men and women, and in every age group including children, states with more firearm restrictions and lower rates of gun ownership have lower rates of overall suicide as well as firearm suicide (Fleegler et al. 2013; Kaufman et al. 2018). States with fewer restrictions on firearm ownership and higher rates of gun ownership have higher rates of firearm suicide (Anestis et al. 2017; Miller et al. 2016). Suicide attempt rates were similar in states with high or low gun ownership, but mortality rates were twice as high in states with high gun ownership. The differences in mortality were entirely attributable to the lethality of firearms. Therefore, even small relative declines in the use of firearms in suicide attempts could result in large reductions in the number of deaths from suicide (Miller et al. 2013).

Broad means restrictions require federal or state legislation regulating access to firearms. Community support for such legislation, although growing, is difficult to mobilize, and even minor proposed changes in firearm laws are politically and socially controversial (Mann and Michel 2016). The use of population-level prevention measures is likely to continue to meet with substantial resistance despite data supporting large population effects. Therefore, although effective, broad implementation of population-level means restrictions strategies in the United States remains problematic.

Individual Strategies

Individual-level interventions require the design and implementation of strategies tailored to individuals and their circumstances and are not means specific. Psychiatrists can work with high-risk patients and their families to remove, even if only temporarily, lethal methods from the immediate environment. Using individual strategies provides the opportunity to include family and friends, a potentially powerful source of social support, in preventing the suicide of a loved one. Reducing the availability of lethal means during a suicidal crisis can prolong the period between the initial decision to attempt suicide and the suicidal act. This provides time during which suicidal impulses and intent may decrease and opportunities to access assistance increase, thereby averting fatal outcomes (Simon and Gold 2016; Yip et al. 2012).

For example, empirical data support the efficacy of safe storage practices as a means of decreasing deaths from firearm suicide. Studies suggest that storing guns locked and unloaded can reduce suicide risk in gun-owning households. A dose-response relationship is consistently found in deaths from suicide that occur in the home, with ease of firearm access creating a hierarchy of suicide risk. Compared to homes without guns, people in homes with loaded firearms were at higher risk of suicide than those in homes with unloaded firearms; people in households in which a gun was stored unlocked were at higher risk than people in homes in which all guns were stored locked (Anestis et al. 2017; Grossman et al. 2005; Miller et al. 2012).

Unfortunately, health care providers, including psychiatrists, do not routinely discuss firearms with patients (Betz et al. 2016; Consortium for Risk-Based Firearm Policy 2017), and patients are not routinely screened for access to firearms (Price et al. 2007; Yip et al. 2012). Similarly, psychiatric residency training does not typically include firearm-injury prevention training (Price et al. 2010), despite the evidence demonstrating the efficacy of teaching empirically based suicide risk assessment (SRA) skills through postgraduate training as well as brief continuing education programs (Consortium for Risk-Based Firearm Policy 2017; Schmitz et al. 2012).

Research indicates that psychiatrists can decrease risk of death from firearm suicide on a case-by-case basis by utilizing two types of individual interventions. The first is implementation of a firearm safety plan that restricts access to firearms when patients are at increased risk of death from suicide. The second is provision of anticipatory patient counseling about the increased risks of keeping firearms in the home in regard to suicide as well as the decrease in suicide risk conferred by safe firearm storage.

Suicide Risk Assessment, Firearms, and Firearm Safety Planning

Lethal means restriction begins with an SRA (see Chapter 1). Questions regarding access to lethal means when assessing risk of suicide should not be limited to firearms. Clinicians who conduct SRAs typically ask patients if they have a plan and, if so, whether they have access to the means identified in the plan. Clinicians will not necessarily ask about access to means that patients do not spontaneously identify. However, given the widespread availability of firearms, their common use as means of suicide, and their high lethality, SRAs should specifically include queries regarding access to firearms regardless of whether patients mention them.

Important questions include whether the patient owns guns, has access to guns owned by someone else in the home, and if not, whether the individual has plans to purchase a firearm (Simon and Gold 2016). If clinicians determine that an individual is at risk of suicide, regardless of degree of that risk, steps should be taken to separate the individual from the firearms. For those at risk of suicide, storing firearms either away from or securely in the home (defined as locked inaccessibly from at-risk persons until risk is mitigated) is a suicide prevention approach that is considered an indispensable part of best practice (Mann and Michel 2016; Weinberger et al. 2015; Yip et al. 2012). Table 29–2 summarizes the key elements of a firearm safety plan.

Discussions regarding firearm safety management should be based on an explicit acknowledgment of concern regarding the patient's safety. A collaborative team approach that includes supportive family members or friends is highly recommended (Simon and Gold 2016). Designing and implementing a firearm safety plan may require one or more meetings with the patient and concerned others. The patient and involved others need to understand that an individual in crisis may be impulsive and reactive and that the presence of a firearm in the home increases the likelihood that a suicide attempt will be fatal. The role of drugs or alcohol in increasing risk of impulsive suicide and fatal outcomes should also be reviewed. If patients at risk refuse authorization for clinicians to speak with others for the purpose of securing firearms, clinicians will have to determine whether the circumstances necessitate a breach of confidentiality.

Safe gun storage at a suicidal patient's home is not possible. Experience has repeatedly demonstrated that an individual who is intent on finding the firearms is likely to be able to do so (Grossman et al. 2005; Simon and Gold 2016). Psychiatrists should communicate these facts to patients and concerned others. If suicide is an identified risk, the safest option is removal of the firearm(s). A supportive family member or friend may be able to effect removal and storage of firearms until the patient's suicide risk decreases. Patients at risk of death from suicide should not be handling firearms, even to remove them from the home.

Clinicians and patients should understand that limiting access to firearms does not have to be permanent. If the decision is made to remove a patient's access to firearms through secured storage outside the home, the firearm safety plan should include dis-

TABLE 29–2.　Sample firearm safety plan

1. Ask patients at risk for suicide (and significant others) whether they have access to guns at home or elsewhere, such as car or workplace. Patients who have a gun at home often have more than one gun.

2. Consider invoking emergency exception to patient confidentiality if a patient at high risk for suicide who has access to firearms or other lethal means withholds consent to contact significant others.

3. Involve significant others and the patient, if possible, in designing a firearm safety plan. Include discussions of clinical criteria to be considered for return of firearms.

4. Use this opportunity to educate all involved of the increased risks of a fatal suicide with access to firearms and use of drugs or alcohol and that the safest option is removal of guns from the home.

5. Designate a willing, responsible individual, usually a family member or partner, to follow through with the agreed-upon gun safety plan.

6. Confirm via callback from the designated person that the gun safety plan has been implemented. For example, confirm that all guns and ammunition were separated, removed from the home, and safely secured in a location unknown to the patient.

7. Document that the designated person implemented the gun removal plan and that a callback was received from that person confirming removal of the guns according to the plan.

8. Repeat suicide risk assessments as often as indicated, particularly before a treatment decision that may restore access to firearms.

Source.　Simon RI, Gold LH: "Decreasing Suicide Mortality: Clinical Risk Assessment and Firearm Management," in *Gun Violence and Mental Illness*. Edited by Gold LH, Simon RI. Washington, DC, American Psychiatric Publishing, 2016, pp 249–289. Used with permission. Copyright © 2016 American Psychiatric Publishing.

cussion of the clinical criteria that will be considered in the decision to restore the patient's access (Simon and Gold 2016). Among other interventions, clinicians should be certain to conduct an SRA prior to any clinical decisions that may result in restoring access to firearms.

Verifying implementation of the plan is an essential element of a firearms safety plan. Clinicians should not assume that patients or family members have followed through with firearm removal or storage. Regardless of the method of safety management, the plan should include a prearranged callback verification from the person responsible for its implementation. If clinicians do not receive the prearranged callback or the patient has refused to comply or otherwise interfered with the agreed-upon firearm safety plan, they should understand that the plan is no longer reliable and that they may need to reassess both level of risk and the plan's feasibility (Simon and Gold 2016).

As a secondary option for patients who may not agree to removal of firearms, clinicians should discuss limiting access through use of safe firearm storage practices. Safe storage requires less effort than removal and allows gun owners to maintain control of their guns, which might be preferable to some patients. Suicide prevention strategies include delaying access to firearms through four specific storage practices:

1. Storing the firearm in a locked container
2. Storing the firearm unloaded
3. Storing ammunition in a separate locked container
4. Storing the locked ammunition container in a separate location

Decreasing levels of risk and mortality were associated with each additional step taken to safely secure firearms. Hiding firearms and ammunition in an unlocked area is the least effective means of restricting access through storage. However, even safe storage in the home does not mitigate risk as effectively as complete removal (McCourt and Vernick 2018).

Anticipatory Guidance

Educating patients about the risks conferred by firearms in the home should not wait until someone in the home is in crisis. Psychiatrists can and should routinely provide information regarding suicide, firearms, and safe storage practices to patients. Many gun owners store at least some guns unlocked and loaded; storage practices vary by the type of gun owned, the reason for ownership, the presence of children in the home, and geographical location (Betz et al. 2016). Studies support the potential to decrease suicide rates among youth by limiting access to lethal means through safer firearm storage (Brent et al. 2013; Rowhani-Rahbar et al. 2016). Gun owners counseled by a physician about safe firearm storage were more likely to improve their storage practices when compared with those who were not counseled (Barkin et al. 2008).

The restriction of access to firearms through safe storage practices is particularly urgent in regard to child and adolescent suicide because storage of firearms locked and unloaded has been associated with lower risk of suicide among children (Betz et al. 2016). The vast majority of child and adolescent deaths from firearm suicide take place in the home using firearms owned by parents or other family members that are more likely to have been stored loaded, unlocked, and within close proximity of ammunition (Choi et al. 2017; Grossman et al. 2005). Investigations of these deaths consistently describe how easily the victims accessed the gun used (Choi et al. 2017). In fact, at least 18 states have "Child Access Prevention" (CAP) laws that mandate that firearms be stored so that a child or teen (the specific ages vary by state) is not able to gain easy access (McCourt and Vernick 2018). Although state CAP laws do not typically mandate a specific storage method, they are associated with lower rates of suicides among teens (Webster et al. 2004).

Physicians have only limited ability to ensure patients comply with recommendations for firearm safety (Simon and Gold 2016). Studies providing data regarding individual-level suicide education and lethal means restriction are needed, particularly for those at higher risk of suicide. Although many patients and their families may not benefit from more routine and proactive physician firearm injury prevention counseling, the benefits of averting even a small number of suicide deaths, especially among children and teens, are incalculable.

Some states, such as Florida, have experimented with physician "gag laws" attempting to bar physicians from asking patients about access to firearms. However, one study of public opinion found that two-thirds of non–firearm owners and more than one-half of firearm owners believe that health care provider discussions about firearms are at least sometimes appropriate (Betz et al. 2016). Regardless, in 2017 the Eleventh Circuit Court of Appeals ruled the Florida law unconstitutional (*Wollschlaeger v. Florida* 2017). Since this ruling, no state has directly prohibited firearm counseling.

Nevertheless, psychiatrists should be aware that certain types of firearm laws can complicate their ability to provide effective counseling about firearms (McCourt and

Vernick 2018). These may include laws restricting temporary transfer of firearms and laws regarding safe firearm storage. Psychiatrists who provide firearm safety counseling, whether as anticipatory guidance or with patients in crisis, should be familiar with their state's specific laws regarding such counseling, temporary transfer of firearms, and safe storage of firearms.

New Approaches to Individual Lethal Means Restriction

Limiting access to firearms on a case-by-case basis requires novel approaches toward public education and community participation. Innovative approaches that mobilize groups other than mental health professionals to be aware of signs of increasing risk in those with access to firearms need to be designed and explored.

In New Hampshire, for example, gun reform advocates, firearm retailers, and public health professionals have collaborated in the design of educational suicide prevention materials, available at stores that sell firearms, that build on the culture of gun safety promoted by many firearms retailers and owners (Vriniotis et al. 2015). The educational materials are based on a social marketing model similar to the "designated driver" and "friends don't let friends drive drunk" public education campaigns. The firearm safety campaign encourages a social norm in which friends and family hold on to one another's guns during a crisis, just as they would hold on to one another's car keys if they were drunk and attempting to drive. This approach demonstrates that areas of agreement, collaboration, and community support can be found between people who own and sell firearms and those who advocate firearm safety when it comes to decreasing rates of firearm suicide. It also avoids the need for any legislation or public policy initiative, which is a considerable advantage.

Another innovative approach uses a combination of population- and individual-level interventions for individual firearms restriction. People at risk may not be in primary care or psychiatric treatment. In addition, mental health and primary care clinicians may not be aware of sudden changes in their patients' level of risk, especially when that level changes in regard to an unexpected personal crisis. Concerned others, family, or friends may be first to become aware of these individuals' increasing risk of suicide as well as their access to firearms.

In response to these circumstances (and also the potential for such individuals to use firearms to harm others), a multidisciplinary group of researchers, medical clinicians, gun safety advocates, and others proposed a new type of legislation, the gun violence restraining order (GVRO; Consortium for Risk-Based Firearm Policy 2013). These are also referred to as an emergency restraining protection order (ERPO) and, more commonly, "red flag laws." Proposed GVRO laws were based on the model of domestic violence restraining orders and allow law enforcement to separate individuals, with or without mental illness, from their firearms during times of crisis. GVRO laws are civil, not criminal; are limited in time and scope; and have been found by researchers to provide the greatest benefit to gun owners by temporarily restricting access to their lethal weapons at a time of high risk of death from suicide (Bonnie and Swanson 2019).

The GVRO is a population-level intervention because it requires a change in state or federal law and applies to everyone equally, but it enables individual-level interventions. The lack of emphasis on whether the individual does or does not have a diagnosis of mental illness reduces the impediment to proactive intervention as well as the stigma associated with a label of mental illness. GVRO laws empower private citizens to petition a court to allow law enforcement to temporarily remove firearms from a family member or intimate partner, whether the individual has a diagnosed mental illness or not, who poses a credible risk of harm to self or others (Consortium for Risk-Based Firearm Policy 2013).

As of July 2019, 17 states and the District of Columbia have enacted such laws, and more states have GVRO legislation pending. At the federal level, the Extreme Risk Protection Order Act of 2019 (U.S. Congress 2019a, 2019b) has been introduced, which would incentivize states to pass GVRO laws by creating a grant program to help fund implementation efforts. Specific features of GVRO laws vary across states. For example, most authorize only law enforcement agencies/officers to petition for an order, but others authorized may include a prosecutor, health care provider, family member or intimate partner, household member, a state's firearm licensing authority, or various combinations of these categories (Bonnie and Swanson 2019).

Connecticut and Indiana implemented their risk-based gun removal laws in 1999 and 2006, respectively. Although more research is needed, limited data from these states (Kivisto and Phalen 2018; Parker 2015; Swanson et al. 2017) indicate that GVROs are most often used in response to concern about suicide risk rather than firearm violence directed toward others. The profile of persons typically subjected to risk-based gun seizure is similar in both states: gun-owning men in their middle years with no known history of mental illness who experienced an emotional crisis, contemplated suicide, and made someone close to them aware of their intent.

Nevertheless, in Connecticut, most individuals whose firearms were seized were also taken to a hospital for psychiatric evaluation, and approximately 30% remained in treatment 1 year later (Swanson et al. 2017). Increased enforcement of the Connecticut law after 2007 was associated with a 14% reduction in the state's firearm suicide rate (Kivisto and Phalen 2018). In Indiana, in the 10 years after the state passed its version of the GVRO law in 2005, the state's firearm suicide rate decreased by 7.5% (Kivisto and Phalen 2018). Another study found that in both Connecticut and Indiana 1 suicide was averted for approximately every 11 gun removals (Swanson et al. 2017).

GVRO laws are primarily directed toward providing families and concerned citizens, not mental health professionals, a means of intervention in difficult circumstances involving an individual at high risk of suicide or violence toward others. In the increasing number of states where such laws have been enacted, clinicians should familiarize themselves with their state's regulations and should communicate information about GVRO laws to patients and their families as part of crisis intervention and anticipatory guidance and counseling. Despite their promise (Mann and Michel 2016), risk-based gun removal laws should be considered as just one part of a larger strategy to manage risk and provide appropriate clinical care for patients at high risk of death from suicide (American Psychiatric Association 2018).

Conclusion

Decreasing the rates of firearm suicide will require multiple interventions on many levels. More research on both population- and individual-level interventions as well as improved training and skills on the part of mental health and primary care providers is needed. In addition, professional organizations need to develop and adopt standardized SRA guidelines that emphasize the need to evaluate access to firearms specifically in addition to general inquiries regarding access to lethal means.

Given the widespread access to and lethality of firearms and the rates of death from firearm suicide, psychiatrists should routinely include questions about firearm access, not ownership, in SRAs and in routine clinical evaluation of patients, particularly those with evidence of psychiatric illness and substance use disorders. Patients at risk for suicide require active implementation of a clinical gun safety management plan. Clinicians should provide counseling regarding the risk of suicide conferred by access to firearms and how to mitigate these risks, to the degree possible, by limiting access to firearms, including the use of safe storage practices.

Key Points

- Firearms are the most commonly used means of suicide in the United States, consistently accounting for approximately 50% of all suicide deaths.

- Suicide risk assessments (SRAs) should include questions about suicide plans and access to lethal means as well as specific inquiries regarding access to, not only ownership of, firearms.

- Safe storage of firearms in the home of an individual at high risk of suicide is not possible. Psychiatrists should work collaboratively with patients determined to be at high risk of death from suicide and their families to implement a plan that at least temporarily removes the patient's access to firearms in the home.

- Firearm safety plans should include agreed-upon clinical indicators of reduced risk before a patient's access to firearms is restored.

- Routine psychiatric evaluations should include patient education regarding the increased risk of suicide conferred by guns in the home, particularly if not stored safely, to the patient and to all members of the household.

- Psychiatrists should routinely provide anticipatory counseling to all patients about safe storage of firearms.

- Psychiatrists should be familiar with the firearm laws in the states in which they practice, including laws regarding storage and transfer of firearms and red flag laws.

References

American Psychiatric Association: Resource Document on Risk-Based Gun Removal Laws. Washington, DC, American Psychiatric Association, 2018. Available at https://www.psychiatry.org/File%20Library/Psychiatrists/Directories/Library-and-Archive/resource_documents/2018-Resource-Document-on-Risk-Based-Gun-Removal-Laws.pdf. Accessed May 3, 2019.

Anestis MD, Houtsma C: The association between gun ownership and statewide overall suicide rates. Suicide Life Threat Behav 48(2):204–217, 2018 28294383

Anestis MD, Khazem LR, Anestis JC: Differentiating suicide decedents who died using firearms from those who died using other methods. Psychiatry Res 252:23–28, 2017 28237760

Anglemyer A, Horvath T, Rutherford G: The accessibility of firearms and risk for suicide and homicide victimization among household members: a systematic review and meta-analysis. Ann Intern Med 160(2):101–110, 2014 24592495

Barber CW, Miller MJ: Reducing a suicidal person's access to lethal means of suicide: a research agenda. Am J Prev Med 47(3 suppl 2):S264–S272, 2014 25145749

Barkin SL, Finch SA, Ip EH, et al: Is office-based counseling about media use, timeouts, and firearm storage effective? Results from a cluster-randomized, controlled trial. Pediatrics 122(1):e15–e25, 2008 18595960

Berman AL, Shepherd G, Silverman MM: The LSARS-II: Lethality of Suicide Attempt Rating Scale—updated. Suicide Life Threat Behav 33(3):261–276, 2003 14582837

Betz ME, Barber C, Miller M: Suicidal behavior and firearm access: results from the second injury control and risk survey. Suicide Life Threat Behav 41(4):384–391, 2011 21535097

Betz ME, Azrael D, Barber C, et al: Public opinion regarding whether speaking with patients about firearms is appropriate: results of a national survey. Ann Intern Med 165(8):543–550, 2016 27455516

Bonnie RJ, Swanson JW: Extreme risk protection orders: effective tools for keeping guns out of dangerous hands. Developments in Mental Health Law 37(2):2–6, 2019

Branas CC, Richmond TS, Ten Have TR, et al: Acute alcohol consumption, alcohol outlets, and gun suicide. Subst Use Misuse 46(13):1592–1603, 2011 21929327

Brent DA, Miller MJ, Loeber R, et al: Ending the silence on gun violence. J Am Acad Child Adolesc Psychiatry 52(4):333–338, 2013 23571100

Centers for Disease Control and Prevention: Injury Prevention and Control: Data and Statistics (search results). Atlanta, GA, Centers for Disease Control and Prevention, 2019. Available at: http://www.cdc.gov/injury/wisqars/index.html. Accessed April 26, 2019.

Choi NG, DiNitto DM, Marti CN: Youth firearm suicide: precipitating/risk factors and gun access. Child Youth Serv Rev 83:9–16, 2017

Conner KR, Huguet N, Caetano R, et al: Acute use of alcohol and methods of suicide in a US national sample. Am J Public Health 104(1):171–178, 2014 23678938

Consortium for Risk-Based Firearm Policy: Breaking Through Barriers: The Emerging Role of Healthcare Provider Training Programs in Firearm Suicide Prevention. Washington, DC, Educational Fund to Stop Gun Violence, 2017. Available at https://efsgv.org/reports. Accessed May 4, 2019.

Consortium for Risk-Based Firearm Policy: Guns, Public Health, and Mental Illness: An Evidence-Based Approach for Federal Policy. Washington, DC, Educational Fund to Stop Gun Violence, 2013. Available at https://efsgv.org/reports. Accessed May 4, 2019.

Fleegler EW, Lee LK, Monuteaux MC, et al: Firearm legislation and firearm-related fatalities in the United States. JAMA Intern Med 173(9):732–740, 2013 23467753

Grossman DC, Mueller BA, Riedy C, et al: Gun storage practices and risk of youth suicide and unintentional firearm injuries. JAMA 293(6):707–714, 2005 15701912

Karp A: Small Arms Survey reveals: more than one billion firearms in the world. Small Arms Survey News, June 2018. Available at http://www.smallarmssurvey.org/de/about-us/highlights/2018/highlight-bp-firearms-holdings.html. Accessed April 26, 2019.

Kaufman EJ, Morrison CN, Branas CC, et al: State firearm laws and interstate firearm deaths from homicide and suicide in the United States: a cross-sectional analysis of data by county. JAMA Intern Med 178(5):692–700, 2018 29507953

Kivisto AJ, Phalen PL: Effects of risk-based firearm seizure laws in Connecticut and Indiana on suicide rates, 1981–2015. Psychiatr Serv 69(8):855–862, 2018 29852823

Liu RT, Trout ZM, Hernandez EM, et al: A behavioral and cognitive neuroscience perspective on impulsivity, suicide, and non-suicidal self-injury: meta-analysis and recommendations for future research. Neurosci Biobehav Rev 83:440–450, 2017 28928071

Mann JJ, Michel CA: Prevention of firearm suicide in the United States: what works and what is possible. Am J Psychiatry 173(10):969–979, 2016 27444796

McCourt AD, Vernick JS: Law, ethics, and conversations between physicians and patients about firearms in the home. AMA J Ethics 20(1):69–76, 2018 29360029

Miller M, Azrael D, Barber C: Suicide mortality in the United States: the importance of attending to method in understanding population-level disparities in the burden of suicide. Annu Rev Public Health 33:393–408, 2012 22224886

Miller M, Barber C, White RA, et al: Firearms and suicide in the United States: is risk independent of underlying suicidal behavior? Am J Epidemiol 178(6):946–955, 2013 23975641

Miller M, Barber C, Azrael D: Firearms and suicide in the United States, in Gun Violence and Mental Illness. Edited by Gold LH, Simon RI. Washington, DC, American Psychiatric Publishing, 2016, pp 31–48

Parker GF: Circumstances and outcomes of a firearm seizure law: Marion County, Indiana, 2006–2013. Behav Sci Law 33(2–3):308–322, 2015 25827648

Pew Research Center: America's Complex Relationship With Guns (website). Washington, DC, Pew Research Center, June 22, 2017. Available at https://www.pewsocialtrends.org/2017/06/22/the-demographics-of-gun-ownership. Accessed April 26, 2019.

Price JH, Kinnison A, Dake JA, et al: Psychiatrists' practices and perceptions regarding anticipatory guidance on firearms. Am J Prev Med 33(5):370–373, 2007 17950401

Price JH, Thompson AJ, Khubchandani J, et al: Firearm anticipatory guidance training in psychiatric residency programs. Acad Psychiatry 34(6):417–423, 2010 21041464

Rowhani-Rahbar A, Simonetti JA, Rivara FP: Effectiveness of interventions to promote safe firearm storage. Epidemiol Rev 38(1):111–124, 2016 26769724

Schmitz WM Jr, Allen MH, Feldman BN, et al: Preventing suicide through improved training in suicide risk assessment and care: an American Association of Suicidology Task Force report addressing serious gaps in U.S. mental health training. Suicide Life Threat Behav 42(3):292–304, 2012 22494118

Shenassa ED, Catlin SN, Buka SL: Lethality of firearms relative to other suicide methods: a population based study. J Epidemiol Community Health 57(2):120–124, 2003 12540687

Simon RI, Gold LH: Decreasing suicide mortality: clinical risk assessment and firearm management, in Gun Violence and Mental Illness. Edited by Gold LH, Simon RI. Washington, DC, American Psychiatric Publishing, 2016, pp 249–289

Swanson JW, Norko M, Lin JH, et al: Implementation and effectiveness of Connecticut's risk-based gun removal law: does it prevent suicides? Law Contemp Probl 80:179–208, 2017

U.S. Congress: Extreme Risk Protection Order Act of 2019, H.R. 1236 (116th Congress) (2019a). Available at: https://www.congress.gov/bill/116th-congress/house-bill/1236/text. Accessed May 6, 2019.

U.S. Congress: Extreme Risk Protection Order Act of 2019, S. 506 (116th Congress) (2019b). Available at: https://www.congress.gov/bill/116th-congress/senate-bill/506/text. Accessed May 6, 2019.

Vriniotis M, Barber C, Frank E, et al: A suicide prevention campaign for firearm dealers in New Hampshire. Suicide Life Threat Behav 45(2):157–163, 2015 25348506

Webster DW, Vernick JS, Zeoli AM, et al: Association between youth-focused firearm laws and youth suicides. JAMA 292(5):594–601, 2004 15292085

Weinberger SE, Hoyt DB, Lawrence HC 3rd, et al: Firearm-related injury and death in the United States: a call to action from 8 health professional organizations and the American Bar Association. Ann Intern Med 162(7):513–516, 2015 25706470

Wollschlaeger v Florida, 848 F.3d 1293 (11th Circ. 2017)

Yip PS, Caine E, Yousuf S, et al: Means restriction for suicide prevention. Lancet 379(9834):2393–2399, 2012 22726520

CHAPTER 30

Suicide Prevention Programs

Peter Yellowlees, M.B.B.S., M.D.

Benjamin Liu, M.D.

Suicide prevention research, a relatively young field, has advanced significantly in the past decade. Early prevention research focused largely on K–12 school-based suicide prevention programs (Pompili et al. 2012). These programs have consistently shown secondary benefits of improved knowledge and attitudes toward and about suicide but minimal impact on reducing rates of death from suicide. Since these early studies, research on other approaches to suicide prevention conducted in multiple countries is proving that certain suicide prevention methods do reduce rates of death from suicide.

Suicide Prevention Methods: Evidence Base

Hundreds of peer-reviewed articles in the literature on suicide prevention have been published, including a robust number of randomized controlled trials (RCTs). Two notable recent reviews of suicide prevention programs that stand out, and which identified numerous key studies discussed in this chapter, are a meta-analysis of RCTs by Riblet et al. (2017) and a 10-year systematic review by Zalsman et al. (2016). Advances in the quantity and quality of assessment of suicide prevention methods over the past decade have allowed the stratification of studies into four major groupings: 1) those with strong evidence supporting their efficacy, 2) those with moderate evidence, 3) those with little evidence, and 4) those that show promise but require more study.

Strong Evidence

Means Restriction

The importance of limiting dangerous means, or access to means, of suicide has been widely acknowledged for years. When access to highly lethal and commonly used methods of suicide is reduced or eliminated, rates of death from suicide decrease. Lethal means restriction has included creating physical barriers to deter jumping; designing facilities to omit hanging points; increasing control of firearm possession, toxic substances, and potentially harmful medicines; and detoxifying natural gas. These interventions have the highest levels of evidence supporting their efficacy (Mann et al. 2005).

Jumping is one of the less common means of suicide, accounting for 5% or less of annual death from suicide (Centers for Disease Control and Prevention 2019). However, jumping from manmade structures and natural points of elevation is associated with a lethality rate of about 35% (Spicer and Miller 2000). Barrier interventions to prevent high-fatality jumping suicides, especially when used at locations or structures that have high notoriety as suicide "hot spots," such as the Golden Gate Bridge, have been shown to be consistently effective.

Pirkis et al. (2013) identified nine interventional studies across more than five countries in which a barrier structure was introduced. The combined results yielded 354 suicides during 57 preintervention study-years (mean 6.2 deaths per year) and 171 deaths during 42 postintervention study-years (mean 4.1 deaths per year). Despite the finding that barrier interventions led to a 44% increase in jumping suicides per year at nearby sites, the total number of deaths due to suicide by jumping decreased overall by 28%. Other experimental studies in Montreal (Perron et al. 2013) and Brisbane (Law et al. 2014) also took into account increased incidence of death from suicide at other jumping sites in the region and found overall benefit in using barriers to decrease jumping suicides from tall and dramatic structures such as bridges and parking garages.

Death from firearm suicide accounts for approximately 50% of all deaths from suicide in the United States (Centers for Disease Control and Prevention 2019). One review (Anglemyer et al. 2014) that pooled 16 observational studies demonstrated significantly elevated odds ratios of death from suicide or homicide in relation to gun ownership or availability. Restricting access to firearms (see Chapter 29, "Suicide and Firearms") is therefore a major area of attention among those researching suicide means-restriction interventions, and evidence continues to build regarding the efficacy of this approach. For example, a retrospective analysis looking across five categories of state-level firearm legislation to generate a "legislative strength score" found that compared with the quartile of states with the fewest gun laws, the quartile with the most gun laws had lower firearm suicide rates (Fleegler et al. 2013).

Congress passed a landmark spending bill in March 2018 that gave the Centers for Disease Control and Prevention the authority to resume gun-related studies, reversing the Dickey Amendment of 1996 (Rostron 2018) that had previously significantly halted research on gun violence. Unfortunately, in 2018 no extra funding was allocated, so research in this area continues to be difficult and depends primarily on nonfederal funding sources.

Poisoning, usually by intentional overdose of medication, is the third leading means used, accounting for about 15% of deaths from suicide (American Association of Suicidology 2019). Controlling access to, and the toxicity of, medications and controlled substances has repeatedly been shown to be effective in suicide prevention. Modifications have ranged from completely removing the hazardous substance to simply decreasing the number of pills in a packet. In 1998, the United Kingdom passed legislation to reduce the pack size of acetaminophen. Packs were restricted to a maximum of 32 tablets through pharmacy sales and 16 tablets for nonpharmacy sales. A comparison of the effect of different pack sizes (Hawton et al. 2013) found that smaller packages resulted in a 43% reduction in rates of death from suicide—that is, an estimated 765 fewer deaths from suicide occurred over the 11.25 years after the legislation. Between 2005 and 2008 in England and Wales, acetaminophen/dextropropoxyphene, a toxic analgesic, was completely phased out of the market. Over the following 6 years, 2005–2010, approximately 500 fewer deaths from suicide occurred, a reduction of 61%, with little observed increase in deaths from suicide using other analgesics (Hawton et al. 2012).

Restrictions in access to high-toxicity or high-absorption nonmedication substances have also been shown to result in a decrease in deaths from suicide. For example, ingestion of widely available pesticides was a common means of suicide in Southeast Asia. Multiple studies in Sri Lanka suggested that restricting pesticides reduces suicide, and restrictions on sales of World Health Organization (WHO) Class-I toxicity pesticides in 1995 and endosulfan in 1998 coincided with 19,800 fewer deaths from suicides in 1996–2005 as compared to 1986–1995 (Gunnell et al. 2007).

Suffocation (i.e., hanging), is the second most common means of suicide in the United States. Notably, although hanging accounts for about 25% of all deaths from suicide annually, this means of death accounts for about 70% of all inpatient deaths from suicide (Williams et al. 2018; see Chapter 16, "Inpatient Treatment"). Implementation of the Mental Health Environment of Care Checklist, which focused on architectural changes, led to an 82.4% reduction in deaths from suicide in Veterans Affairs inpatient mental health units (Watts et al. 2017), suggesting that well-designed quality improvement initiatives can lead to a significant reduction in deaths from suicide in health care settings.

Means restriction for suicide prevention has been a major focus of new elements of performance being introduced by The Joint Commission in 2019 (Table 30–1). As of July 1, 2019, all accredited behavioral inpatient and outpatient facilities in the United States were required to perform environmental risk assessments and mitigation as well as introduce screening tools and evidence-based risk assessments for individuals who are potentially suicidal. The Joint Commission also requires facilities to monitor and ensure follow-up care for individuals who have attempted suicide, the rationale for which is discussed in the next section.

Follow-Up Care After a Suicide Attempt

In a meta-analysis of 72 RCTs and 6 pooled analyses, Riblet et al. (2017) identified the WHO's brief intervention and contact intervention as the most effective suicide prevention method, resulting in a statistically significant reduction in rates of death from suicide. A study by Fleischmann et al. (2008) enacted a treatment protocol in five underresourced nations (Brazil, Sri Lanka, Iran, India, and China) that consisted of providing long-term regular contact with anyone who had been seen in an emergency department after attempting suicide, as well as education and practical advice about alternative constructive coping strategies.

TABLE 30–1.   Joint Commission requirements on suicide prevention, July 2019: elements of performance (EPs)

EP1: Environmental risk assessment and mitigation	Behavioral health care organizations, psychiatric hospitals, and psychiatric units in general hospitals should conduct environmental risk assessments to be ligature resistant.
EP2: Validated screening tool for suicidal ideation	Individuals being treated or evaluated for behavioral health conditions as their primary reason for care need to be screened for suicide risk using a validated tool.
EP3: Evidence-based suicide risk assessment	For individuals who screen positive for suicidal ideation, organizations must use an evidence-based process to conduct a suicide risk assessment that directly asks about suicidal ideation, plan, intent, suicidal or self-harm behaviors, risk factors, and protective factors.
EP4: Document risk level and mitigation plan	Organizations must explicitly document overall level of risk for suicide and the plan to mitigate the risk for suicide to increase clinicians' awareness.
EP5: Address the care of at-risk individuals	Written policies/procedures for monitoring high-risk individuals will include a minimum of training and competence assessment of staff and guidelines for reassessment.
EP6: Care at discharge of at-risk individuals	Organizations must follow written policies/procedures for counseling and follow-up care for individuals identified as being at risk for suicide.
EP7: Performance improvement	Final EP asserts the need for monitoring implementation and effectiveness of screening, assessment, and management of at-risk individuals, with action taken as needed to improve compliance.

Source.   Adapted from Lyons M: "Joint Commission Announces New National Patient Safety Goal to Prevent Suicide and Improve At-Risk Patient Care." *The Joint Commission News Details*, December 5, 2018. © The Joint Commission, 2019. Reprinted with permission. Available at: https://www.jointcommission.org/joint_commission_announces_new_national_patient_safety_goal_to_prevent_suicide_and_improve_at-risk_patient_care. Accessed January 15, 2019.

The relatively minimal costs of the intervention protocol covered the training to administer a 1-hour individual information session near time of discharge and then nine follow-up telephone or in person contacts by a clinically experienced provider such as a nurse or psychologist. Significantly fewer deaths from suicide were found at 18 months after emergency department discharge compared with a treatment-as-usual (TAU) group (0.2% vs. 2.2%, respectively; $P<0.001$). Both intervention and control groups demonstrated similar low rates of usage of mental health services (5.7% vs. 5.0%, respectively). This reinforced the conclusion that the difference in outcomes was likely to be a result of the intervention protocol itself, not the use of mental health services. Although this study was not performed in high-resource Western countries, the results have been influential and have led to this treatment and monitoring approach being required by The Joint Commission, as discussed previously.

Primary Care and Mental Health Provider Education

Primary care physician education has been identified as one of the most promising suicide prevention interventions (Mann et al. 2005; Zalsman et al. 2016). Unfortunately, a direct association has been difficult to confirm, and experimental studies of this suicide prevention strategy are limited. The benefit of physician education is possibly related to an increase in the prescribing of antidepressants, but studies are limited primarily to experimental cohorts. In addition, most studies correlate the increase of improved primary care physician education with increases in antidepressant use and do not demonstrate if one leads to the other or which is more or less effective.

Interactive seminars on depression treatment for general practitioners in a county in Sweden with longstanding high rates of death from suicide between 1995 and 2002 were, however, associated with a reduction in the rate of deaths from suicide in that county to the same level as the national average, while the use of antidepressants increased from 25% below the Swedish average to the national average (Henriksson and Isacsson 2006). In a Hungarian region with a high rate of deaths from suicide, a 5-year depression-management educational program for general practitioners and their nurses, in conjunction with the establishment of a depression treatment clinic and psychiatrist telephone consultation service, led to a decrease in deaths from suicides from 59.7 in 100,000 to 49.9 in 100,000 (Szanto et al. 2007).

These educational interventions need to be expanded to other mental health professionals, including psychiatrists, to see if this may lead to greater impact in terms of suicide prevention.

Moderate Evidence

Pharmacological Interventions and Treatment

Lithium.   Among the numerous pharmacological options for preventing death from suicide in patients with mood disorders, lithium has the most substantial evidence base from a large number of RCTs. A combination of five trials on lithium used in either unipolar or bipolar depression showed lithium was the one pharmacotherapy among all others that had statistical significance in decreasing rates of death from suicide. The adjusted pooled data for the five trials yielded 0 deaths out of 284 patients in the lithium group versus 6 deaths out of 281 in the control group (Riblet et al. 2017). An earlier meta-analysis of 48 RCTs comparing lithium to placebo or active drugs in the treatment of patients with mood disorders showed that lithium was more effective than placebo in reducing the number of deaths from suicide and deaths from any cause (Cipriani et al. 2007).

Lithium has also been shown to be superior to valproate at preventing suicide-related events in patients with bipolar disorder (Song et al. 2017). Lithium and valproate were both administered in a within-individual prospective comparison study over 8 years that included more than 50,000 individuals with bipolar disorder. This study yielded a statistically significant difference in hazard ratios of suicide-related events, which were significantly decreased (by 14%) during lithium treatment but not during valproate treatment.

Antidepressants.   In contrast to lithium, the use of antidepressants has only been demonstrated in national linkage studies, not RCTs, to be associated with decreased rates of death from suicide. An observational cohort study tracking all prescribed antidepressants and recorded deaths from suicide in Denmark from 1995 to 1999 found that patients who continued treatment with selective serotonin reuptake inhibitors (SSRIs; i.e., those who purchased SSRIs twice or more) had a decreased rate of death from suicide compared with patients who purchased SSRIs once only (Søndergård et al. 2006). Another large linkage study across 29 European countries from 1980 to 2009 showed a clear inverse correlation between patient data being converted to defined daily dosage of 1 antidepressant per 1,000 people per day and the standardized death ratio of the group, suggesting an association between appropriate use of antidepressants and reduced risk of suicide (Gusmão et al. 2013).

Although few high-quality reviews assessing the connection between SSRIs and deaths from suicide are available, some RCTs have focused on the connection between SSRIs and deaths from suicide in specific populations, such as elderly or adolescent patients with major depressive disorder. The Treatment for Adolescents with Depression RCT provided reassuring evidence that the benefits of the use of antidepressants outweigh the risk from increased suicidal ideation (March et al. 2007). The authors concluded that suicidal ideation decreased with treatment, but less so with fluoxetine therapy than with combination therapy or cognitive-behavioral therapy (CBT). They noted that suicidal events were more common in patients receiving fluoxetine therapy alone (14.7%) and concluded that combination therapy (8.4%) was superior to monotherapy.

Promising Directions

Psychotherapy.   Psychotherapies, especially those that are CBT based, have strong evidence for their effectiveness in reducing suicidal behavior but not in reducing rates of death from suicide. Cognitive therapies including CBT have been reported to be effective in reducing suicidal ideation and behavior in multiple populations (adolescents, individuals with schizophrenia, individuals with borderline personality disorder) (Zalsman et al. 2016), but the number of RCTs examining CBT in regard to preventing death from suicide is limited. In pooled data from six trials of CBT for suicide prevention, fewer suicide deaths occurred in the intervention group (3 out of 514) compared with the control group (10 out of 526), but these results were not statistically significant (Riblet et al. 2017).

A Cochrane systematic review that assessed psychosocial interventions in adults who engage in self-harm and assessed suicide as a secondary outcome found that 15 RCTs of CBT-based psychotherapy demonstrated no significant treatment effect on rates of death from suicide at the time of final follow-up (Hawton et al. 2016). In another systematic review of 10 RCTs comparing CBT to TAU, CBT was shown to halve the risk of repeated suicide attempt in a population that had engaged in a suicide attempt within 6 months prior to trial entry (Gøtzsche and Gøtzsche 2017). Psychotherapies aimed at reducing suicide attempts were also shown in a recent meta-analysis of 32 RCTs (each of the psychotherapy and TAU arms included more than 2,000 subjects) to have a pooled absolute risk reduction of 6.59% (psychotherapy 9.12%; TAU 15.71%) (Calati and Courtet 2016).

Use of Electronic Medical Records and Depression Questionnaire Screening. The widespread introduction of electronic medical records (EMRs) has led to a number of trials in which attempts have been made to correlate either clinical data or screening tests, such as the Patient Health Questionnaire–9 (PHQ-9), with eventual suicidal thoughts and behaviors or suicide. However, in the assessment of suicide risk, sensitivity tends to be high and specificity low; thus, using these methods as suicide prevention interventions is challenging because the data do not necessarily identify a clear threshold at which to intervene.

In an attempt to assess risk of suicide following outpatient visits, one recent analysis of health record data showed that approximately one-quarter of deaths from suicide occurred in the 5% of patients with highest risk scores (Barak-Corren et al. 2017). Another study evaluated available EMR data combined with PHQ-9 depression data in outpatient clinics across seven health systems in regard to suicide risk. This study found that the patients with the top 5% highest risk scores accounted for a substantially larger proportion of the total deaths from suicide in specialty mental health and primary care, accounting for 48% and 43% of deaths from suicide, respectively (Simon et al. 2018).

The risk factors most highly associated with suicide attempts, as identified by Simon et al. (2018), included prior suicide attempt, mental health and substance use diagnoses, responses to PHQ-9 item 9 on suicidal ideation, and recent inpatient or emergency mental health care. Risk factors for death from suicide were similar to those associated with suicide attempt when comparing primary care with specialty mental health visits. PHQ-9 respondents in outpatient care who reported thoughts of death or self-harm "nearly every day" were six times as likely to die from suicide over the following 90 days compared with patients who did not report having such thoughts. However, all of these studies demonstrate poor specificity, with a high rate of false-positives showing patients who appeared to be at high risk but, fortunately, did not die from suicide.

Another promising area for further investigation concerns the role of social media and apps, especially when used with mobile devices (see Chapter 25, "Social Media and the Internet").

Little Evidence

Many suicide prevention trials have been conducted over the past 30 years, most of which have not been successful in reducing actual rates of death from suicide. Many intervention categories had trials that were too small to be clinically significant and in which the quality of evidence was generally low to moderate. Hawton et al. (2016) summed up the numerous approaches tried in a Cochrane review of RCTs of psychosocial interventions in adults and found no clear evidence supporting the effectiveness of

- Prolonged exposure to dialectical behavior therapy, mixed multimodal interventions (comprising both psychological therapy and remote contact-based interventions)
- Remote-contact interventions (postcards, emergency cards, and telephone contact)
- Case management and approaches to improve treatment adherence
- Interpersonal problem-solving skills training, behavior therapy, provision of information and support, or home-based problem-solving therapy
- Treatment for alcohol misuse
- Intensive inpatient and community treatment, general hospital admission, intensive outpatient treatment, or long-term psychotherapy

The rigorous meta-analysis by Riblet et al. (2017) specific to the outcome of suicide deaths largely agreed with these conclusions.

A number of other recent trials of suicide prevention have not produced encouraging results. For example, clozapine has been considered as a treatment to prevent death from suicide in some patients. However, no placebo-controlled trials of clozapine for suicide prevention are available, nor is there strong evidence to support clozapine's antisuicidal effect. The antisuicidal reputation of clozapine in psychosis largely relies on a single study (Meltzer et al. 2003), but this compared clozapine with olanzapine and found that patients receiving clozapine showed a significant decrease in suicide attempts, not deaths. In a Cochrane meta-analysis of RCTs comparing clozapine with other atypical antipsychotics in the treatment of schizophrenia, fewer clozapine users left the trials early due to inefficacy, but no significant difference in rates of death from suicide was found (Asenjo Lobos et al. 2010).

Similarly, although public awareness campaigns have become increasingly visible in many communities, suicide awareness research has been limited to ecological studies and has generally shown a significant increase in calls to helplines but no reduction in rates of death from suicide (Zalsman et al. 2016). An Austrian state used billboards to depict joyful everyday-life situations and to promote the use of a crisis hotline as part of a suicide awareness campaign (Till et al. 2013) and found that significantly more phone calls were made 3 months after the campaign when compared to the rate of calls 3 months before the campaign, but rates of death from suicide and approaches to improve treatment adherence did not change.

Suicide Prevention Organizations

Over the past decade, a number of organizations have developed specifically to address suicide prevention. Most support research, are involved in policy development, and are a useful source of professional and lay resources that supplement academic publications. Clinicians, patients, family members, and concerned others may find these organizations provide useful advice and information as well as professional and peer support. Some of these organizations include the following.

Suicide Prevention Resource Center.   The Suicide Prevention Resource Center (www.sprc.org) is the only federally supported resource center devoted to advancing the National Strategy for Suicide Prevention (NSSP). It supports multiple initiatives: 1) consultation, training, and resources for providers in settings and organizations that serve populations at risk for death from suicide; 2) the public-private partnerships of the National Action Alliance for Suicide Prevention; and 3) the Zero Suicide initiative for health and behavioral health systems. The website has a search feature that allows access to programs with evidence of effectiveness, defined as having at least one positive outcome related to suicide prevention. This organization propounds five guiding principles, which they refer to as "keys to success" and which include engaging people with lived experience, partnerships and collaboration, safe and effective messaging and reporting, culturally competent approaches, and evidence-based prevention (Suicide Prevention Resource Center 2019).

National Action Alliance for Suicide Prevention (Action Alliance).   The Action Alliance (https://theactionalliance.org) is a public-private partnership for suicide prevention and provides an operating structure to catalyze planning, implementation, and accountability for updating and advancing the NSSP. In its "Prioritized Research Agenda for Suicide Prevention" (National Action Alliance for Suicide Prevention 2014), six key questions ranging from public health approaches to clinical interventions reflect the breadth of the science needed to reduce suicide burden. The intended

TABLE 30–2.   **European Alliance Against Depression four-level approach**

Goal: Improved care for patients with depression and preventing suicidal behavior

Level 1: Education of primary care physicians so they can more effectively recognize and treat depression and explore suicidal tendency.	Level 2: Large-scale public awareness campaigns to improve knowledge and decrease stigma about depression.
Level 3: Education of community facilitators and stakeholders who play an important role in disseminating knowledge about depression.	Level 4: Additional resources for high-risk groups (adolescents in crisis or persons after suicide attempt).

Source.   Adapted from European Alliance Against Depression 2019.

audience for the organization's agenda includes scientists, agencies that support and fund suicide research, survivors of suicide loss or suicide attempt, those at risk for death from suicide, concerned family members, influential leaders who can reach at-risk individuals, and clinicians.

European Alliance Against Depression.   The European Alliance Against Depression (EAAD; www.eaad.net) project was originally based on the experiences of the Nuremberg Alliance Against Depression, which implemented a four-level approach to suicide prevention. This approach, which simultaneously targeted depression and suicidal behavior, was evaluated through a controlled pre/post design and yielded a reduction in the frequency of suicidal acts by 24% at 2 years compared with the baseline year. The four-level approach has been implemented in more than 100 different regions in 17 European countries and is described in Table 30–2.

An additional related project includes the Optimizing Suicide Prevention Programs and Their Implementation in Europe (available at www.eaad.net), which has built upon the EAAD by adding a fifth level of intervention: restricting access to lethal means. Results for the primary outcome of fatal and nonfatal suicidal acts in a controlled, pre/post, cross-country design are pending and, if positive, will substantially strengthen our suicide prevention tools. Some studies have been published of intermediate results such as effectiveness of community facilitator or general practitioner training and public attitudes toward depression and help-seeking (Coppens et al. 2013, 2014, 2017; Kohls et al. 2017; Maloney et al. 2013).

Conclusion

Studies in suicide prevention have undergone substantial updates in the past decade, with burgeoning numbers of high-quality studies showing positive results. National organizations dedicated to decreasing suicide often emphasize a similar set of strategies, many of which have proven in meta-analyses and RCTs to be effective in reducing either suicide attempts or rates of death from suicide. Core strategies that appear successful include close follow-up of individuals who have attempted suicide, means restriction, screening and detection through population data analysis, improved treatment of depression through enhanced primary care physician education, and the use of medications and psychotherapy for mood stabilization.

Key Points

- Means restriction, including firearms restriction, medication packaging, access restriction, and barrier interventions at jumping "hot spots" continue to demonstrate efficacy in reducing rates of death from suicide.

- Follow-up of individuals who have attempted suicide, specifically using the World Health Organization's brief intervention and contact protocol, shows strong statistical evidence for decreasing rates of death from suicide, although study replication in Western countries is needed.

- Increases in systematic precautions particularly for at-risk populations, such as mitigating risks in the physical environment, screening and assessing severity of suicidal ideation, and counseling and follow-up care at discharge, are likely to decrease rates of suicide.

- Pharmacological treatment, especially lithium, has a role in decreasing suicide in mood disorders, but more large-scale randomized controlled trials are warranted involving other mood stabilizers as well as selective serotonin reuptake inhibitors.

- Increased education of primary care physicians about suicide risk assessment and management enables frontline providers to more effectively treat depression and increases antidepressant use, thereby likely reducing risk of death from suicide.

- Electronic medical records combined with screening tests of depression and social media and apps on mobile devices are promising approaches to identifying those at risk of death from suicide.

- Psychotherapy, specifically cognitive-behavioral therapy and dialectical behavior therapy, have been shown to lead to a significant reduction of suicide attempts and self-harm but not actual deaths.

References

American Association of Suicidology: U.S.A. Suicide: 2017 Official Final Data. Washington, DC, American Association of Suicidology, 2019. Available at: https://suicidology.org/wp-content/uploads/2019/04/2017datapgsv1-FINAL.pdf. Accessed March 3, 2019.

Anglemyer A, Horvath T, Rutherford G: The accessibility of firearms and risk for suicide and homicide victimization among household members: a systematic review and meta-analysis. Ann Intern Med 160(2):101–110, 2014 24592495

Asenjo Lobos C, Komossa K, Rummel-Kluge C, et al: Clozapine versus other atypical antipsychotics for schizophrenia. Cochrane Database Syst Rev (11):CD006633, 2010 21069690

Barak-Corren Y, Castro VM, Javitt S, et al: Predicting suicidal behavior from longitudinal electronic health records. Am J Psychiatry 174(2):154–162, 2017 27609239

Calati R, Courtet P: Is psychotherapy effective for reducing suicide attempt and non-suicidal self-injury rates? Meta-analysis and meta-regression of literature data. J Psychiatr Res 79:8–20, 2016 27128172

Centers for Disease Control and Prevention: Leading Causes of Death Reports, 1981–2017. WIS-QARS Database. Atlanta, GA, Centers for Disease Control and Prevention, 2019. Available at: https://webappa.cdc.gov/sasweb/ncipc/leadcause.html. Accessed March 1, 2019.

Cipriani A, Geddes JR, Furukawa TA, et al: Metareview on short-term effectiveness and safety of antidepressants for depression: an evidence-based approach to inform clinical practice. Can J Psychiatry 52(9):553–562, 2007 17953159

Coppens E, Van Audenhove C, Scheerder G, et al: Public attitudes towards depression and help-seeking in four European countries: baseline survey prior to the OSPI-Europe intervention. J Affect Disord 150(2):320–329, 2013 23706876

Coppens E, Van Audenhove C, Iddi S, et al: Effectiveness of community facilitator training in improving knowledge, attitudes, and confidence in relation to depression and suicidal behavior: results of the OSPI-Europe intervention in four European countries. J Affect Disord 165:142–150, 2014 24882192

Coppens E, Van Audenhove C, Gusmão R: Effectiveness of general practitioner training to improve suicide awareness and knowledge and skills towards depression. J Affect Disord 227:17–23, 2018 29049931

European Alliance Against Depression: 4-Level Approach (website). Leipzig, Germany, EAAD, 2019. Available at: http://www.eaad.net/mainmenu/eaad-project/4-level-approach. Accessed January 24, 2019.

Fleegler EW, Lee LK, Monuteaux MC, et al: Firearm legislation and firearm-related fatalities in the United States. JAMA Intern Med 173(9):732–740, 2013 23467753

Fleischmann A, Bertolote JM, Wasserman D, et al: Effectiveness of brief intervention and contact for suicide attempters: a randomized controlled trial in five countries. Bull World Health Organ 86(9):703–709, 2008 18797646

Gøtzsche PC, Gøtzsche PK: Cognitive behavioural therapy halves the risk of repeated suicide attempts: systematic review. J R Soc Med 110(10):404–410, 2017 29043894

Gunnell D, Fernando R, Hewagama M, et al: The impact of pesticide regulations on suicide in Sri Lanka. Int J Epidemiol 36(6):1235–1242, 2007 17726039

Gusmão R, Quintão S, McDaid D, et al: Antidepressant utilization and suicide in Europe: an ecological multi-national study. PLoS One 8(6):e66455, 2013 23840475

Hawton K, Bergen H, Simkin S, et al: Six-year follow-up of impact of co-proxamol withdrawal in England and Wales on prescribing and deaths: time-series study. PLoS Med 9(5):e1001213, 2012 22589703

Hawton K, Bergen H, Simkin S, et al: Long term effect of reduced pack sizes of paracetamol on poisoning deaths and liver transplant activity in England and Wales: interrupted time series analyses. BMJ 346:f403, 2013 23393081

Hawton K, Witt K, Taylor Salisbury T, et al: Psychosocial interventions for self-harm in adults. Cochrane Database Syst Rev (5):CD012189, 2016

Henriksson S, Isacsson G: Increased antidepressant use and fewer suicides in Jämtland county, Sweden, after a primary care educational programme on the treatment of depression. Acta Psychiatr Scand 114(3):159–167, 2006 16889586

The Joint Commission: National Patient Safety Goal for suicide prevention. The R3 Report Requirement, Rationale, Reference 18(27)1–5, 2018. Available at: https://www.jointcommission.org/assets/1/18/R3_18_Suicide_prevention_HAP_BHC_1_2_18_Rev2_FINAL.pdf. Accessed January 15, 2019.

Kohls E, Coppens E, Hug J, et al: Public attitudes toward depression and help-seeking: impact of the OSPI-Europe depression awareness campaign in four European regions. J Affect Disord 217:252–259, 2017 28437762

Law CK, Sveticic J, De Leo D: Restricting access to a suicide hotspot does not shift the problem to another location. An experiment of two river bridges in Brisbane, Australia. Aust NZ J Public Health 38(2):134–138, 2014 24690051

Lyons M: Joint Commission announces new National Patient Safety Goal to prevent suicide and improve at-risk patient care. The Joint Commission News Details, December 5, 2018. Available at: https://www.jointcommission.org/joint_commission_announces_new_national_patient_safety_goal_to_prevent_suicide_and_improve_at-risk_patient_care. Accessed January 15, 2019.

Maloney J, Pfuhlmann B, Arensman E, et al: Media recommendations on reporting suicidal behaviour and suggestions for optimisation. Acta Psychiatr Scand 128(4):314–315, 2013 23590817

Mann JJ, Apter A, Bertolote J, et al: Suicide prevention strategies: a systematic review. JAMA 294(16):2064–2074, 2005 16249421

March JS, Silva S, Petrycki S, et al: The Treatment for Adolescents With Depression Study (TADS): long-term effectiveness and safety outcomes. Arch Gen Psychiatry 64(10):1132–1143, 2007 17909125

Meltzer HY, Alphs L, Green AI, et al: Clozapine treatment for suicidality in schizophrenia: International Suicide Prevention Trial (InterSePT). Arch Gen Psychiatry 60(1):82–91, 2003 12511175

National Action Alliance for Suicide Prevention: A Prioritized Research Agenda for Suicide Prevention: An Action Plan to Save Lives. Washington, DC, National Action Alliance for Suicide Prevention, 2014. Available at: https://theactionalliance.org/our-strategy/research-agenda. Accessed January 24, 2019.

Perron S, Burrows S, Fournier M, et al: Installation of a bridge barrier as a suicide prevention strategy in Montréal, Québec, Canada. Am J Public Health 103(7):1235–1239, 2013 23678905

Pirkis J, Spittal MJ, Cox G, et al: The effectiveness of structural interventions at suicide hotspots: a meta-analysis. Int J Epidemiol 42(2):541–548, 2013 23505253

Pompili M, Innamorati M, Lester D: Suicide prevention programs, in American Psychiatric Publishing Textbook of Suicide Assessment and Management, 2nd Edition. Edited by Simon R, Hales RE. Washington, DC, American Psychiatric Publishing, 2012, pp 593–614

Riblet NBV, Shiner B, Young-Xu Y, et al: Strategies to prevent death by suicide: meta-analysis of randomised controlled trials. Br J Psychiatry 210(6):396–402, 2017 28428338

Rostron A: The Dickey Amendment on Federal Funding for Research on Gun Violence: a legal dissection. Am J Public Health 108(7):865–867, 2018 29874513

Simon GE, Johnson E, Lawrence JM, et al: Predicting suicide attempts and suicide deaths following outpatient visits using electronic health records. Am J Psychiatry 175(10):951–960, 2018 29792051

Søndergård L, Kvist K, Andersen PK, et al: Do antidepressants prevent suicide? Int Clin Psychopharmacol 21(4):211–218, 2006 16687992

Song J, Sjölander A, Joas E, et al: Suicidal behavior during lithium and valproate treatment: a within-individual 8-year prospective study of 50,000 patients with bipolar disorder. Am J Psychiatry 174(8):795–802, 2017 28595491

Spicer RS, Miller TR: Suicide acts in 8 states: incidence and case fatality rates by demographics and method. Am J Public Health 90(12):1885–1891, 2000 11111261

Suicide Prevention Resource Center: Effective Suicide Prevention (website). Waltham, MA, Suicide Prevention Resource Center, 2019. Available at: http://www.sprc.org/effective-suicide-prevention. Accessed January 24, 2019.

Szanto K, Kalmar S, Hendin H, et al: A suicide prevention program in a region with a very high suicide rate. Arch Gen Psychiatry 64(8):914–920, 2007 17679636

Till B, Sonneck G, Baldauf G, et al: Reasons to love life. Effects of a suicide-awareness campaign on the utilization of a telephone emergency line in Austria. Crisis 34(6):382–389, 2013 23942384

Watts BV, Shiner B, Young-Xu Y, et al: Sustained effectiveness of the Mental Health Environment of Care checklist to decrease inpatient suicide. Psychiatr Serv 68(4):405–407, 2017 27842465

Williams SC, Schmaltz SP, Castro GM, et al: Incidence and method of suicide in hospitals in the United States. Jt Comm J Qual Patient Saf 44(11):643–650, 2018 30190221

Zalsman G, Hawton K, Wasserman D, et al: Suicide prevention strategies revisited: 10-year systematic review. Lancet Psychiatry 3(7):646–659, 2016 27289303

CHAPTER 31

Teaching Suicide Risk Assessment in Psychiatric Residency Training

Ashley Blackmon Jones, M.D.

Richard L. Frierson, M.D.

Suicide is a leading cause of death in the United States and a major cause of mortality in the field of psychiatry (Centers for Disease Control and Prevention 2017). Therefore, assessing an individual's suicide risk and subsequently employing treatment strategies with the goal of suicide risk reduction and prevention are key components of clinical practice as a psychiatrist. Because psychiatry residency training programs play a central role in the development of a physician's competence as an independent practicing psychiatrist and must certify that a graduate is capable of practicing independently without supervision, educating psychiatry residents about the principles of suicide risk assessment (SRA) is essential.

Residency is an important time for both didactic learning and the development of practice skills because residents have the unique opportunity to immediately use acquired knowledge under the direct guidance of faculty experts. In light of the increasing number of suicides in the United States, training the next generation of practicing psychiatrists to perform comprehensive SRAs and conceptualize complete risk formulations is imperative in minimizing loss of life due to suicide. SRAs have often been referred to as a "core competency" for residency training (Silverman and Berman 2014; Simon 2012). Although residents are evaluated on their provision of patient care related to assessing suicide risk, no standard teaching curriculum on suicide, SRA, or formulating management strategies for suicidal patients has been developed.

Training Program Requirements in General Psychiatry

The Accreditation Council for Graduate Medical Education (ACGME; 2018a) is a private, not-for-profit organization in the United States that accredits graduate medical programs as well as their sponsoring institutions. The ACGME sets standards for U.S. graduate medical education (residency and fellowship) programs, as well as the institutions that sponsor them, and renders accreditation decisions based on compliance with these standards. The ACGME also develops and implements specialty-specific program requirements, including basic curriculum standards for medical residencies (including psychiatry) and fellowship programs in all specialties. The ACGME monitors the adherence of programs to these standards through annual program self-studies and accreditation site visits every 10 years. As of 2017–2018, more than 11,000 residency programs in 180 specialties and subspecialties voluntarily participated in the accreditation process (Accreditation Council for Graduate Medical Education 2018b). Currently, 248 ACGME-accredited residency programs in psychiatry in the United States provide training to 6,307 on-duty psychiatric residents (Accreditation Council for Graduate Medical Education 2018a).

In order to meet the quality standards of the ACGME, training programs must be in compliance with "Common Program Requirements" as well as the additional requirements specific to their medical specialty. The *ACGME Common Program Requirements*

> set the context within clinical learning environments for development of the skills, knowledge, and attitudes necessary to take personal responsibility for the individual care of patients. In addition, they facilitate an environment where residents and fellows can interact with patients under the guidance and supervision of qualified faculty members who give value, context, and meaning to those interactions. (Accreditation Council for Graduate Medical Education 2018a)

The Common Program Requirements do not contain specific language regarding the inclusion of a suicide curriculum. However, the Common Program Requirements contain standards regarding physician wellness that include recognizing suicidal ideations in colleagues, faculty, or other residents.

In addition to the Common Program Requirements, each specialty or subspecialty has specific program requirements. The *Program Requirements for Graduate Medical Education in Psychiatry* (Accreditation Council for Graduate Medical Education 2017) never mention the word *suicide*. However, they state that "resident experience in forensic psychiatry must include experience evaluating patients' potential to harm themselves or others, appropriateness for commitment" (Accreditation Council for Graduate Medical Education 2017, p. 20). Furthermore, the psychiatry program requirements also call for a training experience in emergency psychiatry that must include "crisis evaluation and management." So, by inference, although clinical experience must include potentially suicidal patients, the methods and curriculum used to train residents in SRA are left to the individual training programs to decide.

Resident Evaluation

Assessment of individual resident progress in preparation for practice and evaluation of the overall educational outcomes of the training program are another required

TABLE 31–1.   **Milestones containing suicide risk assessment components**

Milestone	Description
Patient Care 1C: Psychiatric evaluation	"Safety assessment"
Patient Care 2 Footnotes: Psychiatric formulation and differential diagnosis	"Identifying risk and protective factors"
Medical Knowledge 2B: Psychopathology	"Knowledge to assess risks and determine level of care"
Systems-Based Practice 3C: Prevention	"Employs risk reduction in clinical practice"

component for ACGME accreditation. In 1999, the ACGME developed six general "core competencies" in which residents in all medical specialties must be assessed: 1) patient care, 2) medical knowledge, 3) practice-based learning and improvement, 4) interpersonal and communication skills, 5) professionalism, and 6) systems-based practice (Humphrey et al. 2013). Over time, modifications have been made regarding how the six core competencies are used when evaluating residents.

In 2015, the ACGME and the American Board of Psychiatry and Neurology published the "Psychiatry Milestone Project" outlining key developmental tasks for psychiatry residents (Accreditation Council for Graduate Medical Education and American Board of Psychiatry and Neurology 2015). Residents are evaluated twice annually on each of the 22 specialty-specific milestones by a Clinical Competency Committee established by the residency or fellowship training program. The milestones are used to monitor a resident's progression over time, and the completion of these evaluations is an ACGME requirement. Several milestones include aspects of SRAs (Table 31–1).

In addition to resident and program evaluations, the Psychiatry Resident-in-Training Examination (PRITE), an individual self-assessment examination developed by the American College of Psychiatrists and provided to all psychiatric residents annually, includes questions related to suicide (Silverman and Berman 2014). Even with the requirement for evaluation of residents' ability to perform an SRA and the incorporation of questions related to suicide on the PRITE, no standard educational curriculum or specific guidelines for residency programs is available for teaching suicide risk assessment and management (Cornette et al. 2014).

Educational Curriculum

Psychiatry residency programs are tasked with creating and teaching a comprehensive curriculum to include diverse aspects of psychiatric practice, with the goal of developing competent psychiatrists who can transition into independent practice. As mentioned previously, a standard educational curriculum for suicide assessment, prevention, and intervention does not currently exist. On a broad scale, many models for assessing suicide risk are available; however, no specific method that will reliably predict who will die from suicide exists (Simon 2012). Although guidelines from national organizations and specialists on suicide risk assessment and management share certain common elements, discrepancies between suggested models still exist. This leads to a lack of consensus and the absence of a gold standard for suicide risk assessment and management for psychiatric residency training purposes (Bernert et al. 2014).

Only limited data are available regarding the content and efficacy of existing curricula. A handful of surveys of training programs were conducted from 1983 to 2005, two of which reported that about 90% of programs have formal teaching on suicide (Melton and Coverdale 2009; Silverman and Berman 2014). Since the 1980s, surveys of the psychiatry residency training directors have indicated the most common form of teaching SRA occurred in an informal or passive method, with supervision, didactics, case discussions, or journal clubs. Workshops designed to foster skill development were reported in just over 25% of the programs. Didactic content was often embedded within other courses and not necessarily part of an established suicide curriculum (Silverman and Berman 2014).

However, with the lack of standard requirements for teaching and training, resident and fellowship programs appear to have different approaches in teaching SRA. In a 2005 survey of chief residents regarding the existing suicide curriculum in their programs, all reported that identifying the risk factors for suicide is included in their existing educational content, with an average number of 3.6 seminars devoted to this topic. Other topics covered in seminars reported by at least 90% of the respondents were early recognition of the warning signs for suicide, clinical care standards, and the ethics of hospitalization. Only 25% of respondents reported that postvention (responding to suicide deaths) was covered in their training, and 70% indicated that this area needs attention by their program (Melton and Coverdale 2009).

Implementing a Suicide Risk Assessment and Management Training Curriculum

Many of the crucial concepts of risk management can be incorporated into the existing six ACGME core competencies (Frierson and Campbell 2009). Most psychiatry residency programs provide instruction on risk factors associated with suicide. The evidence for psychotherapy, social interventions, pharmacotherapy, and crisis strategies (included in other chapters in this text) should be provided to residents in order to create a well-rounded curriculum.

With the significant volume of administrative work required from academic leaders, reimagining, developing, and implementing curriculum changes can be daunting. This task can become much more manageable by using existing resources. Several options include actively participating in established educational programs through workshop attendance or partnerships with other organizations, adapting existing effective suicide training programs for use, and referencing national organizations for inclusion of evidence-based teaching content. Unfortunately, limited data regarding the efficacy of many of these educational training programs are available.

Several reputable leaders in the field of suicide have established training experiences and workshops. These types of programs can be important references for content, implementation strategies, and training resources. A list of programs for suicide prevention, including specific notations for those with evidence for efficacy, can be found online at the Suicide Prevention Resource Center (SPRC; www.sprc.org).

Pisani et al. (2011) published a review of 12 suicide risk assessment and management workshops for mental health professionals that aimed to enhance clinical competence; one of them included psychiatry residents as participants. This publication included several well-known workshops and listed the various areas of clinical competence that each program aimed to address. Many programs reported the number of clinicians they had trained up until 2008, program outcomes, teaching format, number of hours, and the training required for instructors (Pisani et al. 2011).

Due to the high number of suicides encountered among active-duty U.S. military personnel and combat veterans, the U.S. Department of Veterans Affairs (VA) has developed a comprehensive approach to suicide prevention and risk management. The VA can offer both clinical and informational resources and can also serve as a potential collaboration partner to assist psychiatry residency programs with training (Pheister et al. 2014). Educational leaders may wish to consult with these resources, because they can be helpful in a multitude of ways.

Referencing and using nationally recognized groups dedicated to suicide prevention provides an additional opportunity for educational leaders to find and develop curriculum content. The Centers for Disease Control and Prevention (CDC), American Foundation for Suicide Prevention, Substance Abuse and Mental Health Services Administration, American Association of Suicidology, VA, and the National Strategy for Suicide Prevention are examples of potentially accessible resources on suicide (Office of the Surgeon General and National Action Alliance for Suicide Prevention 2012; Silverman and Berman 2014). Guidelines can also be found in the American Psychiatric Association's (2003) practice guidelines for treating suicidal patients, the Zero Suicide model (Brodsky et al. 2018), and the SPRC. Programs can provide residents and fellows access to quick reference tools for use in the clinical setting to reinforce concepts during active patient care.

The American Psychiatric Association's *Practice Guideline for the Assessment and Treatment of Patients With Suicidal Behaviors* and *Assessing and Treating Suicidal Behaviors: A Quick Reference Guide* were originally developed in 2003, not as a standard of care but as guidelines that can assist psychiatrists who frequently work with suicidal patients. This set of guidelines outlines strategies for assessment and management, lists specific treatment modalities, and provides guidance on considerations for risk management and documentation (American Psychiatric Association 2003, 2004). Also, the National Action Alliance for Suicide Prevention developed the Zero Suicide program, which has 10 clinical interventions aimed at helping clinicians incorporate suicide prevention into routine practice (Brodsky et al. 2018; Retamero et al. 2014). Additionally, the SPRC adapted existing models into a "Comprehensive Approach to Suicide Prevention" that includes nine broad areas that can each incorporate a multitude of programs and interventions (Retamero et al. 2014; Suicide Prevention Resource Center 2018). An outline of the models can be found in Table 31–2.

It has been suggested that psychiatry residents be taught "best practices" for prevention, early detection, pharmacotherapy strategies, and psychotherapy interventions (Zisook et al. 2013). Instead of applying a "one-size-fits-all" method for assessing and preventing suicide, these methods can be applied more specifically and purposefully for the populations at risk (Silverman and Berman 2014). Residents should also be taught how to use validated suicide assessment tools in conjunction with other assessment methods in an evidence-based manner (see Chapter 1, "Suicide Risk Assessment"). However, clinicians, including residents, who are learning SRA should not rely solely on these structured SRA tools because they cannot replace clinical judgment and their positive predictive value is low (Simon 2012; Tanguturi et al. 2017).

TABLE 31–2.   **Models for suicide assessment and management**

Name	Components

American Psychiatric Association 2003, 2004	Assessment
	  1. Psychiatric evaluation
	  2. Inquiry for specific thoughts, plans, and behaviors related to suicide
	  3. Development of comprehensive list of diagnoses, psychosocial stressors, and level of functioning*
	  4. Estimation of suicide risk
	Management
	  1. Therapeutic alliance
	  2. Assessment and intervention for patient's physical safety
	  3. Treatment setting determination
	  4. Treatment plan development
	  5. Collaboration and coordination of care
	  6. Adherence promotion
	  7. Psychoeducation
	  8. Safety and risk reassessments over time
	  9. Monitoring
	  10. Consultations if needed

Suicide Prevention Resource Center 2018	1. Identify and assess 2. Increase help-seeking 3. Effective treatment 4. Transitions of care 5. Crisis response 6. Postvention 7. Access to means reduction 8. Resilience and life skills 9. Connectedness

National Action Alliance for Suicide Prevention's Zero Suicide Model (Brodsky et al. 2018)	Assess, Intervene and Monitor for Suicide Prevention (AIM-SP):
	  Assess (steps 1–3): risk assessment, screening
	  Intervene (steps 4–6): suicide-specific psychosocial interventions (coping/psychotherapy, restricting access to lethal means, safety planning)
	  Monitor (steps 7–10): ongoing monitoring and support, increase support during high risk times

Note.   *Updated description created for the purposes of this chart because original wording in practice guidelines is "establish multiaxial diagnosis."

SRA training should absolutely begin in the first year of residency. In the vast majority of general psychiatry residency programs, the bulk of on-call coverage of psychiatric emergency departments, where persons with active suicidal thoughts are likely to be encountered, is relegated to the postgraduate-year (PGY)-1 and PGY-2 residents. Going from the role of medical student to physician in a short timeframe can create anxiety regarding clinical responsibilities, especially those conducted after hours when a faculty supervisor may not be readily available. Without such early training in SRA, newly graduated physicians entering psychiatry residency may be ill equipped to deal with and distinguish between acutely suicidal patients who present in crisis and chronically suicidal patients for whom psychiatric commitment might not be indicated.

Teaching residents to incorporate strategies that emphasize a systematic and comprehensive approach to SRAs to inform and enhance clinical management is ideal (Simon 2012). The acquisition of knowledge in risk assessment and the development of skills in determination of risk and creating management plans are two distinct learning objectives. Residents must achieve competency in both knowledge and skill. In addition to didactic content, this could be addressed by adding more active strategies, such as case discussions, clinical vignettes, roleplay, and active experiences providing care for suicidal patients under supervision (Silverman and Berman 2014). A clinician's own culture, beliefs about suicide, and experience with mental health problems with friends and family can also affect clinical judgment. Therefore, including an educational forum to discuss these issues may be beneficial (Foster et al. 2015). As with any educational initiative, establishing a method for monitoring the efficacy and adequacy of the curriculum is important.

Beyond developing suicide curriculum content, residency programs can include creative teaching strategies and consider implementation of changes within their sponsoring institution or within a larger health care system to aid in SRA. Virtual patients, online modules, live simulations, and workshops are all potential ways to solidify clinical skills by incorporating a variety of educational modalities. Seemingly simple changes to electronic medical record resources, such as including pop-up notifications or clickable scales that incorporate SRA questions, could also potentially make positive impacts across health systems. Although not a comprehensive review of these interventions, several examples of nontraditional educational activities are outlined in Table 31–3.

Sample Curriculum

Practical aspects of residency training such as the number of residents in a specific program and the schedule of clinical rotations will likely inform the development and implementation of a comprehensive suicide curriculum in a general psychiatry residency training program. Using an approach based on level of training is a simple way to organize content that can be applied broadly and subsequently adjusted on an individual programmatic basis. The most common patient population and work locations will significantly influence the knowledge and skills that residents need for that particular year of training and therefore should be part of a curriculum consideration. As seen with the milestones, residents are expected to gradually develop skills over the course of 4 years. Given the significant impact of suicide and the high likelihood of residents

TABLE 31–3.   Nontraditional educational strategies for a suicide curriculum

Targeted skill	Reference	Method	Learners	Purpose	Outcomes
Skill and interview	Foster et al. 2015	Virtual patient simulation Video teaching module	Medical students	Teach SRA	88.2% asking about suicide in virtual simulation and 75.8% in video module; a feasible method for both acquiring knowledge and practicing skills
Documentation	Tanguturi et al. 2017	Paper documentation EMR documentation	Psychiatry residents	Examine deficiencies in documenting SRAs in paper vs. EMR (based on the C-SSRS)	Use of EMR with selectable risk and protective factors adapted from the C-SSRS showed improved documentation
Documentation	Reshetukha et al. 2018	Brief educational instruction session and prompt for risk assessment in the ED	ED residents Psychiatry residents	Determine if brief teaching session and prompt in the EMR that includes risk assessment information can lead to improved SRA documentation in the ED	Documentation of suicide risk factors improved after intervention and was maintained at 6 months
Evidence-based review	Zisook et al. 2013	Team-based learning	Psychiatry residency Training directors	Demonstrate a team-based learning approach to teach evidence-based review of SRA	80% indicated a favorable likelihood of using the information back at their home program
Overall understanding of suicide	Retamero et al. 2014	Film	Medical students	Assess the use of film in augmenting instruction on suicide	Better understanding of risk factors and stigma; receptive to the idea of using film as an addition to the curriculum

Note.   C-SSRS=Columbia-Suicide Severity Rating Scale; ED=emergency department; EMR=electronic medical record; SRA=suicide risk assessment.

encountering patients at risk for suicide during all years of training, a curriculum must begin in the first year and continue longitudinally. The sample curriculum that follows represents one potential way to organize a suicide curriculum.

Postgraduate Year 1

During the first year of general psychiatry residency, inpatient and emergency-based psychiatry rotations (and often on-call experiences) make up the majority of the psychiatry experiences. In a suicide curriculum, this year should emphasize the importance of building a solid knowledge base and developing practical skills related to the common clinical situations encountered. Basic topics include SRA purpose and content, methods for performing a risk assessment, basic management of an acute crisis or times of high risk, and support in obtaining additional supervision if needed.

Initially, during orientation, a "crash course" or "intern boot camp" is often used as an introduction to important themes, including suicide. This course can include an observational experience where the first-year resident interviews and presents a standardized patient to a faculty member. Didactic content should occur throughout the academic year with particular emphasis in the beginning on what may be the most immediately needed skill. Specific topics include introductory information about the impact of suicide, diseases associated with suicide, interview strategies for suicidal patients, risk factors (modifiable and nonmodifiable), protective factors, documentation of risk assessment, criteria for inpatient hospitalization (voluntary and involuntary), and basic management of patients in an acute crisis.

Lecture content should be relevant to mostly inpatient and emergency settings and be enhanced when possible by case discussion, roleplay, and practice in involuntary commitment procedures. PGY-1 residents should be allowed and encouraged to attend case conferences or other opportunities to observe interviews, discussions, and treatment planning for suicidal patients. Rotation evaluations that include milestone language related to basic risk assessments and determining level of care should be developed. Also, dedicated teaching faculty should be tasked with the role of observing interviews during rotations to reinforce important suicide-related concepts and discuss medical decision making with the resident.

Postgraduate Year 2

Second-year general psychiatry residents should continue to have the same topics emphasized in the didactic curriculum, with inclusion of more active discussion and skills practice. Assigning readings prior to didactics can refresh the resident on the information presented during the first year of training and also provide a more substantial amount of didactic time for active teaching strategies. Risk assessment seminars and clinical teaching should be more advanced and comprehensive to match the knowledge, skill, and autonomy level of a PGY-2 resident. An introduction to the management of outpatients who are at risk of dying from suicide should also be included. Public health models and progressive management strategies for discharge planning, safety planning, and referrals to comprehensive community programs should be reviewed and residents provided with the opportunity to teach medical students and other residents about suicide.

Postgraduate Year 3

As residents enter the final 2 years of training, emphasis should be placed on advanced skill development and clinical management decisions. Although some programs may begin outpatient work earlier, most programs use the third year of training as the dedicated time for a yearlong clinical experience in the outpatient setting. Seminars should focus on treating suicidal patients on an outpatient basis—including crisis management, contingency plan development, and psychotherapeutic interventions. Residents should be taught procedures for increasing the level of care for clinic outpatients, documenting an SRA in the record, monitoring risk factors over time, managing countertransference in treating suicidal patients, handling crisis phone calls, and navigating the therapeutic relationship in the context of suicidal ideations or hospitalizations. Individual caseload supervision should include verbal discussions, session observations (live or recorded), and documentation reviews of patients at significant suicide risk.

Postgraduate Year 4

Residents in their final year of training in general psychiatry should be filling knowledge gaps and focusing on clinical skills with the impetus of preparing for independent practice. Rotations can be considered "junior attending" experiences where the resident serves as team leader and has more autonomy than any other time in residency, including taking on the responsibility to supervise early level residents with attending backup. During this time, teaching faculty continue to provide supervision and give feedback on clinical management decisions with suicidal patients to provide guidance and have the resident gain additional clinical confidence prior to graduation. Residents can also participate on an administrative level with postvention procedures or quality improvement planning to enhance patient safety in a variety of work systems.

Public Health Models

Suicide is associated with increased health care costs, loss of productivity, morbidity, and mortality, making it a significant public health concern (Centers for Disease Control and Prevention 2017). Proposed public health–based programs for suicide emphasize prevention instead of prediction (Pisani et al. 2016). Overall, the public health approach to decreasing disease burden is accomplished by identification, implementation, and evaluation. For suicide, this would mean identifying risk and protective factors, implementing interventions to address these factors, and evaluating the efficacy of these interventions (Cornette et al. 2014).

In a review of the evidence for several existing public health approaches to suicide intervention, those that demonstrated some empirical support included means restriction (firearms, medications, bridge barriers, chemical mandates); pharmacology (psychiatric medications and monitoring); media practices (guidelines for suicide coverage); emergency department practices (training for parents, patients, and staff); community-based strategies (schools and military); and follow-up contacts (postdischarge contacts, help-seeking encouragement while hospitalized) (Cornette et al. 2014).

A potential assessment model based on the public health emphasis on suicide prevention recommends examination of "risk status," "risk state," "available resources," and "foreseeable changes" (Pisani et al. 2016). *Risk status* is defined as an individual's risk compared with a certain population or subpopulation, including a broad examination of evidence-based risk factors. *Risk state* is the current risk for the individual as compared to their own risk at baseline or other times. *Available resources* include assessment of an individual's internal and external resources and safety planning, with particular emphasis on individual treatment planning. *Foreseeable changes* refers to reviewing potential future changes that could increase or decrease the suicide risk of that individual. All of these should be included to inform management decisions, keeping in mind that these aspects of a public health model of risk assessment may be fluid (Pisani et al. 2016).

The CDC recommends that risks be studied from a social ecological model, including risk factors, protective factors, and interventions supported by research that demonstrates significant impact on suicide. These interventions include the following strategies: promoting connectedness, strengthening economic supports, lessening harms and preventing future risk, identifying and supporting people at risk, teaching coping and problem-solving skills, creating protective environments, and strengthening access and delivery of suicide care (Centers for Disease Control and Prevention 2017). In addition to having a strong, evidence-based curriculum on risk assessment and intervention strategies for suicidal patients, training programs should also consider curriculum related to handling a patient's death from suicide.

Resident Response to Suicide

Between 31% and 69% of psychiatry residents experience patient suicide during residency training (Puttagunta et al. 2014). Having a patient die from suicide is one of the most difficult occupational events to deal with during a psychiatric career (see Chapter 32, "Psychiatrist Reactions to Patient Suicide and the Clinician's Role"). However, psychiatric residents in training may have increased difficulty coping because residents commonly blame themselves and experience a myriad of emotional responses. These responses may include the initial reactions of shock, disbelief, denial, and depersonalization followed by grief, shame, guilt, fear of blame, and anger (American Psychiatric Association 2018).

As with other poor outcomes, patient death from suicide may have profound effects on the trainee's developing sense of a professional self and may trigger feelings of personal and professional failure. At the very minimum, residents experiencing the loss of a patient to suicide should receive direct individual support from their immediate supervisor and training director.

Unfortunately, only around one-third of psychiatry residents receive formal education on the impact that a patient suicide may have on them during their career (Pilkinton and Etkin 2003). However, model curricula for teaching residents how to cope with a patient's death from suicide are available, and many training directors advocate that such instruction should be a standard part of psychiatric training (Lerner et al. 2012; Prabhakar et al. 2013). Some discussion of patient suicide and available support systems should be provided at intern orientation because the experience of a patient's death from suicide can be particularly difficult for new trainees (Whitmore et al. 2017).

Practical considerations that may be helpful to psychiatric residents after a patient's death from suicide include allowing the resident to take time off to process the full range of emotions associated with such an event, encouraging the resident to engage in mindfulness regarding personal wellness, and encouraging the resident to talk about the experience and personal reactions with colleagues and supervisors (American Psychiatric Association 2018). It may also be useful for the resident to discuss the patient with a supervisor not involved in the case. Healthy defenses to such a tragedy could also include reading additional literature on SRA, reading literature on dealing with the death of a patient, or writing a paper about the experience of losing a patient to suicide during residency training.

Conclusion

With the variability in methodology that exists for teaching and training suicide risk assessment and management strategies, developing a standard model curriculum for trainees can be challenging. Programs should consider using and integrating multiple instructional methods in a comprehensive longitudinal curriculum that includes opportunities for practical skill acquisition. A suicide curriculum should also include formal instruction on how to cope with patient death from suicide and a model plan to provide support, mentorship, and a compassionate response to residents who have experienced such a tragic event. Both faculty and residents should be diligent in reading the most evidence-based literature on suicide and stay abreast of the emerging guidelines and recommendations from national organizations. Given the importance of suicide, programs should be thoughtful and purposeful in creating and maintaining a solid evidence-based curriculum for psychiatry residents.

Key Points

- Psychiatry residency training programs should develop goals and objectives for an independent longitudinal suicide curriculum and should educate faculty, residents, and fellows about these goals and procedures.

- Psychiatric residents should be taught suicide risk assessment and clinical management consistent with the most updated evidence from the extant literature about suicide.

- Opportunities for skills assessments that include knowledge of suicide risk assessment and management should be developed.

- A suicide curriculum should be enhanced with active teaching strategies, partnerships, or educational workshops.

- Residency programs should implement strategies to assess efficacy of the suicide educational program.

- As part of a comprehensive suicide curriculum, residency programs should provide instruction on coping with patient death from suicide and develop a plan to provide support to residents who have experienced a patient suicide.

References

Accreditation Council for Graduate Medical Education: ACGME Program Requirements for Graduate Medical Education in Psychiatry. Chicago, IL, Accreditation Council for Graduate Medical Education, 2017. Available at: https://www.acgme.org/Portals/0/PFAssets/ProgramRequirements/400_psychiatry_2017-07-01.pdf. Accessed November 18, 2018.

Accreditation Council for Graduate Medical Education: ACGME Common Program Requirements. Chicago, IL, Accreditation Council for Graduate Medical Education, 2018a. Available at: https://www.acgme.org/What-We-Do/Accreditation/Common-Program-Requirements. Accessed November 18, 2018.

Accreditation Council for Graduate Medical Education: ACGME Data Resource Book, 2017–2018. Chicago, IL, Accreditation Council for Graduate Medical Education, 2018b. Available at: https://www.acgme.org/About-Us/Publications-and-Resources/Graduate-Medical-Education-Data-Resource-Book. Accessed December 1, 2018.

Accreditation Council for Graduate Medical Education, American Board of Psychiatry and Neurology: The Psychiatry Milestone Project. 2015. Available at: https://www.acgme.org/Portals/0/PDFs/Milestones/PsychiatryMilestones.pdf?ver=2015–11–06–120520–753. Accessed November 18, 2018.

American Psychiatric Association: Practice Guideline for the Assessment and Treatment of Patients With Suicidal Behaviors. Arlington, VA, American Psychiatric Association, 2003. Available at: https://psychiatryonline.org/pb/assets/raw/sitewide/practice_guidelines/guidelines/suicide.pdf. Accessed November 20, 2018.

American Psychiatric Association: Assessing and Treating Suicidal Behaviors: A Quick Reference Guide. Arlington, VA, American Psychiatric Association, 2004. Available at: https://psychiatryonline.org/pb/assets/raw/sitewide/practice_guidelines/guidelines/suicide-guide.pdf. Accessed November 20, 2018.

American Psychiatric Association: Helping Residents Cope With a Patient Suicide. Washington, DC, American Psychiatric Association, 2018. Available at: https://www.psychiatry.org/residents-medical-students/residents/coping-with-patient-suicide. Accessed December 1, 2018.

Bernert RA, Hom MA, Roberts LW: A review of multidisciplinary clinical practice guidelines in suicide prevention: toward an emerging standard in suicide risk assessment and management, training and practice. Acad Psychiatry 38(5):585–592, 2014 25142247

Brodsky BS, Spruch-Feiner A, Stanley B: The zero suicide model: applying evidence-based suicide prevention practices to clinical care. Front Psychiatry 9:33, 2018 29527178

Centers for Disease Control and Prevention: Preventing suicide: a technical package of policy, programs, and practice, 2017. Available at: https://www.cdc.gov/violenceprevention/pdf/suicidetechnicalpackage.pdf. Accessed November 18, 2018.

Cornette MM, Schlotthauer AE, Berlin JS, et al: The public health approach to reducing suicide: opportunities for curriculum development in psychiatry residency training programs. Acad Psychiatry 38(5):575–584, 2014 24923779

Foster A, Chaudhary N, Murphy J, et al: The use of simulation to teach suicide risk assessment to health profession trainees—rationale, methodology, and a proof of concept demonstration with a virtual patient. Acad Psychiatry 39(6):620–629, 2015 25026950

Frierson RL, Campbell NN: Commentary: core competencies and the training of psychiatric residents in therapeutic risk management. J Am Acad Psychiatry Law 37(2):165–167, 2009 19535552

Humphrey HJ, Marcangelo M, Rodriguez ER, et al: Assessing competencies during education in psychiatry. Int Rev Psychiatry 25(3):291–300, 2013 23859092

Lerner U, Brooks K, McNiel DE, et al: Coping with a patient's suicide: a curriculum for psychiatry residency training programs. Acad Psychiatry 36(1):29–33, 2012 22362433

Melton BB, Coverdale JH: What do we teach psychiatric residents about suicide? A national survey of chief residents. Acad Psychiatry 33(1):47–50, 2009 19349444

Office of the Surgeon General; National Action Alliance for Suicide Prevention: 2012 National Strategy for Suicide Prevention: Goals and Objectives for Action: A Report of the U.S. Surgeon General and of the National Action Alliance for Suicide Prevention. Washington, DC, U.S. Department of Health and Human Services, 2012. Available at: https://www.ncbi.nlm.nih.gov/books/NBK109917/. Accessed November 18, 2018.

Pheister M, Kangas G, Thompson C, et al: Suicide prevention and postvention resources: what psychiatry residencies can learn from the Veteran's Administration experience. Acad Psychiatry 38(5):600–604, 2014 24800730

Pilkinton P, Etkin M: Encountering suicide: the experience of psychiatric residents. Acad Psychiatry 27(2):93–99, 2003 12824109

Pisani AR, Cross WF, Gould MS: The assessment and management of suicide risk: state of workshop education. Suicide Life Threat Behav 41(3):255–276, 2011 21477093

Pisani AR, Murrie DC, Silverman MM: Reformulating suicide risk formulation: from prediction to prevention. Acad Psychiatry 40(4):623–629, 2016 26667005

Prabhakar D, Anzia JM, Balon R, et al: "Collateral damages": preparing residents for coping with patient suicide. Acad Psychiatry 37(6):429–430, 2013 23653109

Puttagunta R, Lomax ME, McGuinness JE, et al: What is the prevalence of the experience of death of a patient by suicide among medical students and residents? A systematic review. Acad Psychiatry 38(5):538–541, 2014 24664601

Reshetukha TR, Alavi N, Prost E, et al: Improving suicide risk assessment in the emergency department through physician education and a suicide risk assessment prompt. Gen Hosp Psychiatry 52:34–40, 2018 29549821

Retamero C, Walsh L, Otero-Perez G: Use of the film The Bridge to augment the suicide curriculum in undergraduate medical education. Acad Psychiatry 38(5):605–610, 2014 24699837

Silverman MM, Berman AL: Training for suicide risk assessment and suicide risk formulation. Acad Psychiatry 38(5):526–537, 2014 25059537

Simon R: Suicide risk assessment, in The American Psychiatric Publishing Textbook of Suicide Assessment and Management, 2nd Edition. Edited by Simon RI, Hales RE. Washington, DC, American Psychiatric Association, 2012, pp 3–28

Suicide Prevention Resource Center: A Comprehensive Approach to Suicide Prevention (website). Waltham, MA, Suicide Prevention Resource Center, 2018. Available at: http://www.sprc.org/effective-prevention/comprehensive-approach. Accessed November 21, 2018.

Tanguturi Y, Bodic M, Taub A, et al: Suicide risk assessment by residents: deficiencies of documentation. Acad Psychiatry 41(4):513–519, 2017 28083763

Whitmore CA, Cook J, Saig L: Supporting residents in the wake of patient suicide. Am J Psychiatry 12(1):5–7, 2017

Zisook S, Anzai J, Ashutosh A, et al: Teaching evidence-based approaches to suicide risk assessment and prevention that enhance psychiatric training. Compr Psychiatry 54(3):201–208, 2013 22995449

PART VII

Aftermath of Suicide

CHAPTER 32

Psychiatrist Reactions to Patient Suicide and the Clinician's Role

Michael Gitlin, M.D.

Katrina DeBonis, M.D.

The suicide of a patient in ongoing treatment has been and continues to be among the most traumatic events in the professional life of a psychiatrist. Despite the occasional paper urging more attention to this area, systematic examinations of the prevalence of psychiatrists' reactions to patient deaths from suicide, the specific reactions that are typically seen, predictors of these responses, and recommendations for optimal coping mechanisms in these situations continue to be remarkably sparse in the psychiatric literature.

A number of potential reasons for our field's relative silence in considering what are frequently traumatic events for psychiatrists have been proposed. Even though a substantial percentage of psychiatrists will experience a patient's death from suicide, it remains a relatively very-low-frequency event. As an example, in a study from Scotland with the highest percentage of surveyed psychiatrists having experienced a patient's death from suicide, 87% had experienced six or fewer patients' deaths from suicide over an average career of 17.5 years, yielding an average of fewer than one patient death every 3 years (Alexander et al. 2000). In another study of private practitioners and hospital-based psychiatrists and psychologists, no private practitioners had experienced more than one patient death from suicide in the previous 5 years (Wurst et al. 2010).

In contrast, those working in institutional settings such as hospitals or academic medical centers were more likely to experience multiple patient deaths from suicides, with two-thirds having had more than one patient death during the same time frame. (This would include recently treated patients after discharge from inpatient units.)

Overall, with relatively few patient deaths per psychiatrist, the topic never becomes one that demands an agreed-upon set of coping skills that has been shaped and taught over generations. Finally, with death a more common outcome in most of the other medical specialties, medical schools treat it as a natural outcome of disorders that physicians treat and generally do not focus on death from suicide as playing a unique role as a stress-generator for the treating physicians.

Nonetheless, a substantial proportion of psychiatrists, estimated to range from 15% to 68%, has experienced at least one patient death from suicide (Alexander et al. 2000; Chemtob et al. 1988; Wurst et al. 2010). A substantial number of psychiatric trainees also experience patient death from suicide (see Chapter 31, "Teaching Suicide Risk Assessment in Psychiatric Residency Training"). Thus, despite the relative infrequency of patient deaths over a psychiatrist's professional lifetime, it occurs with regularity, especially with psychiatric residents. It behooves us to better understand our own reactions and potential coping mechanisms and to incorporate this knowledge into enhanced education and support for ourselves, our colleagues, and psychiatric trainees.

General Reactions to Patient Suicide

The few surveys that have examined psychiatrists' reactions to patient death from suicide consistently show that, in general, a significant proportion of those affected show strong negative reactions affecting professional and personal lives at levels of distress that are frequently comparable with those seen in clinical populations. In one study using an ordinal scale, 38% of psychiatrists rated their distress after patient death from suicide as 7 out of 10 or higher, classified as severe by Hendin et al. (2004). Similarly, one-third of psychiatrists and psychologists in another study rated their distress as severe (visual analogue scale score >70) (Wurst et al. 2010).

Finally, consideration of discontinuing the practice of psychiatry would be a clear and rather dramatic expression of distress. In one survey of psychiatrists in Great Britain, one-third described patient death from suicide as having affected their personal lives; they became more irritable at home and coped less well with family problems. Fifteen percent of these psychiatrists considered taking early retirement; however, only 3% considered it seriously (Alexander et al. 2000). Finally, in a qualitative study of psychoanalytic clinicians who experienced patient death from suicide, one clinician reported that she "longed for a job with the least amount of interpersonal contact and responsibility…and laughed about her fantasy of working as a forest ranger" (Tillman 2006, p. 166).

After patient death from suicide, many psychiatrists develop rather classic symptoms of anxiety, depression, or acute or posttraumatic stress symptoms. These include sleep difficulties, suicidal thoughts, accident proneness, intrusive thoughts, and exaggerated startle responses (Alexander et al. 2000; Chemtob et al. 1988; Gitlin 1999; Ruskin et al. 2004; Sacks 1989; Tillman 2006). At least three papers (Gitlin 1999; Hendin et al. 2004; Sacks 1989) have noted that some psychiatrists show an exaggerated startle response to late-night telephone calls or pages for up to 1 year or more afterward, with the reflexive assumption that news about another patient death from suicide is impending.

Finally, a few surveys have noted the remarkable vividness of feelings, specific memories, and dreams/fantasies surrounding a patient's death from suicide, even

TABLE 32–1.	**Reactions to patient suicide**

Initial reactions
  Shock
  Disbelief
  Denial
  Depersonalization
Second-phase reactions
  Grief
  Shame
  Guilt
  Fear of blame
  Anger
  Relief
  Finding of omens and subsequent behavioral changes
  Conflicting feelings of specialness

years or decades later (Brown 1987; Gitlin 1999; Hendin et al. 2000; Tillman 2006). This indicates that despite the general healing that occurs over time, the experience often remains deeply etched in clinicians' psyches. In a descriptive study, half the interviewed clinicians cried during the research interview when recalling their experience of the patient's death from suicide, often years after the event (Tillman 2006).

For most clinicians, however, distress levels diminish over time. As an example, in one study, distress scores declined over time such that by 6 months after the suicide, most psychiatrists' scores had decreased to nonclinical levels (Chemtob et al. 1988). In another study, the high levels of distress seen immediately after a patient death from suicide had decreased significantly by 2 weeks later and after 6 months had decreased even more (Wurst et al. 2010).

Specific Reactions to Patient Suicide

Beyond the general intensity of psychiatrists' reactions to patients' deaths from suicide, a characteristic set of psychological responses, shown in Table 32–1, can be identified (Brown 1987; Gitlin 1999; Hendin et al. 2000; Sacks 1989; Sacks et al. 1987; Tillman 2006; Wurst et al. 2010).

Of course, not every psychiatrist exhibits each of the typical reactions, nor is the evolution or order of the responses invariant. In general, these responses reflect universal responses to the death of another with whom we have deep emotional ties, altered by the special role of psychiatric physicians in our society. Compared with other physicians, psychiatrists generally have deeper ties with their patients, reflecting a more emotionally intimate knowledge of them given that the medium of discussion is psychological feelings or symptoms rather than the more distanced physical symptoms. This may be true even with patients seen only in psychopharmacological treatment with whom discussions of mood or cognitions may still be experienced as intimate. This is especially relevant because psychiatrists who identify themselves as biologically oriented are more likely to experience patient death from suicide either because they see higher volumes of patients or because they treat patients with more severe illness (Ruskin et al. 2004).

Initial Responses: Shock, Disbelief, Denial, Depersonalization

Typically, initial responses revolve around the difficulties assimilating the new information about the patient's death from suicide, the intense affective arousal that the suicide engenders, and the internal mechanisms used to diminish that intensity. Initial responses include convictions such as "There must be a mistake" (Sacks et al. 1987). The dissociative symptoms of depersonalization and derealization—numbness, a sense of unreality, or spaciness—frequently accompany or follow the initial shock. These descriptors are entirely consistent with the symptoms described in DSM-5 as acute stress disorder (American Psychiatric Association 2013).

Second-Phase Responses: Grief, Shame, Guilt, Fear of Blame

Typically following, but often intermingling with, the initial disbelief responses are those reactions related to grief, shame, and guilt commonly associated with fear of blame. The experience has been described as consistent with an acute grief reaction (Tillman 2006). Grief can be related to a number of different simultaneous losses. First, losing a patient with whom the psychiatrist has had a deep, meaningful relationship may be experienced as a personal loss. This type of grief encompasses both the loss of the person and the loss of the possibility of the patient achieving the hoped-for positive goals of treatment.

Another type of grief, however, reflects a different type of loss—that of the psychiatrist's own fantasies of power, influence, and ability to make a difference in patients' lives (Gitlin 1999; Sacks 1989). One psychiatrist acknowledged his own primitive fantasy that "with his skill, empathy, and good training, he would make a positive difference in all his patients' lives. That [his patient] could kill himself despite [the psychiatrist's] best efforts and judgments made the practice and outcome of psychiatric treatment far less certain" (Gitlin 1999, p. 1631). Another psychiatrist expressed almost identical thoughts and feelings: "I really thought if you were good enough you could help almost everybody. That these things only happen to clinicians who miss something, and I learned that this is not true....This was a turning point, a reorienting point" (Tillman 2006, p. 164).

The loss of this youthful grandiosity is, in the long run, appropriate and necessary for optimal professional development. It is presumed (but not studied) that this second type of grief is more likely to occur when the treating psychiatrist is young and has been practicing for a relatively short period of time. Thus, although traumatic, this type of grief ultimately serves a larger, necessary purpose. The mourning of unrealistic youthful fantasies is analogous to the effect of other losses in one's personal life, leading to a deeper appreciation of the finiteness of life. Of course, as with other losses, timing is critical, and it can be postulated that losses at a too-early stage of development can be deeply scarring.

Shame and guilt are also very common reactions to patient death from suicide, with at least one observer suggesting these as the most universal responses (Sacks

1989). Questions/thoughts arise such as "Did I listen to him?" and "wracking my brain for what I missed" (Tillman 2006). Among the four factors identified in one study as the most common sources of severe distress, two related to technical decisions made regarding the patient's care with subsequent feelings of (presumably) guilt (Hendin et al. 2004). The aforementioned fantasies of moving to another city or retiring are linked to the deep shame and guilt that some psychiatrists experience after patient death from suicide.

At times, severe guilt has led to false confessions of wrongdoing. In one example, a psychiatrist "confessed" to having prescribed an incorrectly low dosage (which was not true) of an antidepressant with the (incorrect) implication of his having treated the patient inadequately (Sacks 1989). The shame and guilt reactions are inextricably linked to fear of blame or reprisal.

Foremost among these is the fear of a potential malpractice suit (Gitlin 1999; Hendin et al. 2000, 2004; Tillman 2006; Wurst et al. 2010). Even in Germany and Switzerland, two countries generally considered to be less litigious than the United States, overall distress levels after patient death from suicide correlated significantly with fear of lawsuit (Wurst et al. 2010).

A corollary of this is the fear that even without a malpractice suit, colleagues will be deeply critical of a psychiatrist who has had a patient die from suicide and will stop referring patients. Clinicians who lose a patient to suicide may fear that their reputations and careers will be ruined. Implied in these concerns is the common fantasy that a patient death from suicide, with or without subsequent litigation, is a very public event to colleagues, potential patients, and the community. Concerns about public exposure and humiliation are common and very powerful despite the fact that public discussions of these issues are rare. In one survey, only 9% of patient deaths from suicide eventuated in a lawsuit, and only 2% (2/120) went to trial. Consistent with these themes, one study found that after a patient death from suicide, 79% of psychiatrists felt professionally devalued and were concerned that they would no longer be respected professionally (Ruskin et al. 2004).

Anger

Although not as universal as grief, guilt, and shame, anger is a common and, in many ways, more difficult psychological response for psychiatrists after a patient death from suicide. What differs among individuals is the object of the anger and the rationale for the anger. Among those treating outpatients, the likely objects of anger are the patients and their families. If an inpatient dies from suicide, however, the list of potential objects lengthens to include nurses and administrators. If the treating psychiatrist is a trainee, others to be angry at might include supervisors and residency directors or the institution itself.

Rationales for anger are similarly diffuse. Feelings of betrayal toward the patient who did not, for example, honor a therapeutic contract, such as calling the psychiatrist if intense suicidal feelings erupted, may emerge (Hendin et al. 2000). Some psychiatrists feel angry at the waste of the previous therapeutic work. Others feel angry at the patient for engendering such painful feelings in them as guilt and shame or for making them look stupid in their own eyes. In one detailed case report, a young psychiatrist focused his anger on the patient's having died from suicide, overdosing on the antidepressant medications prescribed. It felt unfair to the psychiatrist that the patient had killed himself and caused great psychological pain to the psychiatrist using the "personal healing ministrations of the doctor, the actual means of his healing" (Gitlin 1999, p. 1632).

When the patient dies from suicide in an institutional setting, the theme of the anger in these cases is that of receiving inadequate support, help, or guidance from other professional staff or of being pressured by hospital administrators or utilization reviewers to discharge a patient from a more protected setting such as an inpatient unit. As in so many other situations in which anger is a dominant affect, the anger often serves to protect the individual against excessive guilt or blame ("It's their fault, not mine"). In the United States, anger may also be directed at those who dictate availability of care for financial, not clinical reasons, such as insurance companies who may deny further inpatient days despite the pleading of the treating psychiatrist.

Relief

Less common, yet still conflictual when they arise, are feelings of relief. Relief is likely to be experienced after the death of a chronically suicidal patient who has exhausted those around him or her by endless threats or attempts. These feelings may also arise in the family members of chronically suicidal individuals who, like the treating psychiatrists, have often lived in dread of the late-night phone calls surrounding either suicidal threats or self-destructive behavior. In these cases, the mixture of the more classic feelings—sadness, grief, guilt, and self-blame—with feelings of anger and relief can make for a very difficult internally conflicted brew.

Missed Signals and Behavioral Changes

Among the more interesting psychological sequelae of patient death from suicide is the "finding of omens" (Sacks 1989)—that is, retroactive identification of often subtle changes in behavior that psychiatrists consider to be missed signals indicating an impending suicide attempt. These would not rise to the level of a recognized suicide risk factor but in retrospect seem significant. For example, these typically include rather trivial differences in nuance, such as an ending greeting of "goodbye" instead of "so long" or a different look at the end of the last session. Identifying these subtle behavioral changes provides an illusory sense of control to an event that makes the psychiatrist feel helpless. If signs existed, even if they were missed, then the suicide risk would have been more evident and therefore the psychiatrist would have taken action to mitigate risk and will do so in the future.

The finding and examination of potentially missed signals of impending suicide and identifying high-risk situations based on a patient who died from suicide typically lead to behavioral changes. On the surface, as with the finding of missed signals, the purpose of these behavioral changes is to learn from the patient's death from suicide and to mitigate the risk of suicide in current and future patients. In fact, more frequently these behavioral changes simply serve as rituals, repetitive behaviors that bind the caregivers' anxiety and reduce the feelings of helplessness that accompany patient death from suicide.

For example, after a patient death from suicide, one outpatient psychiatrist began ritualistically asking all patients (even those who had never had suicidal ideation) about the presence of suicidal thoughts at every visit. Because his patient had died from suicide via an overdose of prescribed antidepressants, the psychiatrist also be-

TABLE 32–2.	Potential predictors of distress after patient suicide

Younger age

Less experience

Intensity of involvement with patient

Treatment setting

Gender of psychiatrist

Clinician's personality

Clinician's history of depression and anxiety

came excessively anxious about all his other patients and began ritualistically quizzing them about the exact amounts of medications at home and their thoughts of overdosing. He continued to do this, even with those patients for whom overdosing had never been raised or considered, until a patient confronted him on his anxious questioning (Gitlin 1999). In another example, after a patient death from suicide, one psychiatrist demanded that some of her suicidal patients be hospitalized far more quickly than was typical for her while another psychiatrist acknowledged attempting to have a patient with suicidal thoughts and behaviors terminate with him because he could not bear to lose another patient (Tillman 2006).

Conflicting Feelings of Specialness

In some situations, especially in institutional settings where psychiatrists are in frequent contact with other professionals, a psychiatrist experiencing a patient death from suicide develops feelings of isolation and specialness (Gitlin 1999; Sacks 1989; Tillman 2006). The isolation feelings reflect the irrational conviction that no one else has had the same experience—that one is "branded" as different by the patient's death from suicide. If the patient death from suicide is not discussed openly, the treating psychiatrist may feel shunned.

In association with these feelings, however, is also a sense of specialness, of having gone through a rite of passage, of becoming a member of a very special club in which only those who have had a similar experience could really understand, similar to that described by war veterans; "to survive it is testimony to one's hardiness, endurance, and being a 'real' physician" (Sacks 1989, p. 568). Although overall the feelings of specialness generate isolation and shame, it is important to acknowledge the positive and adaptive, albeit defensive, nature of these feelings.

Predictors of Distress

Among the predictors of increased distress in psychiatrists who experience a patient suicide, shown in Table 32–2, the most consistent are age and experience (which are, of course, highly correlated), with older age and more years of experience predicting somewhat less distress.

This finding can be seen in most, but not all, of the few data-based papers examining the topic (Chemtob et al. 1988; Hendin et al. 2004; Ruskin et al. 2004; Wurst et al. 2010) as well as in most impressionistic papers. That age and experience are the most important factors in predicting distress is deeply intuitive. Psychiatrists develop perspectives over time that buffer them from greater pain after the loss of a patient, as they do when coping with other and perhaps personal losses or tragedies. A number of papers have highlighted the greater vulnerability of trainees who experience a patient death from suicide. Trainees, the youngest and least experienced of our field, are uniquely vulnerable because they typically have not yet been able to internalize a self-image as competent professionals who can successfully treat some patients despite the tragedy of a patient death from suicide (see Chapter 31; Sacks 1989).

Another factor commonly assumed to predict greater distress after patient death from suicide is the intensity of involvement between the professional and the patient. Surprisingly, no data exist to support this assumption. (In the one study that examined this issue systematically, a patient's length of time in treatment did not contribute to ratings of therapist distress [Hendin et al. 2004].) Nonetheless, greater *emotional* involvement with the patient is likely to be associated with greater distress. The involvement may not always be measurable by simply establishing the length of treatment time. Related factors might also be the sheer volume of time spent with the patient, with the possibility that the suicide of a therapy patient may have a deeper effect than that of a patient seen in medication management. At the same time, however, remarkably deep ties often develop between patients and psychiatrists who work purely as psychopharmacologists.

Work setting—inpatient versus outpatient, private practice versus institutional setting—has also not been shown to be related to distress after patient death from suicide. However, the type of treatment setting will certainly dictate the reaction of others to the suicide and will therefore have an impact on the treating psychiatrist. As noted earlier, in a private practice setting, only the psychiatrist and the patient's family are ordinarily involved in the aftermath of the death. In an institutional setting, especially if the patient was either an inpatient or a partial hospital (day treatment) patient, other professionals and administrators become involved. If the treating physician is a trainee, supervisors and other faculty may be added to the list. In these situations, either greater support and cohesion or projected anger and blame could emerge. In one study, negative reaction by the therapist's institution was one of four factors identified as sources of severe distress (Hendin et al. 2004). The different ways in which institutions respond to the patient's death from suicide may play a role in explaining the inconsistent relationship between treatment setting and individual clinicians' responses to patient death from suicide.

In the three studies examining the issue, female psychiatrists were almost twice as likely to experience severe distress as their male counterparts after patient death from suicide in one study (Hendin et al. 2004) or more likely to experience more severe distress (Wurst et al. 2010) and exhibited higher rates of shame, guilt, and self-doubt (Grad et al. 1997). Of course, greater distress should not always be considered as a negative finding. Emotional denial and excessive repression may interfere with optimal learning from experience and could negatively impact the treatment of future patients.

Finally, among the most important factors in predicting reactions to patient death from suicide is the individual clinician's personality and own psychiatric history. In one study, psychiatrists who were less distressed after a patient death from suicide were more likely to identify changes in treatment they might consider in the future, a possible marker for flexible thinking and the ability to learn from the death as opposed to feeling dominated by guilt and self-blame (Hendin et al. 2004). Although

TABLE 32–3.	Optimal coping methods after patient suicide

Decreasing isolation

Using philosophical and cognitive approaches

Effecting temporary behavioral changes

Instituting reparative, constructive behaviors

never studied, overall resilience—with its roots in both temperament/biology and prior experience—might be the single most important factor in predicting response to patient death from suicide. Other psychological factors, such as tendencies for introjection versus projection, are also likely to be important.

Finally, the individual psychiatrist's potential past history of depression and anxiety might also play a role in predicting individual vulnerability to greater distress. Although speculative, the finding of greater distress among female psychiatrists could reflect the greater likelihood of depressive disorders and most anxiety disorders among women versus men in general. In one study, a past personal experience with death from suicide in close friend or family member did not predict greater distress after patient suicide (Ruskin et al. 2004).

Coping With Patient Suicide

A number of methods for optimal coping with patient suicide have been suggested. These methods, shown in Table 32–3, may be broadly divided into four categories (Gitlin 1999).

Decreasing Isolation

Despite a lack of data, reducing the feelings of isolation is the most commonly recommended method of combating the negative effects of a patient's death from suicide (Alexander et al. 2000; Brown 1987; Gitlin 1999; Hendin et al. 2000, 2004; Sacks 1989; Sacks et al. 1987). This coping method, which can be accomplished in a broad variety of ways, is perfectly analogous to the suggestions we make to our patients after tragedies in their own lives. Talking to others one trusts and respects, whether lovers, friends, family, or colleagues, is likely to be helpful. Discussion with former or current supervisors (assuming they know something about this area) can be exceedingly helpful. It is surprising how few papers comment on the use of the psychiatrist's own individual psychotherapy as a useful method of decreasing isolation (Tillman 2006 is an exception). Colleagues sharing their own experiences with a patient's death from suicide may be more helpful than the soothing comments about the inevitability of the death or of reflexive reassurance ("you did nothing wrong") (Hendin et al. 2004; Tillman 2006).

A specific method of decreasing isolation is meeting with the significant others of the person who died from suicide or going to the person's funeral or memorial service. In one case series, 59% of psychiatrists contacted their patients' relatives after the suicides (Ruskin et al. 2004). Although meeting with family members is typically described as positive, this is not always the case. Fear of relatives' reactions correlated with greater degrees of distress in one study (Wurst et al. 2010). Psychiatrists must be aware of the possibility that relatives will be angry because of the feeling that they do not know enough about the specifics of their relative's psychopathology, because of projected anger, or because of well-meaning decisions by the psychiatrist that may indeed have not prevented or may even have contributed to the suicide. Therefore, a psychiatrist meeting with the relatives of a patient who died from suicide must be prepared for anger and must be able to respond in a nondefensive manner while not being too quick to accept blame caused by guilt feelings. Care must also be taken in these meetings with regard to patient confidentiality, which extends beyond the death of a patient. It is possible, although delicate, to provide sufficient feedback and discussion with family members without violating the core of the patient's privileged information.

Each family will have specific and differing needs after the tragedy of a suicide within the family. Some families will simply need support for their loss. Others will want exoneration for their feeling of not having done enough to save their relative or not having been involved enough during the last crisis. (This will be especially true when the patient has withdrawn or alienated family members). Still other families will want more understanding about their relative's psychiatric problems, bringing the delicate balance of confidentiality to the fore. In this last situation, generalizations may be provided without exposing intimate details that emerged during the therapy.

As noted earlier, deaths from suicide within institutional settings provide unique opportunities for decreasing isolation *or* engaging in blaming behaviors. In many situations, the group setting provides greater support. A psychological autopsy often occurs as a mandated suicide review in certain psychiatric hospitals. Its goal is to review the patient's death from suicide, understand its causes, and learn so as to treat patients better in the future. When done properly, it should be a supportive, constructive learning experience.

However, the psychological autopsy can too easily become a public shaming by blaming the treating professional (Sacks 1989). If the suicide occurred in an inpatient setting, a review of the method used, staffing levels, and environmental contributors such as ligature points may be useful in identifying ways to improve the safety of the inpatient environment and prevent future suicides (see Chapter 16, "Inpatient Treatment"). In today's environment in which the concern/threat of lawsuits psychologically dominates many situations, it is particularly important that the perceived institutional response not be dominated by projecting blame away from the institution and toward one or more treating professionals.

Using Philosophical and Cognitive Approaches

Understanding a patient's death from suicide using philosophical and cognitive approaches is a second useful strategy. These approaches may sound trite but may be powerful when presented in interactive discussion. In many ways, they may be most helpful if they are inculcated during psychiatric training and *before* a patient's death from suicide instead of after one.

The first of these approaches acknowledges that psychiatrists who treat patients with serious psychiatric disorders—depression, bipolar disorder, drug and alcohol abuse, schizophrenia, borderline personality disorder—must embrace the expectation that some of their patients will die because of the natural course of their disorder. It must be understood that we cannot prevent the worst outcome of every case any more than can our colleagues in cardiology or oncology. Additionally, it must be understood that although demographic and clinical risk factors for suicide are clear among groups of patients, the field is unable to predict death from suicide for any individual patient (Pokorny 1983). These statements must not be used to foster a passivity, fatalism, or therapeutic nihilism in our therapeutic work; rather, they should be used to understand the inherent inconsistent effect of our best efforts (implied in the earlier discussion of the loss of omnipotence or grandiosity in young psychiatrists after a patient's death from suicide).

Effecting Temporary Behavioral Changes

Because of the frequency with which patient death from suicide adversely affects psychiatrists, a number of relatively simple, temporary behavioral changes can be effected to help diminish distress and ensure that the psychiatrist continues to practice optimal care. In the immediate aftermath of a patient death from suicide, most psychiatrists, especially younger ones, feel distinctly less trusting of their own judgment. This typically leads to an overly conservative set of decisions and behaviors, such as more aggressively querying patients about suicide (in ways that are neither appropriate nor therapeutic) or too quickly hospitalizing other suicidal patients (Tillman 2006). If possible, psychiatrists who have recently experienced a patient's death from suicide should consider avoiding treating patients with complex behavioral issues and psychiatric disorders until they have regained a sense of balance and confidence in their own judgment.

Instituting Reparative, Constructive Behaviors

Although rarely used in the immediate aftermath of a patient's death from suicide, helping others cope with similar incidents may be a remarkably effective and constructive long-term behavior. Such help would include being available to other, younger colleagues who have had a first patient die from suicide, presenting about the topics at conferences, or writing about the experience (Biermann 2003; Gitlin 1999). Because this type of activity requires some distance from the traumatic event itself, it usually becomes a viable option only months or even years later and typically in those who have achieved some maturity and experience in the field. Of course, being more open about personal experiences with patient death from suicide decreases isolation in both the presenter and the audience, thereby effectively using two of the most important techniques of coping.

Conclusion

A substantial proportion of psychiatrists will experience a patient's death from suicide at some point in their careers. Inpatient psychiatrists, trainees, and those who work in academic centers may be at higher risk to have a patient die from suicide because they treat the patients with the greatest psychopathology.

Responses to the death from suicide are similar to those seen in others who have lost an important person in their life, exacerbated by the shame, guilt, and fear of reprisal given the current climate of blame and malpractice threats in the United States. In the immediate aftermath of a patient's death from suicide, many psychiatrists will exhibit psychiatric distress and symptoms comparable with clinical populations. Typically, these symptoms diminish over the next few months. The most important predictor of greater distress after a patient's death from suicide is the psychiatrist's age and experience, with younger clinicians exhibiting greater difficulty.

Optimal coping with a patient's death from suicide involves a number of different interactions and techniques. First and foremost is to decrease the (irrational) feelings of isolation. This can be accomplished in a number of ways, no one of which is superior to the others. In institutional settings such as hospitals with training programs, group discussions should be handled in a constructive, supportive manner while still attempting to learn from the death from suicide. In these situations, care must be taken not to use the group discussions to establish blame for the event (typically directed toward the youngest, least experienced clinician involved).

Anticipating patient deaths from suicide during one's career, especially during training, would help psychiatrists prepare psychologically. Given how frequently residents experience patient death from suicide and how vulnerable they are to negative effects from these suicides, more attention needs to be paid to formal instruction in this area in training programs (see Chapter 31). It would also be helpful if senior psychiatrists were more open about their experiences in this area, modeling for younger psychiatrists and decreasing the sense of isolation common after patient suicides.

Key Points

- A substantial proportion of psychiatrists will experience the death from suicide of a patient at some point in their careers.

- Responses to patient death from suicide resemble reactions to other meaningful losses including denial, grief, and anger, exacerbated by shame, guilt, and fear of blame.

- The most important predictors of distress in psychiatrists after a patient's death from suicide are younger age and lesser experience.

- The most important coping technique after patient death from suicide is decreasing isolation of the treating psychiatrist.

- There may be a role, albeit a limited one, for the treating psychiatrist to assist family members who are confronted with a patient's death from suicide.

References

Alexander DA, Klein S, Gray NM, et al: Suicide by patients: questionnaire study of its effect on consultant psychiatrists. BMJ 320(7249):1571–1574, 2000 10845964

American Psychiatric Association: Diagnostic and Statistical Manual of Mental Disorders, 5th Edition. Washington, DC, American Psychiatric Association, 2013

Biermann B: When depression becomes terminal: the impact of patient suicide during residency. J Am Acad Psychoanal Dyn Psychiatry 31(3):443–457, 2003 14535612

Brown HN: Patient suicide during residency training, I: incidence, implications, and program response. J Psychiatr Educ 11:201–216, 1987

Chemtob CM, Hamada RS, Bauer G, et al: Patients' suicides: frequency and impact on psychiatrists. Am J Psychiatry 145(2):224–228, 1988 3341466

Gitlin MJ: A psychiatrist's reaction to a patient's suicide. Am J Psychiatry 156(10):1630–1634, 1999 10518176

Grad OT, Zavasnik A, Groleger U: Suicide of a patient: gender differences in bereavement reactions of therapists. Suicide Life Threat Behav 27(4):379–386, 1997 9444733

Hendin H, Lipschitz A, Maltsberger JT, et al: Therapists' reactions to patients' suicides. Am J Psychiatry 157(12):2022–2027, 2000 11097970

Hendin H, Haas AP, Maltsberger JT, et al: Factors contributing to therapists' distress after the suicide of a patient. Am J Psychiatry 161(8):1442–1446, 2004 15285971

Pokorny AD: Prediction of suicide in psychiatric patients. Report of a prospective study. Arch Gen Psychiatry 40(3):249–257, 1983 6830404

Ruskin R, Sakinofsky I, Bagby RM, et al: Impact of patient suicide on psychiatrists and psychiatric trainees. Acad Psychiatry 28(2):104–110, 2004 15298861

Sacks MH: When patients kill themselves, in American Psychiatric Press Review of Psychiatry, Vol 8. Edited by Tasman A, Hales RE, Frances AJ. Washington, DC, American Psychiatric Press, 1989, pp 563–579

Sacks MH, Kibel HD, Cohen AM, et al: Resident response to patient suicide. J Psychiatr Educ 11:217–226, 1987

Tillman JG: When a patient commits suicide: an empirical study of psychoanalytic clinicians. Int J Psychoanal 87(Pt 1):159–177, 2006 16635866

Wurst FM, Mueller S, Petitjean S, et al: Patient suicide: a survey of therapists' reactions. Suicide Life Threat Behav 40(4):328–336, 2010 20822359

Index

Page numbers printed in **boldface** type refer to tables or figures.